the big book of
juices

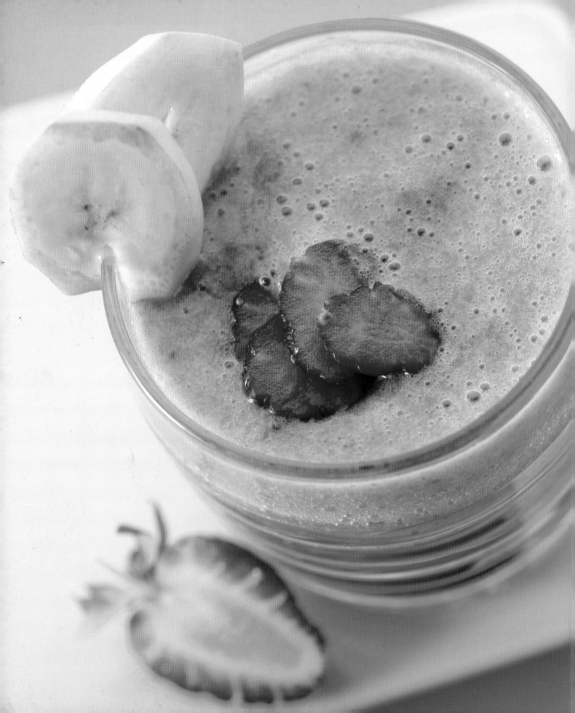

NATALIE SAVONA

the big book of juices

more than 400 natural blends for health and vitality every day

DUNCAN BAIRD PUBLISHERS

LONDON

The Big Book of Juices
Natalie Savona

Distributed in the USA and Canada by
Sterling Publishing Co., Inc.
387 Park Avenue South
New York, NY 10016-8810

This edition first published in the UK and USA in 2011
by Duncan Baird Publishers, an imprint of
Watkins Publishing Limited
75 Wells Street
London W1T 3QH

A member of Osprey Group

Savona, Natalie.
  The big book of juices : more than 400 natural blends
for health and vitality every day / Natalie Savona. -- 1st
paperback ed.
    p. cm.
Includes index.

ISBN 978-1-84483-973-5

1. Vegetable juices. 2. Fruit juices. 3. Smoothies
(Beverages) I. Title.
TX811.S288 2010
641.3'4--dc22

                                    2010015247
10 9 8 7 6

Typeset in Frutiger and Apollo MT
Color reproduction by Scanhouse, Malaysia
Printed in China

For information about custom editions, special sales,
premium and corporate purchases, please contact
Sterling Special Sales Department at 800-805-5489
or specialsales@sterlingpub.com.

Publisher's Note: The information in this book is not
intended as a substitute for professional medical advice
and treatment. If you are pregnant or breastfeeding
or have any special dietary requirements or medical
conditions, it is recommended that you consult a
medical professional before following any of the
information or recipes contained in this book. Watkins
Publishing Limited, or any other persons who have
been involved in working on this publication, cannot
accept responsibility for any errors or omissions,
inadvertent or not, that may be found in the recipes or
text, nor for any problems that may arise as a result of
preparing one of these recipes or following the advice
contained in this work.

Follow either the imperial or the metric measurements
when making the recipes. The measurements are not
interchangeable.

Author's acknowledgments
Thank you... to nutritionist Jane Windsor-Smith for
her consultation work on the recipe properties; to my
parents for giving me, amongst everything else, one of
the best juicers money can buy; to Amanda Bluglass for
being my juicing buddy and so much more.

Juicer supplied by Theolife Ltd: Samson 6 in 1
Multipurpose Juice Extractor GB9001

contents

introduction

The mouthwatering tang of freshly squeezed orange juice straight from squeezer to mouth within minutes — my early experiences of fresh juice came, as for most of us, from this staple citrus fruit. My first venture into the more alien world of vegetable juices came on a beach in Thailand: a large glass of frothy, deep orange carrot juice. This sublime taste in an exotic location marked the beginning of a culinary adventure.

First, using a basic, modestly priced juicer salvaged from the depths of my parents' kitchen, I turned out concoctions of almost anything I had in the fruit bowl or refrigerator. As I became bolder, I requested an expensive, high-powered juicer as a present a few years ago and haven't looked back since.

The overriding selling point for all juices and smoothies is that they attain the magical quality, so elusive in so much of what we eat and drink today, of tasting sensational and being supremely good for you. Raw fruit and vegetables are laden with vitamins, minerals, enzymes and other ingredients that give us a boost in energy, help ward off illness and keep our bodies' cleansing processes working optimally.

Once you have developed the habit of making your own fresh juice combinations each morning, nothing else will do. I wager you will become so convinced that

you would no sooner go without your daily juice than
without brushing your teeth. Ahead of you are the
recipes for more juices and smoothies than you could
ever ask for, not to mention a selection of frozen drinks
and some refreshing teas. My breakfast is regularly
fresh, home-made juice and a creamy smoothie. You really
couldn't get a much better start to the day.

how to use this book

This book provides you with over 400 recipes to
guide and inspire you to begin a daily juicing habit.
It is organized into chapters of juices, smoothies and
quenchers. For further information on their specific
health benefits, the recipes also list the main vitamins,
minerals and other key nutrients in each drink. In
addition, each recipe has a star-rating system giving the
drink marks out of five for its energy-boosting, detoxing
and immunity-boosting properties, and its benefits to the
digestive system and the skin.

   At the end of the book, there is a nutrient chart
providing further information on vitamins and minerals,
and an ailments chart with suggested juices and smoothies
to drink to help combat a range of common illnesses, as
well as a comprehensive index that will help you pinpoint a
juice, smoothie or quencher according to ingredient.

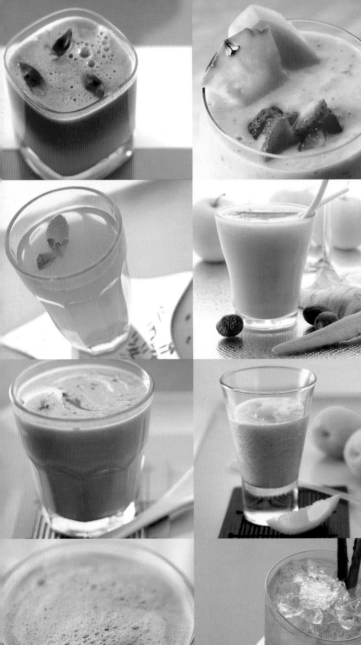
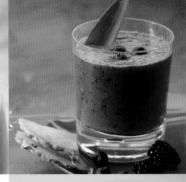
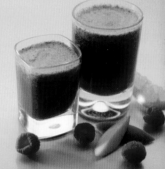
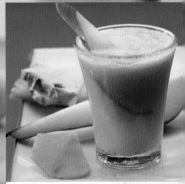
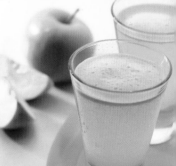

juicing
basics

You're sold on the idea that juicing is a good thing: you know that fresh juices are not only delicious but also packed with healthy ingredients. But before you go rushing out to buy a state-of-the-art juicer, take some time to absorb the advice presented in this chapter. This will help you get the most out of your juicing.

Over the following pages we look at the different kinds of juice drinks you can make and offer some suggestions on the basic kit you'll need. We explore why juices really are so good for you – we examine the many benefits of drinking juice daily and reveal how the body uses this direct source of nutrients for optimum health. We discover that there are few fruit and vegetables that cannot be consumed in the form of a nutritious drink, and learn how best to choose and prepare them. Finally, we look at some of the optional extras, such as flaxseed (linseed) and wheatgerm, that can add a healthy bonus to your glass.

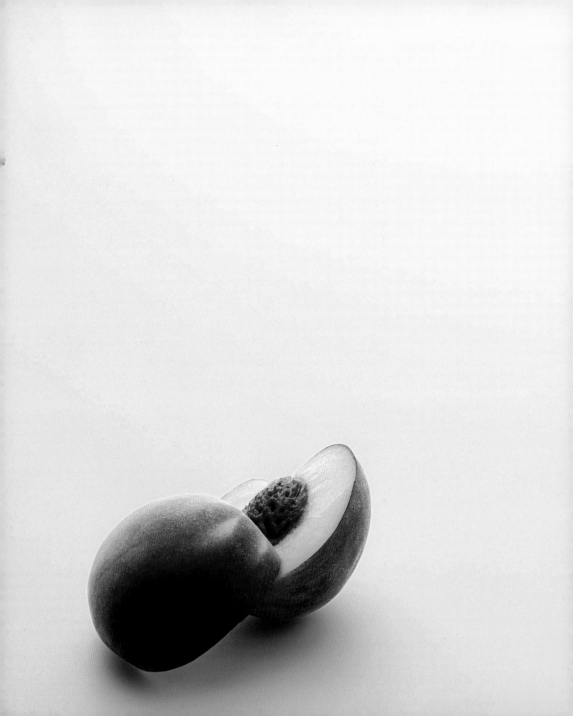

why juice?

First of all, let us not forget that one of the most important aspects of anything we eat or drink is pleasure. Savouring a home-made, fresh juice is, for anyone who has tried it, an immensely pleasurable experience. Not only does it taste truly delicious, it also invigorates your body and mind, and gives you the added satisfaction of having created it yourself.

Following on from the pleasure principle comes the effect that food and drink has on our body and mind. Raw, fresh juice is probably one of the most health-affirming, rejuvenating substances we can take. Drinking a fresh juice provides the body with nutrients on a superhighway – it's a fast delivery of vitamins, minerals, enzymes, carbohydrates, chlorophyll and countless other phytonutrients (nutrients derived from plants), which increasingly are being shown to boost health. And all of this contained in pure, fresh water. These natural blends of nutrients work together to enhance immunity, helping to protect us from not just colds and coughs but cancer and cardiovascular disease too. Juices are powerhouses of antioxidants – nutrients such as vitamins A, C and E that fight oxidants (sometimes called free radicals) in our bodies which contribute to cancer, heart disease and aging. Other substances present in a juice, such as green chlorophyll, are particularly cleansing.

Even the least health-conscious person is now aware that we are supposed to have at least five servings of fruit and vegetables a day. Officially, a glass of juice counts as a single portion, although immediately I'd say that a fresh, unadulterated, home-made juice, drunk straight from the jug, easily rates higher than your average shop-bought juice. A fresh juice also delivers the nutrients straight into your body within minutes, as it does not need to be digested in the way that fruit and vegetables do. And, given that some of your fruit, and probably all of your vegetables, are eaten at the same time as other foods, they are digested pretty slowly, and perhaps not too efficiently, so the nutrients may not be well absorbed.

So, in drinking your daily juice, you are not only fuelling yourself with energy, but you are also supporting your body's natural cleansing processes and helping stave off all manner of diseases. A home-made juice stands in a league of its own compared with off-the-shelf processed juices, not to mention coffee, tea, cordials, fizzy and so-called "energy" drinks, and is simply the best liquid refreshment that a body can have.

juice or smoothie?

So what is the difference? It's really a question of semantics – you can call your juice drinks what you like, but for the sake of clarity I have chosen to make a distinction. Simply, a juice is a drink made using a special juice extractor or citrus press and a smoothie is a drink made by mixing whole ingredients into a pulp in a blender. This book divides smoothies into two basic categories, fruity and creamy – where a creamy smoothie has a richer, creamier texture owing to the addition of yogurt to the mix. Some further variations on the smoothie theme appear in Chapter 4, Making Quenchers. Here, frozen fruit, ice and sparkling water are added for an extra-chilled, refreshing taste.

Now that we've got the semantics clear, there is actually a great deal of difference in the consistency and properties of the end products. With a juice you are getting just that – the juice from the fruit or vegetable as it is pushed through the extractor or press and the fibre is left behind. Because a smoothie is made by simply blending the fruit to a pulp, you get the whole fruit, including the fibre, merely in a different form. A smoothie can be breakfast in itself; a juice may be just the first course.

There are particular benefits associated with both the juice and the smoothie group of drinks. Juices provide nutrients at top speed – our body absorbs their goodness with maximum efficiency, unhindered by any need to break down and digest bulkier foodstuffs. The lack of any fibre (left behind in the juicing process) means that our body can assimilate the nutrients from a juice in a matter of minutes rather than hours.

This is a sure-fire way of getting the most out of the vitamins, minerals, enzymes, cleansing elements and other nutritional goodness from a fruit or vegetable. After drinking a fresh juice, you feel invigorated almost immediately. By doing this daily, you provide your body with a high dose of naturally derived nutrients that boosts your health and helps keep you well protected against toxins and disease.

Unlike juices, smoothies contain a good amount of fibre, something that is an important nutrient in itself. Indeed, fibre is an essential and all-too-often lacking ingredient in our diet. Not only does it help keep our gut moving, but it also helps it to stay healthy and to maintain the right levels of good bacteria. In addition to this, any drink using yogurt or milk, such as our creamy smoothies, becomes an important source of protein, another essential in a healthy diet.

getting ready

equipment

To make a variety of the recipes from this book, you will need a juice extractor, a citrus press and a blender. All of the juice recipes can be made using a juice extractor alone, although citrus fruits are best squeezed on a proper citrus press; they tend to clog up a juicer and leave behind a lot of their precious juice. For the purposes of this book, when I say "juice", I mean put the fruit into an electric juicer, and when I say "squeeze", I mean extract its juice by squeezing it on a citrus press.

When choosing your first juicer, buy one at the lower end of the price range which will give you a perfectly good introduction to the joy of juicing. Most juicers are what are called "centrifugal extractors", which means they grate the fruit and quickly spin it out towards a mesh which catches the pulp and sends the juice down into a jug. This can make quite a mess in the machine and I suggest cleaning it immediately, before you've even allowed yourself a sip of the end product. It really doesn't take more than a couple of minutes.

Once you are converted to the delights of juicing, you may want to invest in one of the more expensive machines. As with most things in life, you tend to get what you pay for – the more expensive juicers have a hardier motor and extract more juice per piece of fruit.

Citrus presses can be bought for a reasonable price in most kitchen accessory shops or department stores. They usually take the form of a stainless-steel structure around which you squeeze halved fruit, although electric ones are also available.

The essential piece of smoothie kit is a blender. Most kitchens already have one, though often little-used, but, again, you can buy one quite cheaply and it will soon become a smoothie-making machine, creating breakfast or a refreshing drink in a flash.

storing juices and smoothies

In my book, there really is no such thing as storing a juice or smoothie – you can't beat drinking them the moment you've made them. However, you may like to take them out to work or on a picnic. In that case, the best way to store them is to put a teaspoon of vitamin C powder or a squeeze of lemon juice in the bottom of the jug attached to the juicer. The vitamin C acts as an anti-oxidant, preventing the juice from turning brown. The same goes for smoothies. Also, keep the drinks covered and cool – in a sealed container in the refrigerator, or in a vacuum flask.

ingredients

choosing the best

Where possible, always choose fresh, local, organic produce that is in season. Organic fruits and vegetables provide you with all the goodness you need and none of the agrochemicals you don't. Buying locally supports your local economy, too, and avoids adding to the economic and environmental costs of long-distance transport and storage of goods. That said, you sometimes can't beat a delicious tropical mango or pineapple that has come all the way from India or Thailand!

The following pages list information and preparation details for the fruits and vegetables used in the order in which blends based on them appear in the book.

fruits

Apple — The best apples are sharp, crisp ones such as Granny Smith, Braeburn, Egremont Russet or Discovery. Apples make a fantastic base juice and are laden with health properties from their vitamin, mineral, malic acid and fibre content. They are not only detoxifying but also good for lowering cholesterol, aiding digestion and improving the condition of the skin. *Preparation: Wash well. For juicing, simply remove the stalk and cut into pieces small enough to fit through your juicer. For smoothies, core and chop.*

Grapefruit — The sharp flavour of even the sweetest grapefruit is remarkably refreshing. White, pink, red is the order of increasing sweetness. Grapefruits are packed with vitamin C, so good for immunity. The pith contains the bioflavonoids (powerful antioxidants which work alongside vitamin C), so don't peel that off when juicing grapefruits. However, squeezing the fruit using a citrus press actually produces more juice, but you lose the bioflavonoids. *Preparation: If juicing, peel and cut to fit. If squeezing, cut in half.*

Orange — The classic fruit juice, and of course the best way to get the most out of the fruit is to cut it into quarters, suck out the juice and nibble the flesh from the skin. However, you simply can't beat fresh, home-made orange juice. Oranges, with their high vitamin C and bioflavonoid content, are a famous immune-booster, but they are also rich in minerals and very cleansing. You get the most juice by squeezing them, but juicing means you benefit from the bioflavonoids in the pith too. *Preparation: If juicing, peel and chop into chunks. If squeezing, cut in half.*

Raspberry — Plump, summer raspberries may warrant popping into the mouth as is, but they do make a wonderful addition to a juice or blended drink. Like all berries, they are a rich source of nutrients, especially antioxidants. *Preparation: Wash well. Pick out any that are mouldy or still attached to the hull.*

Peach — Good peaches yield a fantastic, rich nectar, ideal for blended drinks. Because of their high beta-carotene content, peaches help protect against lung, skin and digestive problems. With countless varieties of colour, it's best to choose a peach by its tenderness and its smell. A good peach will yield to a gentle squeeze and have a sweet scent, but an under-ripe specimen will be hard and barely smell of anything. *Preparation: Wash well. Halve, remove the stone and chop into chunks.*

Nectarine — The bald relatives of peaches, good nectarines also burst with an orange, sweet nectar. They are a rich source of beta-carotene, as well as vitamin C and a spectrum of minerals. Use nectarines only when they are tender to a gentle squeeze in the palm. *Preparation: Wash well. Halve, remove the stone and chop into chunks.*

Apricot — You're likely to get sweeter apricots in mid- and late-summer rather than earlier in the year. Choose them slightly soft to the touch and smelling sweet as they're unlikely to ripen further. Also, the riper they are, the higher their beta-carotene content. As a winter alternative, soaked, dried apricots make a delicious, sweet addition to a smoothie. *Preparation (fresh apricots): Wash well. Halve and remove the stone.*

Cherry — A luxury inasmuch as you need time and patience to yield a decent quantity of stoned, fresh fruit. But you will be grateful not only for the intense flavour of the juice; cherries contain rich antioxidant nutrients as well as highly alkaline properties, particularly good for arthritis and gout. *Preparation: Wash well. Slice in half and prise out the stone or use an olive stoner.*

Pear — As with many fruits, I hesitate to hand ripe Williams pears to my juicer rather than eat them straight up. While a juicy, ripe pear is best for blending, use a slightly under-ripe pear for juicing, even Comice or

Conference varieties, and you will get a surprisingly thick yield. Similar to apples, pears are very cleansing and full of a range of vitamins, minerals and fibre. *Preparation: Wash well. For juicing, simply remove the stalk and cut the fruit into pieces small enough to fit through your juicer. For smoothies, core and chop.*

Pineapple — The delicious flesh of the pineapple is a perfect juice or smoothie ingredient. It is rich in a range of vitamins and minerals, but is particularly known for an alkaline substance called bromelain, which aids digestion and is linked to a reduction of inflammation in arthritis and other inflammatory disorders. Choose a pineapple that is a deep yellow colour and gives off a sweet scent from the bottom. *Preparation: Chop off the top and bottom of the fruit, and slice down the sides to remove the skin. If blending, remove any remaining eyes (there's no need if you are juicing).*

Banana — Completely unjuiceable, but a wonderful staple for blended drinks, turning a smoothie into a meal in itself. As with most fruit, the riper the banana, the richer the flavour, and they're even good in a drink when they are past their eating best. A banana is a nutritional powerhouse – full of fibre, vitamins and minerals, as well as carbohydrates, which are a key source of energy. *Preparation: Peel and break or slice into pieces.*

Mango — Mangoes, one of nature's most sumptuous fruits, come in a variety of colours and sizes, although my favourite is the amber Alfonse variety from India (available in late spring). Otherwise, choose your mango carefully to avoid disappointment: look out for one that yields slightly to the thumb and smells sweet (don't be fooled by the colour, as some green mangoes are perfectly ripe). Mangoes are extremely rich in beta-carotene, as well as minerals such as magnesium. *Preparation: Peel and slice the flesh away from the stone. (Then chew and suck it unashamedly!)*

Papaya — One of the Tropics' wonderfoods, the papaya (or paw paw) is packed with beta-carotene, enzymes that help digestion, vitamin C and fibre. It comes in several varieties, although the most common is the more squat, pear-shaped type. Papayas are ripe when they are fully amber in colour and yield to gentle pressure. *Preparation: Peel, remove the seeds, and slice into chunks.*

Blackberry — One of the few fruits that we can continue to pick wild. All the scratches are worth the effort for a pile of freshly picked, plump blackberries. Otherwise, nip down to the local fruit and veg store. Blackberries are rich in antioxidants, especially vitamin C. *Preparation: Wash well. Discard any berries that are mouldy or still attached to the hull.*

Blackcurrant — Sharp but not sour, perfectly ripe blackcurrants add a strong flavour to any drink. They are an extremely rich source of vitamin C and other antioxidant nutrients. Crunch their seeds well in a blended drink as they contain healthy essential fats. *Preparation: Wash well. Remove any stalks and discard any berries that are mouldy.*

Blueberry — Small in size, big in flavour and goodness, blueberries are laden with antioxidant nutrients such as vitamins A and C, as well as bioflavonoids. They yield a rich, sweet flavour and give a blended drink blue specks. The berries are good for overcoming bladder problems, as well as boosting immunity and protecting the eyes and blood vessels. *Preparation: Wash well. Remove any stalks and discard any berries that are mouldy.*

Cranberry — Cranberries are excellent therapy for male and female urinary-tract problems, but only in their pure, unsweetened form – the sweeteners often present in commercial drinks can aggravate such conditions. Because they are rather tart, cranberries are best mixed with other fruits. Like all berries, they are rich in a range of antioxidant nutrients. *Preparation: Wash well. Remove any stalks and discard any berries that are spoiled.*

Cantaloupe/Honeydew melon — These are the most widely available varieties of melon. The orange-fleshed cantaloupe is particularly high in beta-carotene, but both kinds are rich in a range of vital nutrients, especially vitamin C. They have diuretic properties, meaning that they help eliminate excess fluid from the body. Choose melons that are firm, but yield slightly to pressing, and that smell sweet. *Preparation: Halve, slice and cut the flesh away from the rind. Chop into chunks.*

Watermelon — Loaded with water and minerals, watermelon is one of the easiest healthfoods to digest. Its redness indicates its high levels of beta-carotene, although it is also rich in minerals, especially potassium, and is a great cleanser. Blitz the seeds in the blender too, for extra zinc and vitamin E. Choose a watermelon that feels heavy for its size and makes a hollow sound when tapped. *Preparation: Cut out a wedge from the whole fruit and cut the flesh away from the rind. Chop to fit.*

Strawberry — Probably the most abundant and popular berry in the West, the strawberry is one of the richest food sources of vitamin C. It is also abundant in a range of beneficial minerals, especially calcium, which is good for bones and teeth. *Preparation: Wash well and, if blending, remove the hulls (no need if juicing).*

The following fruits appear in the recipes, but not as base ingredients. It is worth noting their nutritional value.

Date — Clearly not for juicing, but give a rich, natural sweetness to a smoothie and load it with energy from the sugar. They're also a useful source of vitamin C. The best are the large, soft, sticky Medjool variety. *Preparation: Wash, halve and remove the stones.*

Grape — The grape is a very cleansing, alkaline, nutritious fruit, which is why grape-juice diets have been used for many years to heal chronic illnesses. The seedless varieties of either green or red grapes should be used for drinks, although red grapes are richer in antioxidants, notably those which can help reduce the threat of heart disease. *Preparation: Wash well.*

Guava — Not easy to get hold of, but if you do come across guavas, they make a fantastic addition to a drink. Choose fruits with a green-yellow skin – the fruit and the juice will be white to pink. Many stores sell guava nectar, but be sure to buy unsweetened brands. *Preparation: Peel, halve, remove the seeds and chop into chunks.*

Kiwi — The brown, hairy exterior of the kiwi fruit belies its beautiful green interior with magically patterned black seeds. One of the richest sources of vitamin C, kiwis are also laden with beneficial minerals, especially potassium. Unfortunately, like much fresh produce these days, they are usually picked too early, but will ripen at home – just make sure they don't get too soft and develop a sweet acetone flavour. *Preparation: Peel and chop into chunks.*

Lemon — Too tart ever to be drunk neat, lemon juice is perfect for toning down the sweetness or saltiness of other juices, or even for being diluted with hot or cold water. Rich in vitamin C and bioflavonoids (mainly in the pith), lemons are also high in a range of minerals and are a particularly good source of potassium. To extract the maximum amount of juice, choose lemons that are heavy given their size and feel slightly soft. *Preparation: If juicing, peel and chop into chunks. If squeezing, cut in half.*

Lime — Smaller, green relatives of lemons, limes have similar health properties and add a wonderful tropical tang to juices. *Preparation: If juicing, peel and chop into chunks. If squeezing, cut in half.*

Passion fruit — The uglier and wrinklier the passion fruit, the more likely it is to be full and juicy. Each fruit should have orange flesh, grey seeds and a pink inner lining. Passion fruit is a good source of vitamin C and has a richly perfumed flavour that stands out in almost any drink. *Preparation: Cut in half and scoop out the flesh.*

Tangerine — Similar to the orange, but sweeter and with a far looser skin, any one of the tangerine/clementine family produces a refreshing, milder alternative to orange juice. Although you get the most juice by squeezing tangerines, putting them through a juicer will give you bioflavonoids from the pith. *Preparation: If juicing, peel and chop into chunks. If squeezing, cut in half.*

vegetables

There are few vegetable juices, other than carrot, that are drinkable neat: most are simply not palatable enough. They are also generally too strong and should be diluted with other juices.

Carrot — Producing the sweetest and best-tasting of vegetable juices, carrots are packed with vitamins and minerals, not least the antioxidant beta-carotene. The carrot's overall nutrient value makes it an immune-boosting, skin-clearing, digestion-supporting drink. *Preparation: Scrub well, top and tail and cut to fit your juicer.*

Cucumber — Cucumber juice is surprisingly flavourful, given the bland nature of the vegetable. Because of its mineral balance and high water content, cucumber is one of the best natural diuretics. Choose firm, dark cucumbers. *Preparation: Wash well and chop to fit.*

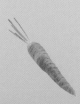

Watercress — Watercress is a very powerful cleanser owing to its high chlorophyll and sulphur contents. It is good for digestion, the skin, the circulation and the bladder, and is an exceptional, all-round juice. Because it is so potent, watercress is best well-diluted with other juices. Choose only green leaves, discarding any that have started to go yellow. *Preparation: Wash well.*

Broccoli — With even more vitamin C than oranges (weight for weight), broccoli is loaded with important antioxidant and cleansing nutrients, some of which have been shown to protect against cancer. Choose compact, green heads for the freshest, most nutritious juice. *Preparation: Wash well and cut to fit your juicer.*

Cabbage — Although on its own it is not particularly palatable as a juice, cabbage is worth slipping into other juices for its far-reaching health properties. Like other members of its family (broccoli, kale and so on), cabbage is full of vitamins, minerals and anti-cancer nutrients. It is also soothing for stomach problems, including ulcers. *Preparation: Remove outer leaves, cut off pieces to fit.*

Kale — One of nature's wonderfoods, kale is full of vitamins (especially A and C) and minerals as well as anti-cancer nutrients. As such it is a very cleansing, immune-boosting, skin-healing, bone-building, generally excellent all-round health bonanza. *Preparation: Wash well.*

Lettuce — Choose the darker varieties, which tend to be richer in all minerals and vitamins. Lettuce is cleansing because of the combination of nutrients and high water content, but it is also known for its sedative properties and is best added to juices as a relaxant or sleep aid. *Preparation: Wash well.*

Parsley — Parsley is one of the top ingredients in the health stakes. Its dark green colour comes from its rich chlorophyll content, which makes it highly cleansing. Parsley is also good for aiding digestion and for generally providing the body with a stack of minerals and vitamins. *Preparation: Wash well.*

Spinach — Exceptionally rich in vitamin C, beta-carotene and iron, spinach is also highly cleansing and is laden with health-boosting, regenerative properties. These tone the digestive system, the liver and the circulation. However, it is high in oxalic acid, which interferes with calcium absorption, so spinach juice should not be drunk in large quantities. Choose small, bright green leaves. *Preparation: Wash well.*

Beet (beetroot) — The wonderful juice of beet has a distinctly "soily" taste to it. This earthiness gives a hint of the very rich mineral and vitamin content, and, as such, beet is one of the most cleansing, blood-boosting, tonic-like juices there is. Juice the greens too, if you can get hold of them, as they add an even greater health dimension. *Preparation: Top and tail, scrub well and cut to fit.*

Parsnip — This white relative of the carrot provides a sweet, earthy touch to a juice, as well as an all-round dose of minerals and vitamins for the body. Parsnip is rich in the trace elements sulphur and silicon, good for healthy hair, skin and nails. *Preparation: Scrub well, top and tail and cut to fit.*

Sweet potato — Not related to the potato, the sweet potato is generally easier to digest and higher in fibre than its namesake. It is also a rich source of beta-carotene. Sweet potatoes are soothing to the digestive tract, cleansing, and have an alkalizing effect on the body. *Preparation: Scrub well and cut to fit.*

Tomato — Although strictly speaking a fruit, the tomato is commonly classed as a vegetable as it has a savoury rather than a sweet taste. Tomatoes taste quite acidic, but, in fact, have a soothing effect on the body. They offer nutrients which can ease problems with digestion, the liver and the skin. Tomatoes also contain lycopene, an antioxidant shown to help prostate problems. *Preparation: Wash well and slice to fit.*

Celery — A refreshing, salty juice, celery complements other vegetable-juice flavours by cutting through the richer, sweeter tastes. Celery is a very cleansing, soothing juice, with diuretic properties (helping to rid the body of excess water). Juice the whole stick, including the leaves. *Preparation: Scrub well.*

Other ingredients used in some of the recipes include:

Bell peppers — Also called simply peppers or capsicums, red, green and yellow bell peppers add a sweet flavour to juice and are an excellent source of antioxidants, particularly vitamin C and beta-carotene. *Preparation: Wash well and slice.*

Ginger — An age-old natural remedy, the root of the ginger plant helps improve digestion and circulation, and relieves nausea, bloating, colds, sore throats and inflammation of any sort. *Preparation: Wash well, peel if shrivelled and slice.*

Mint — This aromatic herb is a refreshing, soothing addition to a drink. It helps to enhance digestion and calm the digestive tract, quell nausea and relieve cramps. The menthol in mint can also soothe congestion in the respiratory tract. Choose fresh, deep green leaves. *Preparation: Wash well.*

healthy additives

You can enhance the health properties of your juice or smoothie even further by adding certain vitamin and mineral supplements, and other health-enhancing foods. Some of the additives are best blended with smoothies only, as they don't mix well in a pure, liquid juice.

additives for juices or smoothies

Vitamin and mineral drops/powder — Some companies make excellent vitamins and minerals in the form of liquid drops or powders. Adding them to your daily juice or smoothie is a good way of taking them, especially for children.

Herbal drops — If you take herbal medicines, such as echinacea or a blend from your herbalist, mixing them with a juice may be a more palatable option. (Check with your herbalist whether or not mixing with just water may be better.)

Spirulina/Barleygrass/Wheatgrass powder— Dense forms of nutrients especially rich in cleansing chlorophyll, these three are nature's wonderfoods in a green powder. If you're mixing one with juice, it is best to shake it with a little juice in a jar before blending it with the rest.

smoothie-only additives

Wheatgerm — Most of the goodness in a grain of wheat is found in the germ: a great additive to smoothies for an extra boost of vitamins and minerals, particularly vitamins B and E.

Flaxseeds — Also known as linseeds, these are one of the richest vegetarian sources of essential fatty acids, as well as being packed with vitamins and minerals.

Pumpkin/sunflower seeds — These not only give smoothies a nutty, crunchy taste and texture, but also increase their vitamin, mineral and essential fatty acid content.

Cold-pressed seed oils — Far from the usual commercial varieties, cold-pressed oils, such as from sunflower or pumpkin seeds, are unadulterated sources of essential fatty acids.

Tahini — This creamed sesame seed paste adds a distinctive flavour to any smoothie, as well as boosting its nutrient content.

Blackstrap molasses — Derived from the whole cane from which sugar is extracted, syrupy sweet molasses is laden with minerals (particularly iron and calcium) and B-vitamins.

Lecithin — Part of every cell of the body, lecithin is particularly important for the digestion of fats and for healthy nerve and brain cells. Add it to your smoothie in powder form.

Brewer's yeast — This is one of the best sources of B-vitamins available, and also contains a host of vital minerals.

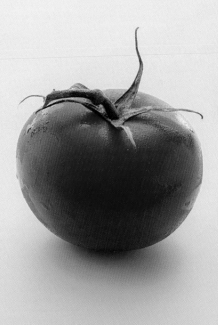

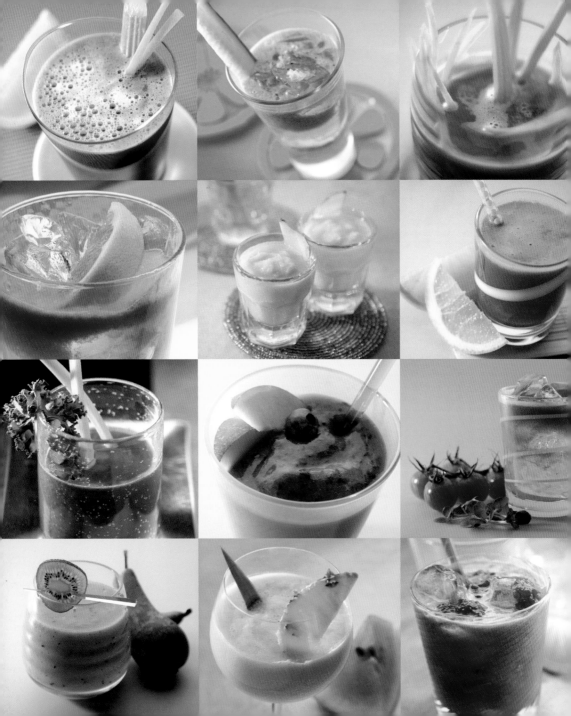

making
juices

Once you start on the adventure of making a fresh juice every day, you will be hooked. By now you are aware of the delights and benefits of pressing your own juice and here's where the actual process begins. You've got the juicer (you may even have used it); on the following pages are hundreds of blends to stimulate both your palate and your imagination.

We begin with juices based on fruits (blends 1–132), followed by juices based on vegetables (blends 133–228). Each recipe makes two portions unless otherwise stated. If you feel you'd like some guidance on which recipes to try first, you may like to experiment with The Basic Intro Week (see page 706) which will gently introduce you to the idea of blending different fruits and a few vegetables. Guidelines for preparing the ingredients are given on pages 16–30, so simply get them ready and juice away!

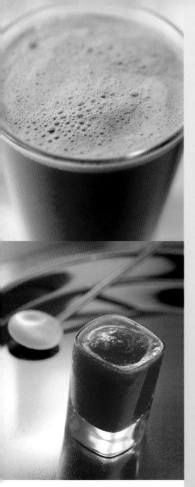

top tips

Below are a few reminders and helpful hints, tips and suggestions to enable you to get the most from your juicing.

1 When selecting fruit to juice, choose pieces that are almost but not quite ripe, as these tend to yield the maximum amount of juice and the best taste from your juicer.

2 Avoid juicing fruits that are over-ripe or too soft as these generally do not pass well through a juicer.

3 Get into the habit of always washing your juicer immediately after use, when it is much easier to clean.

4 To get the most out of citrus fruits, extract the juice using a citrus press rather than a juicer.

5 While all fruit and veg must be washed well before use, avoid soaking them as this can weaken their nutrient content.

6 If you do peel your fruit or veg, do it as finely as possible so as to preserve as many of the vital nutrients as you can.

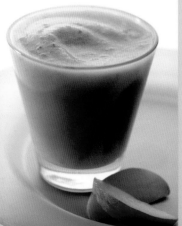

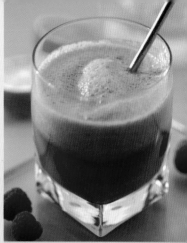

7 To prevent juices from going even slightly brown (signifying oxidation, which damages their nutrient content), drink them immediately or pour them into a jug containing a squeeze of lemon juice or a spoon of vitamin C powder.

8 Dilute your vegetable juices with a little water if you find them too strong-tasting. Always dilute vegetable juices for children.

9 If you find that your energy levels fluctuate throughout the day, emphasize vegetable juices, and dilute any fruit juices you do have with water. Fruit juices contain high levels of natural sugar which give an immediate energy boost but this can be followed by a dip in your energy level.

10 Although you won't ever be stuck for recipes using this book, be experimental and create your own blends using whatever you have in the refrigerator and fruit bowl.

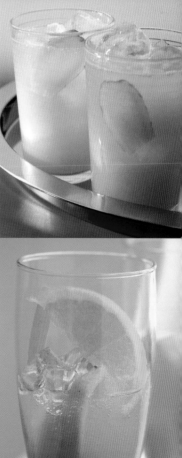

001 eve's downfall

4 apples

I always have a sense that if you're going to make the
effort to make a juice, then make it interesting – but
pure, freshly pressed apple juice is exquisite and
you can't beat the home-made, frothy, delicate green
version. My favourite apples are Granny Smith and
Egremont Russet but you could use any type you like.

NUTRIENTS
Beta-carotene, folic acid, vitamin C;
calcium, magnesium, phosphorus,
potassium, sulphur

ENERGY	★★★★★
DETOX	★★★★☆
IMMUNITY	★★☆☆☆
DIGESTION	★★★☆☆
SKIN	★★★☆☆

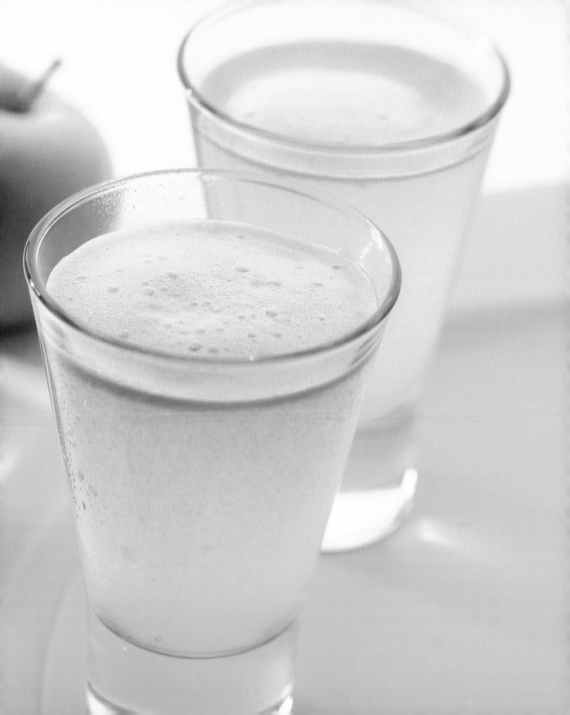

002   apple basic

3 apples

2 carrots

Most of us can rustle up a few apples from the fruit bowl and carrots from the refrigerator. This delicious but simple combination is a good way to introduce carrot to your juice repertoire if you're not used to vegetable juices.

NUTRIENTS
Beta-carotene, folic acid, vitamin C;
calcium, magnesium, phosphorus,
potassium, sodium, sulphur

ENERGY	★★★★☆
DETOX	★★★★☆
IMMUNITY	★★☆☆☆
DIGESTION	★★☆☆☆
SKIN	★★★★☆

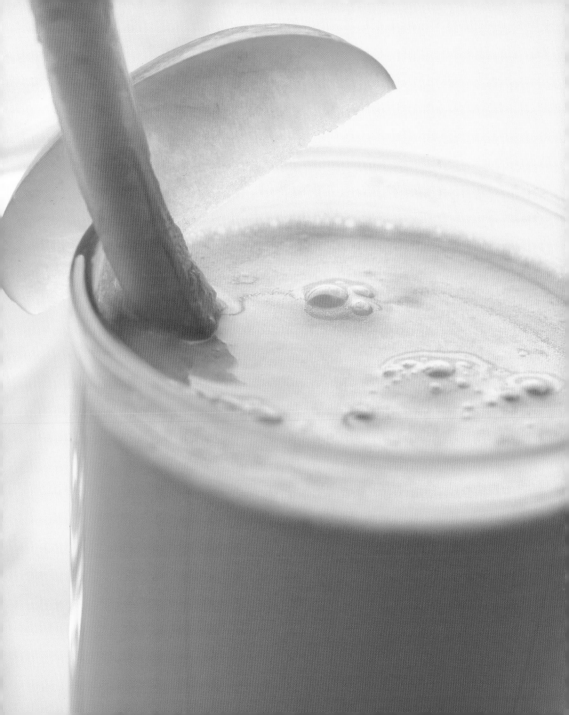

003 ocean deep

4 apples

1 teaspoon spirulina

The combination of the pale green apple juice and dark green spirulina powder makes this power-packed juice look like the deep, green sea. Shake the spirulina with a little of the juice in a jar before mixing it with the rest of the juice.

NUTRIENTS
Beta-carotene, folic acid, vitamins B1, B2, B3, B5, B6 and C; calcium, magnesium, phosphorus, potassium, sulphur; protein; essential fatty acids

ENERGY ★★★★☆
DETOX ★★★★☆
IMMUNITY ★★★☆☆
DIGESTION ★★☆☆☆
SKIN ★★★★☆

004 basic with a boost

3 apples

2 carrots

½ inch (1 cm) ginger root

1 teaspoon spirulina

The addition of spirulina sends the nutritious value of this juice on to another plane. Stir or shake in the spirulina powder after you have made the juice.

NUTRIENTS
Beta-carotene, folic acid, vitamin C; calcium, magnesium, phosphorus, potassium, sulphur; protein; essential fatty acids

ENERGY ★★★☆☆
DETOX ★★★★☆
IMMUNITY ★★★☆☆
DIGESTION ★★★☆☆
SKIN ★★★☆☆

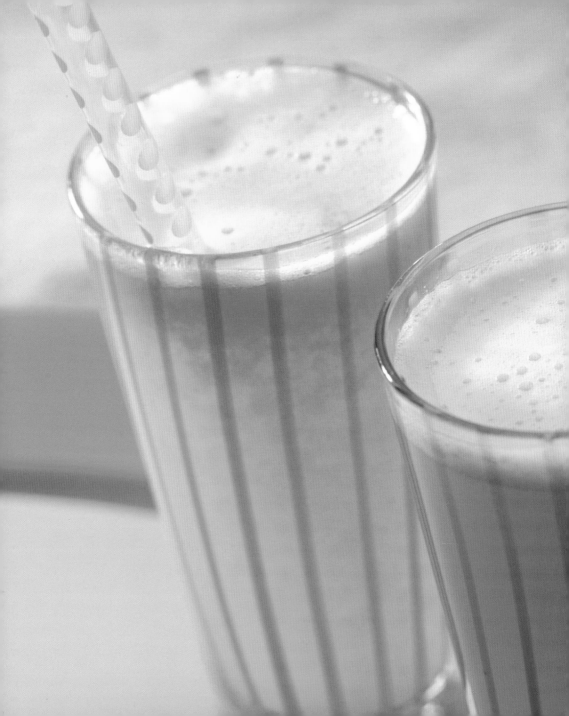

005 orchard blend

3 apples

1 pear

Made with classic orchard fruits, this sweet juice really makes you realize why apples and pears are the staples of a fruit bowl and not so boring after all.

NUTRIENTS

Beta-carotene, folic acid, vitamin C; calcium, magnesium, phosphorus, potassium, sulphur

ENERGY	★★★★☆
DETOX	★★☆☆☆
IMMUNITY	★★☆☆☆
DIGESTION	★★★☆☆
SKIN	★★★☆☆

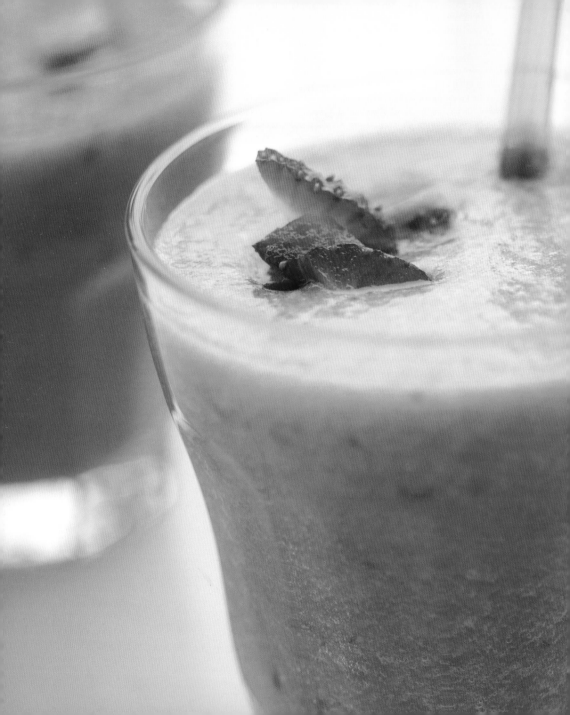

006 apple blush

3 apples

1 nectarine

8 strawberries

The delicate colour of this juice gives only the slightest indication of the sensational taste, especially if you use a tangy variety of apple such as Granny Smith combined with sweet, ripe strawberries and nectarines.

NUTRIENTS
Beta-carotene, biotin, folic acid, vitamin C; calcium, magnesium, phosphorus, potassium, sulphur

ENERGY	★★★★★
DETOX	★★☆☆☆
IMMUNITY	★★★☆☆
DIGESTION	★☆☆☆☆
SKIN	★★★★☆

007 sweet 'n' savoury

3 apples

2 sticks celery

The saltiness of the celery nicely offsets the sweetness of the apples in this refreshing juice. It's a perfect thirst-quencher, especially if you use a sharp apple variety such as Granny Smith.

NUTRIENTS
Beta-carotene, folic acid, vitamin C; calcium, magnesium, manganese, phosphorus, potassium, sodium, sulphur

ENERGY	★★☆☆☆
DETOX	★★★☆☆
IMMUNITY	★☆☆☆☆
DIGESTION	★★★☆☆
SKIN	★★★☆☆

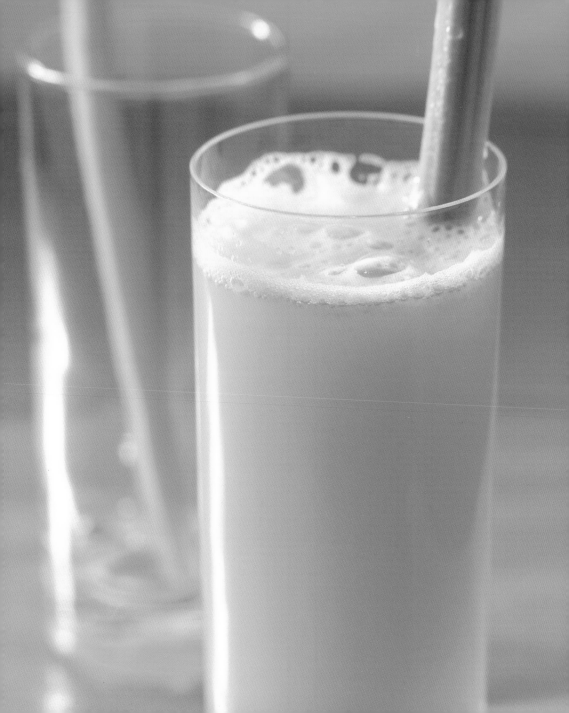

008   sweet c

3 apples

2 guavas

This is one of the few recipes for which I suggest using a sweeter variety of apple, such as Cox, to offset the tangy guava, which is a phenomenally rich source of vitamin C.

NUTRIENTS
Beta-carotene, folic acid, vitamin B3, vitamin C; calcium, magnesium, phosphorus, potassium, sodium, sulphur

ENERGY ★★★★☆
DETOX ★★★☆☆
IMMUNITY ★★★★★
DIGESTION ★☆☆☆☆
SKIN ★★★★☆

009 sweet c too

2 apples

2 oranges

You may think that oranges would completely overwhelm the delicate juice of the apples, but actually they really enhance it and make this drink a simple, refreshing start to the day. Remember that oranges are best juiced on a citrus press and added to the apple juice made in the extractor, although you can push peeled orange pieces through the juicer.

NUTRIENTS
Beta-carotene, folic acid, vitamin C;
calcium, magnesium, phosphorus,
potassium, sodium, sulphur

ENERGY	★★★★☆
DETOX	★★★☆☆
IMMUNITY	★★★★☆
DIGESTION	★☆☆☆☆
SKIN	★★★☆☆

010 apple tropics

3 apples

½ pineapple

½ lime

½ passion fruit

An extra tang and taste of the tropics is evident in this apple recipe. It's best to stir the passion fruit into the juice once it's made, rather than passing it through the blender.

NUTRIENTS
Beta-carotene, folic acid, vitamin C; calcium, magnesium, manganese, phosphorus, potassium, sulphur

ENERGY ★★★★☆
DETOX ★★☆☆☆
IMMUNITY ★★★☆☆
DIGESTION ★★★★☆
SKIN ★★★☆☆

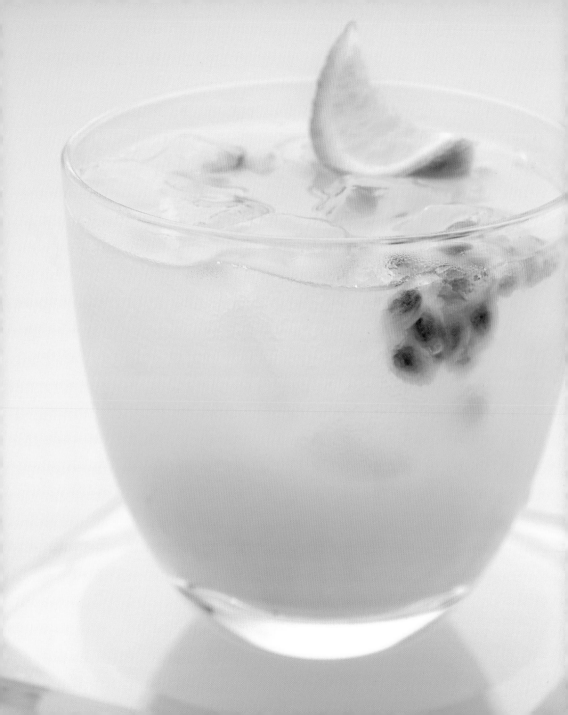

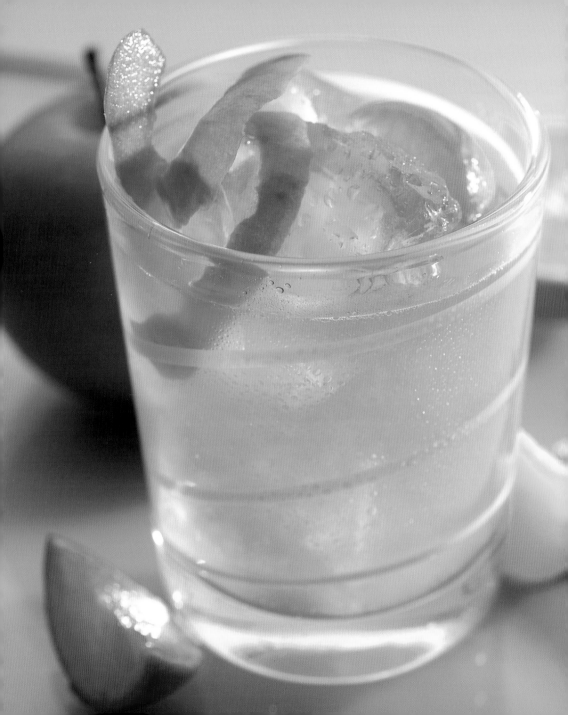

011 citrus apples

3 apples

2 tangerines

½ lime

The more delicate flavour of tangerines
(or clementines or other such fruits, rather than
oranges) adds a subtle layer around the apple,
while the lime gives it a great afterbite.

NUTRIENTS
Beta-carotene, folic acid, vitamin C;
calcium, magnesium, phosphorus,
potassium, sodium, sulphur

ENERGY	★★★☆☆
DETOX	★★☆☆☆
IMMUNITY	★★★★☆
DIGESTION	★☆☆☆☆
SKIN	★★★☆☆

012 apple cleanser

2 apples

2 kale leaves

1 stick celery

⅓ long cucumber

½ beet (beetroot)

The fruitiness of the apples offsets the more challenging taste of the greens to produce this beautifully red detoxifying juice.

NUTRIENTS
Beta-carotene, folic acid, vitamin B3,
vitamin C; calcium, iron, magnesium,
manganese, phosphorus, potassium,
sulphur

ENERGY	★★☆☆☆
DETOX	★★★★☆
IMMUNITY	★★★☆☆
DIGESTION	★★☆☆☆
SKIN	★★★☆☆

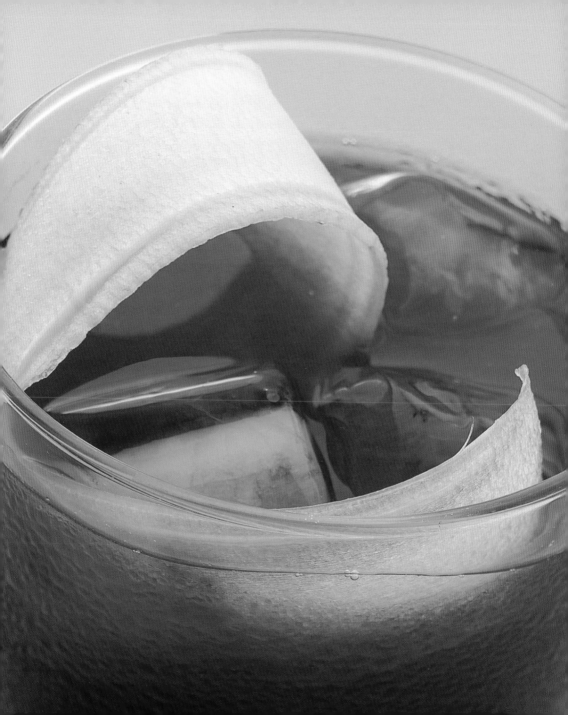

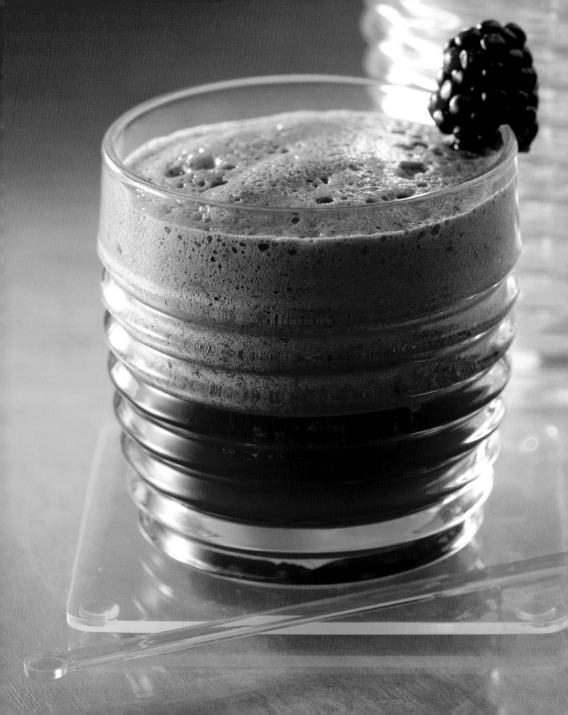

013 winter crumble

2 apples

2 handfuls blackberries

I can't help but think of a hot pie or crumble when I make this juice. You could actually heat it up (but don't let it boil) after you've made it, for a warm drink on a cold night, but personally I like my juices cold.

NUTRIENTS
Beta-carotene, folic acid, vitamin B3, vitamin C; calcium, iron, magnesium, manganese, phosphorus, potassium, sodium, sulphur

ENERGY	★★★★★
DETOX	★★☆☆☆
IMMUNITY	★★★★☆
DIGESTION	★☆☆☆☆
SKIN	★★★★☆

014 apple pie

4 apples

½ teaspoon ground cinnamon

It's quite hard to stir in the cinnamon powder – instead I suggest putting the juice in a jar and shaking it up to add the spicy kick.

NUTRIENTS
Beta-carotene, folic acid, vitamin B3,
vitamin C; calcium, magnesium,
phosphorus, potassium, sodium,
sulphur

ENERGY	★★★★☆
DETOX	★★★☆☆
IMMUNITY	★★☆☆☆
DIGESTION	★★★☆☆
SKIN	★★★☆☆

015 apple blues

3 apples

2 good handfuls blueberries

If your blueberries are particularly sweet, choose a crisp, tangy apple such as Granny Smith; otherwise, use a sweeter type like Jonagold or Empire.

NUTRIENTS
Beta-carotene, biotin, folic acid,
vitamins B1, B2, B6, C and E; calcium,
chromium, magnesium, sodium

ENERGY ★★★★★
DETOX ★★★☆☆
IMMUNITY ★★★★☆
DIGESTION ★☆☆☆☆
SKIN ★★★★☆

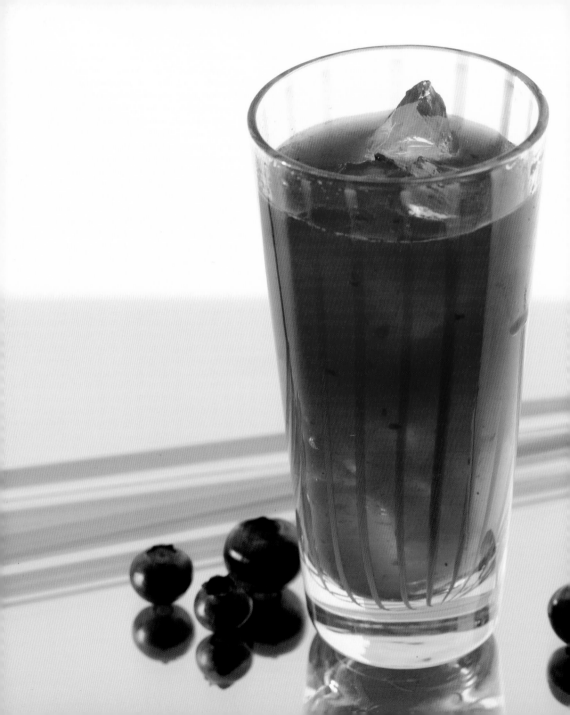

016 black orchard berry buster

3 apples

2 good handfuls dark berries such
as blueberries, blackcurrants
or blackberries

It may seem a waste to juice plump,
sweet berries, but I can't resist it
sometimes. In the winter you can
throw a few canned berries into the
juicer but it's not quite the same thing.

NUTRIENTS
Beta-carotene, folic acid,
vitamins B1, B2, B6, C and E; calcium,
chromium, magnesium, manganese,
phosphorus, potassium, sodium,
sulphur

ENERGY	★★★★★
DETOX	★★★☆☆
IMMUNITY	★★★★☆
DIGESTION	★☆☆☆☆
SKIN	★★★★☆

017   pink orchard berry buster

3 apples

2 good handfuls red berries such as raspberries or strawberries

Another treat, using fresh, sweet berries in the summer to turn tangy
apple juice into a pastel thirst-quencher.

NUTRIENTS
Beta-carotene, biotin, folic acid,
vitamin C; calcium, magnesium,
manganese, phosphorus, potassium,
sodium, sulphur

ENERGY	★★★☆☆
DETOX	★☆☆☆☆
IMMUNITY	★★★★☆
DIGESTION	★☆☆☆☆
SKIN	★★★★☆

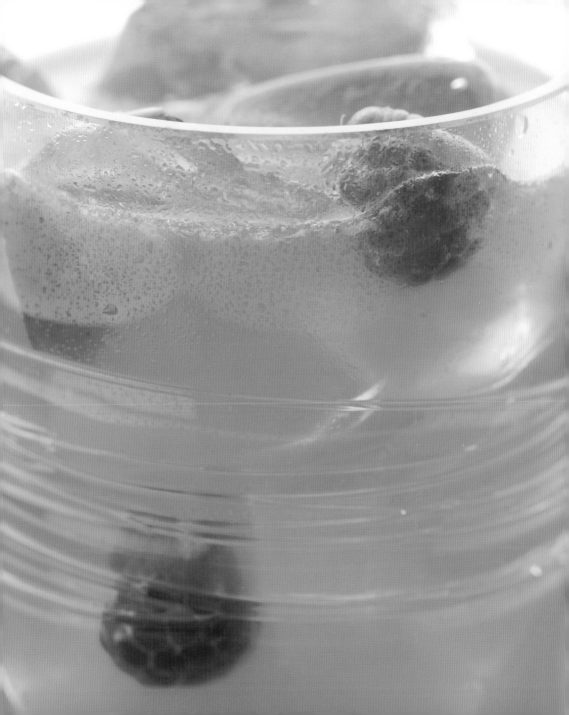

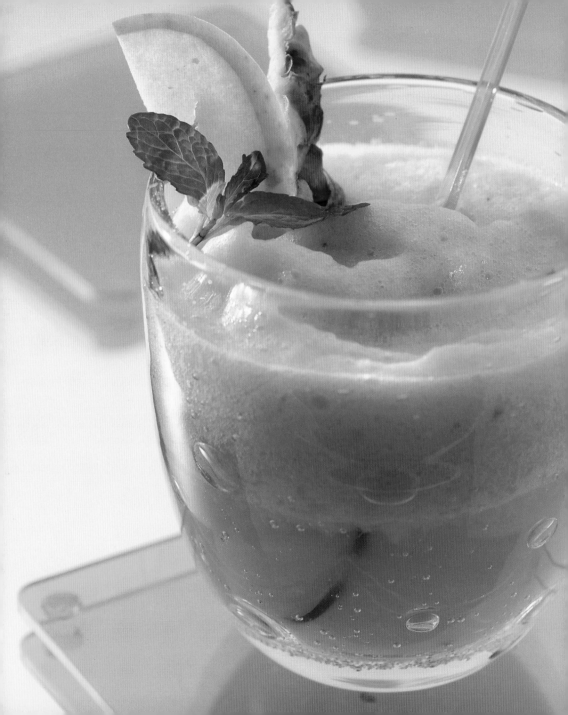

018 double apple

2 apples

⅓ pineapple

1 small bunch fresh mint

When I was living in Bangkok, apples were a luxury, unlike the ubiquitous pineapple. Unfortunately, it's completely the other way around in most other parts of the world. Use sweeter apples such as Cox to match with the amazing juicy tang of the pineapple, which is particularly helpful for digestion.

NUTRIENTS
Beta-carotene, folic acid, vitamin B3, vitamin C; calcium, magnesium, manganese, phosphorus, potassium, sodium, sulphur

ENERGY	★★★☆☆
DETOX	★☆☆☆☆
IMMUNITY	★★★☆☆
DIGESTION	★★★★★
SKIN	★★☆☆☆

019 waldorf salad

2 apples

2 sticks celery

1 tablespoon (15 ml) cold-pressed hemp-seed oil

This one reminds me of a Waldorf salad, without the walnuts – the hemp-seed oil will give you a similar benefit of omega-3 fatty acids. The oil will blend best if it's shaken with the juice in a jar.

NUTRIENTS
Beta-carotene, folic acid, vitamin C; calcium, magnesium, manganese, phosphorus, potassium, sodium, sulphur; essential fatty acids

ENERGY	★★★★☆
DETOX	★★★☆☆
IMMUNITY	★★★☆☆
DIGESTION	★★★☆☆
SKIN	★★★☆☆

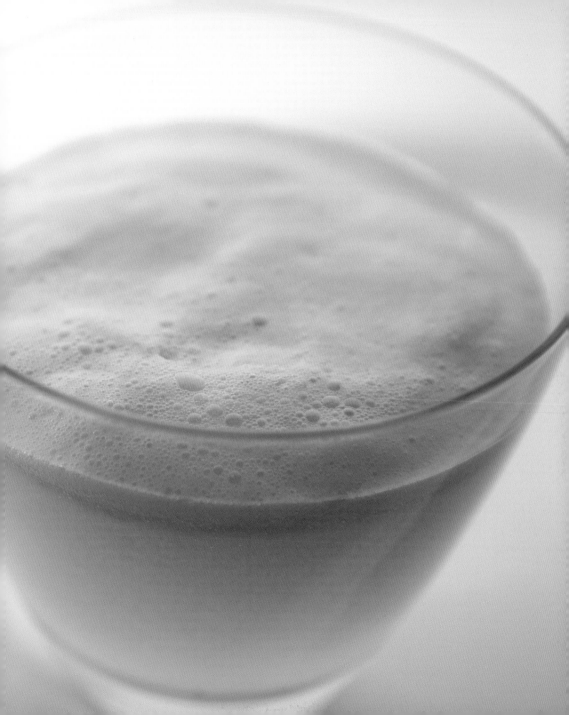

020 bleeding apples

3 apples

½ beet (beetroot)

The colour of beet overtakes that of any other juice and it gives a deep, earthy flavour. This recipe is a gentle introduction to the powerful juice of this root vegetable. For heftier doses, see blends 187–90.

NUTRIENTS
Beta-carotene, folic acid, vitamin C;
calcium, magnesium, phosphorus,
potassium, sodium, sulphur

ENERGY	★★★★☆
DETOX	★★★★★
IMMUNITY	★★☆☆☆
DIGESTION	★★☆☆☆
SKIN	★★★☆☆

021 apple tang

3 apples

1 grapefruit

1 lime

The sweetness of the apple – best to use a sweet variety – combines well with the grapefruit and lime.

NUTRIENTS
Beta-carotene, folic acid, vitamin C;
calcium, magnesium, phosphorus,
potassium, sodium, sulphur

ENERGY	★★★★☆
DETOX	★★☆☆☆
IMMUNITY	★★★☆☆
DIGESTION	★☆☆☆☆
SKIN	★★★☆☆

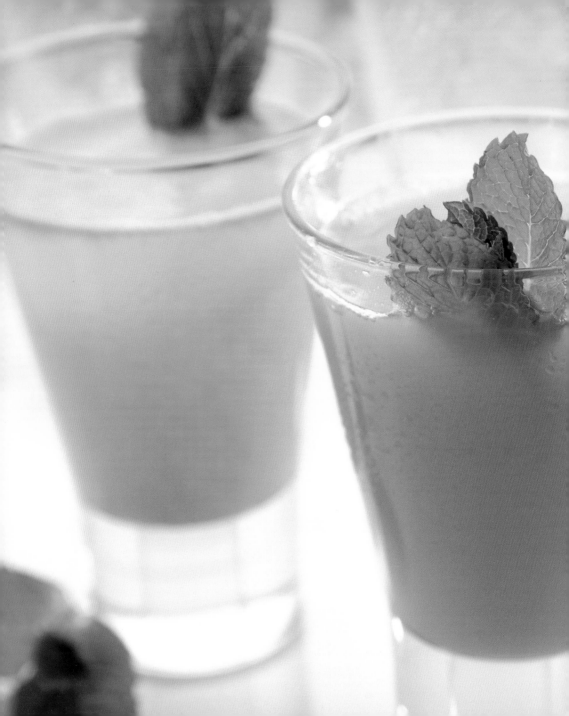

022 apple gone loupey

3 apples

2 thick slices melon

1 small bunch fresh mint

To contrast with the sweetness of a ripe melon, it's best to use a sharper apple variety such as Egremont Russet or Granny Smith.

NUTRIENTS
Beta-carotene, folic acid, vitamin C; calcium, magnesium, phosphorus, potassium, sodium, sulphur

ENERGY	★★★★★
DETOX	★★★☆☆
IMMUNITY	★★★☆☆
DIGESTION	★☆☆☆☆
SKIN	★★★★☆

023   waterapple

3 apples

2 thick slices watermelon

1 lime

I would usually use watermelon to make a smoothie (see blends 288–90), but this combination is irresistible. Use a sharp type of apple.

NUTRIENTS
Beta-carotene, folic acid, vitamin C;
calcium, magnesium, phosphorus,
potassium, sulphur

ENERGY	★★★★★
DETOX	★★★★☆
IMMUNITY	★★★☆☆
DIGESTION	★☆☆☆☆
SKIN	★★★★☆

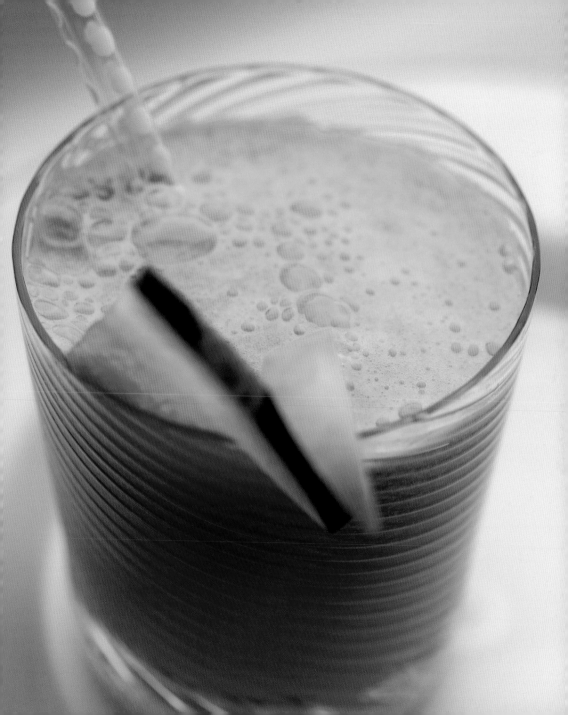

024 apple lullaby

2 apples

¼ lettuce

½ lemon

(makes 1 glass of juice)

The lettuce is the key sleep-inducing ingredient in this juice.
Best drunk just as you plan to hit the pillow. You can use any
variety of lettuce.

NUTRIENTS
Beta-carotene, folic acid, vitamin C;
calcium, magnesium, phosphorus,
potassium, sulphur

ENERGY	★☆☆☆☆
DETOX	★★★☆☆
IMMUNITY	★★★☆☆
DIGESTION	★☆☆☆☆
SKIN	★★★☆☆

025 grape ape

3 apples

1 bunch red grapes

1 nectarine

Very cleansing and refreshing. Choose a variety of apple that contrasts with the level of sweetness of the grapes, and use a nectarine (or peach) that is ripe enough to yield to a gentle press of your thumb.

NUTRIENTS
Beta-carotene, folic acid, vitamin C,
vitamin E; calcium, magnesium,
manganese, phosphorus,
potassium, sulphur

ENERGY ★★★★★
DETOX ★★★☆☆
IMMUNITY ★★★☆☆
DIGESTION ★☆☆☆☆
SKIN ★★★★☆

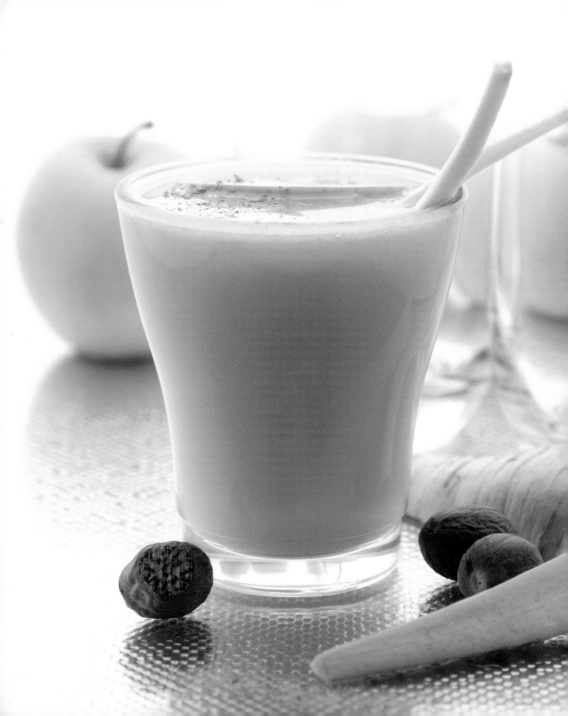

026 parsnapple

3 apples

2 parsnips

sprinkling of grated nutmeg

I certainly turned my nose up when I first heard of the concept of juicing a parsnip, but actually it's deliciously sweet. Blend it with a sharp apple variety. You can leave out the nutmeg if you don't feel like shaking it all up, otherwise it'll just sit on top.

NUTRIENTS
Beta-carotene, folic acid, vitamin C; calcium, magnesium, phosphorus, potassium, sodium, sulphur

ENERGY	★★★☆☆
DETOX	★★★☆☆
IMMUNITY	★★☆☆☆
DIGESTION	★☆☆☆☆
SKIN	★★★☆☆

027 apple zing

3 apples

2 carrots

½ inch (1 cm) ginger root

Basic with a bite – the ginger gives a sharp snap to an otherwise sweet juice. Just break or slice off a piece of ginger root and juice it with the other ingredients.

NUTRIENTS
Beta-carotene, folic acid, vitamin C;
calcium, magnesium, phosphorus,
potassium, sulphur

ENERGY	★★★★☆
DETOX	★★★☆☆
IMMUNITY	★★★☆☆
DIGESTION	★★★★☆
SKIN	★★★★☆

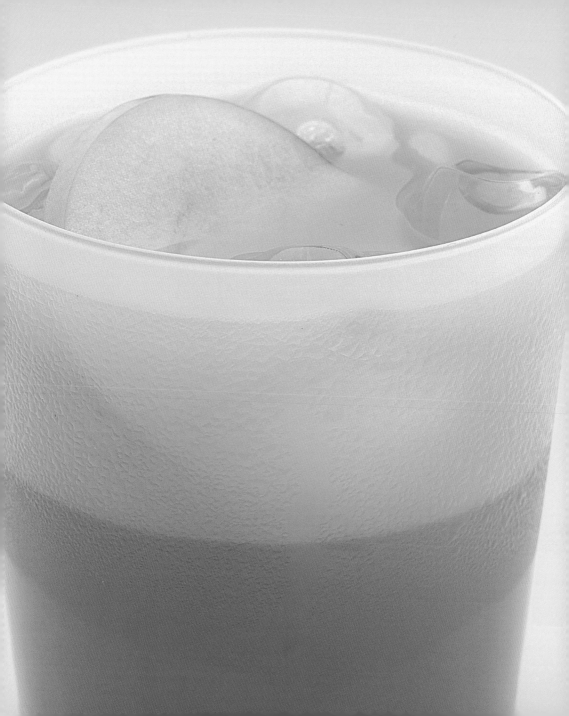

028   cranapple

3 apples

1 handful cranberries

1 handful grapes

Although cranberries are best known for combating urinary tract infections, they are also delicious, tangy and great for the immune system in general. Use sweet varieties of apples and grapes to offset the sharpness of the cranberries.

NUTRIENTS
Beta-carotene, folic acid, vitamin C, vitamin E; calcium, iron, magnesium, manganese, phosphorus, potassium, sulphur

ENERGY	★★★★★
DETOX	★★☆☆☆
IMMUNITY	★★★★☆
DIGESTION	★★☆☆☆
SKIN	★★★★☆

029 prime cooler

3 apples

½ long cucumber

1 inch (2.5 cm) ginger root

1 small bunch fresh mint

There are few juice blends which are quite so refreshing – the sweetness of the apple is offset by the watery cucumber and sharpened by the ginger and mint.

NUTRIENTS
Beta-carotene, folic acid, vitamin C; calcium, magnesium, phosphorus, potassium, sodium, sulphur

ENERGY	★★☆☆☆
DETOX	★★★☆☆
IMMUNITY	★★☆☆☆
DIGESTION	★★★☆☆
SKIN	★★★☆☆

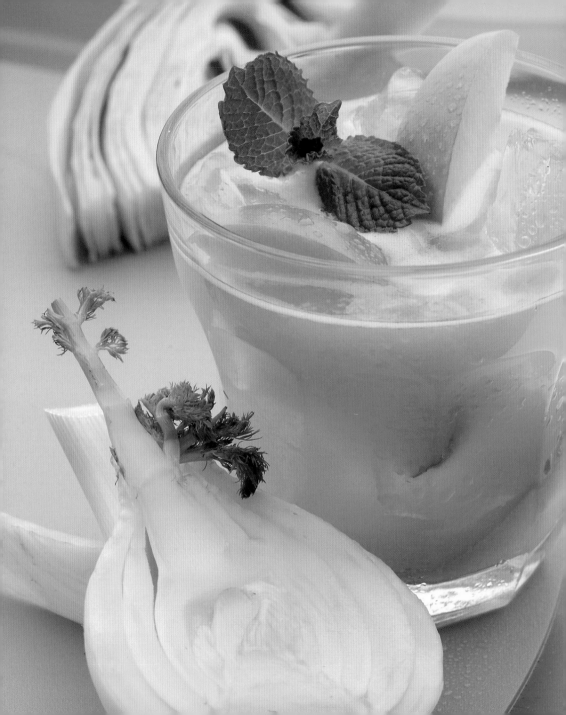

030 bellyful

3 apples

¼ white cabbage

¼ small fennel bulb

1 small bunch fresh mint

This combination is an excellent one for soothing the digestive system. The cabbage is especially good for the stomach.

NUTRIENTS
Beta-carotene, folic acid, vitamin C, vitamin E; calcium, magnesium, phosphorus, potassium, sodium, sulphur

ENERGY	★★☆☆☆
DETOX	★★★☆☆
IMMUNITY	★★☆☆☆
DIGESTION	★★★★★
SKIN	★★★☆☆

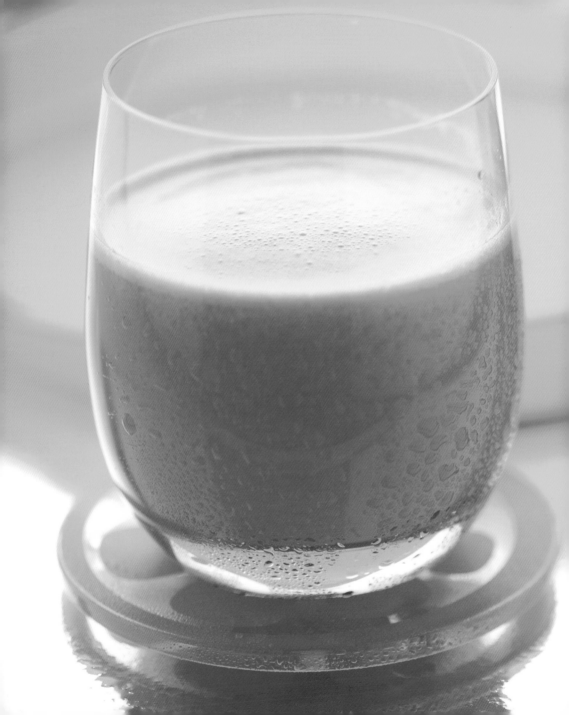

031 pure grapefruit

3 grapefruits

Another firm favourite all on its own, whether you prefer it made with sharper white fruit or the sweeter pink or ruby varieties.

NUTRIENTS
Beta-carotene, folic acid, vitamin C; calcium, magnesium, phosphorus, potassium, sulphur

ENERGY	★★★★★
DETOX	★☆☆☆☆
IMMUNITY	★★★★☆
DIGESTION	☆☆☆☆☆
SKIN	★★☆☆☆

032 grapefruit sharp

2 grapefruits

1 lemon

1 lime

You really will want to use sweet pink grapefruits for this one, unless you enjoy that eye-watering sourness.

NUTRIENTS
Beta-carotene, folic acid, vitamin C; calcium, magnesium, phosphorus, potassium, sodium, sulphur

ENERGY ★★★★☆
DETOX ★☆☆☆☆
IMMUNITY ★★★★★
DIGESTION ★☆☆☆☆
SKIN ★★☆☆☆

033 grapefruit sweet

2 grapefruits

2 tangerines

I prefer using white grapefruits for this one to contrast with the sweetness of tangerines (or clementines).

NUTRIENTS
Beta-carotene, folic acid, vitamin C; calcium, magnesium, phosphorus, potassium, sodium, sulphur

ENERGY	★★★★☆
DETOX	★☆☆☆☆
IMMUNITY	★★★★☆
DIGESTION	★☆☆☆☆
SKIN	★★☆☆☆

034 grapefruit basic

1 grapefruit

1 apple

2 carrots

1 stick celery

Another one of my stock blends for a good wake-up call in the morning.

NUTRIENTS
Beta-carotene, folic acid, vitamin C; calcium, magnesium, manganese, phosphorus, potassium, sodium, sulphur

ENERGY ★★★★☆

DETOX ★★★☆☆

IMMUNITY ★★★★☆

DIGESTION ★☆☆☆☆

SKIN ★★★☆☆

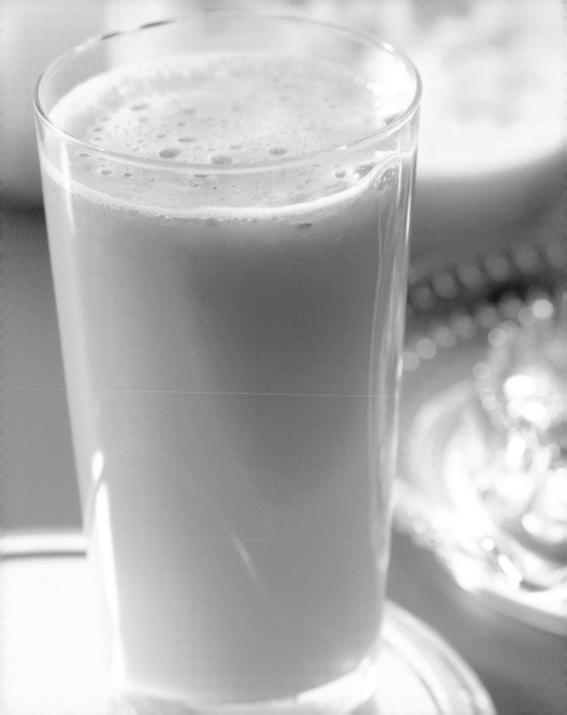

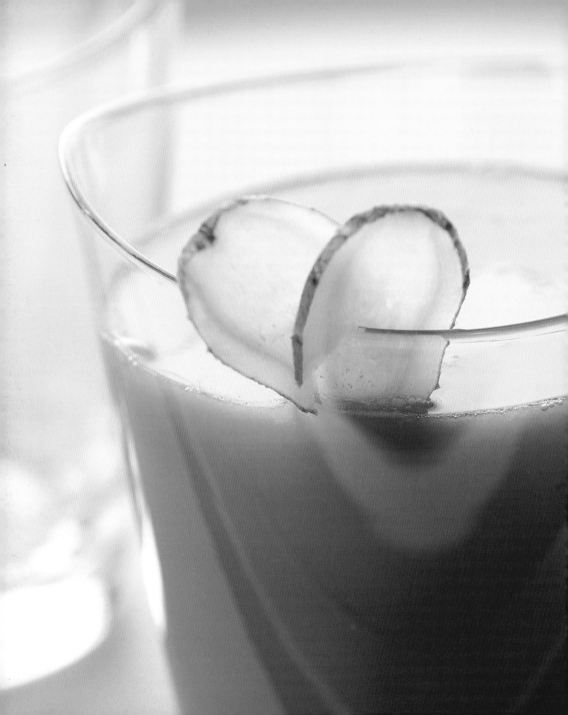

035 grapefruit basic with a bite

1 grapefruit

1 apple

2 carrots

1 stick celery

½ inch (1 cm) ginger root

This is the basic with a sharp kick from the ginger, particularly good if you've got a cold.

NUTRIENTS
Beta-carotene, folic acid, vitamin C; calcium, magnesium, manganese, phosphorus, potassium, sodium, sulphur

ENERGY	★★★★☆
DETOX	★★★☆☆
IMMUNITY	★★★☆☆
DIGESTION	★★☆☆☆
SKIN	★★★☆☆

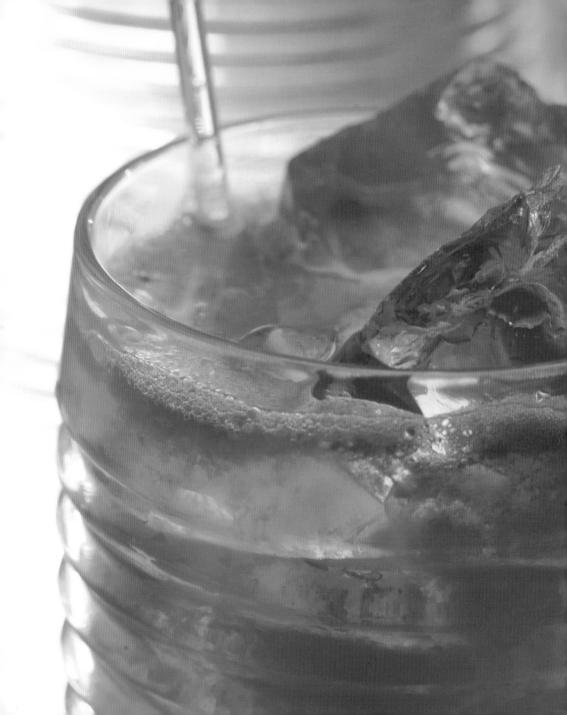

036   water cooler

2 grapefruits

1 thick slice watermelon

I have a slight preference for this over Water Cooler II (see blend 072) because the contrast of flavours and textures is even better.

NUTRIENTS
Beta-carotene, folic acid, vitamin C; calcium, iron, magnesium, phosphorus, potassium, sodium, sulphur

ENERGY	★★★★☆
DETOX	★★☆☆☆
IMMUNITY	★★★★☆
DIGESTION	☆☆☆☆☆
SKIN	★★★☆☆

037 grapefruit blues

2 grapefruits

1 large handful blueberries

Whether you choose a tangy white grapefruit or the sweeter pink variety, the addition of the blueberries will transform the colour and give an extra antioxidant lift.

NUTRIENTS

Beta-carotene, biotin, folic acid, vitamins B1, B2, B6, C and E; calcium, chromium, magnesium, phosphorus, potassium, sodium, sulphur

ENERGY	★★★★☆
DETOX	★★☆☆☆
IMMUNITY	★★★★★
DIGESTION	☆☆☆☆☆
SKIN	★★★★☆

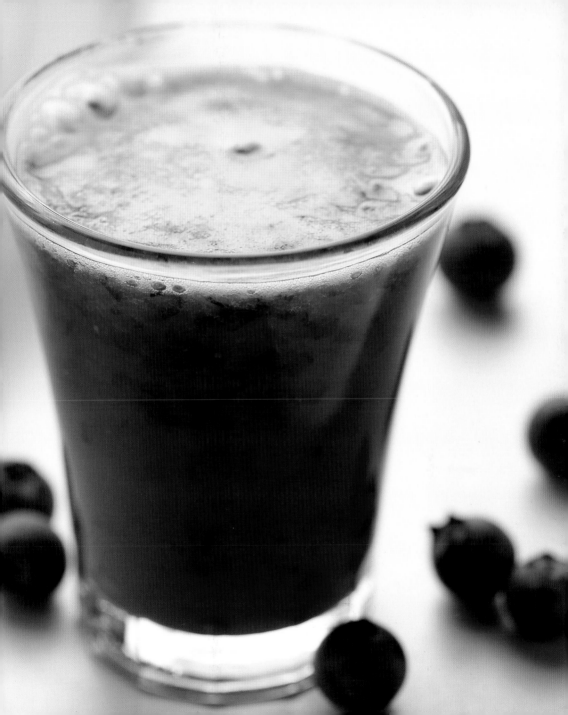

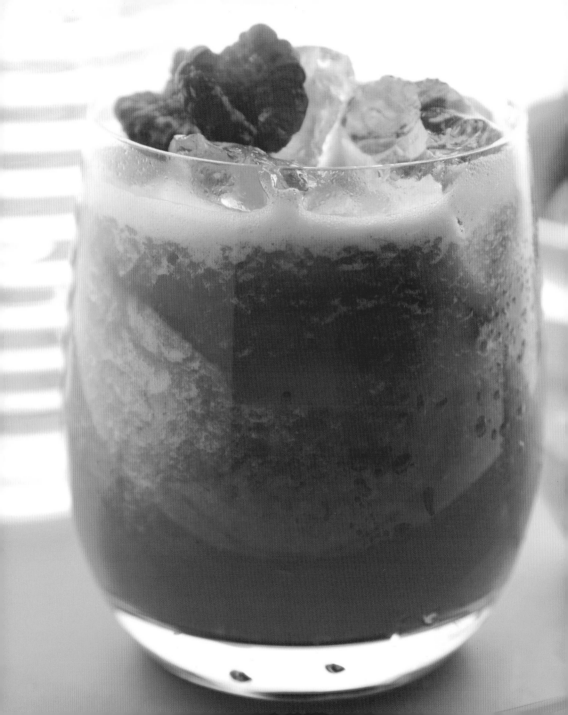

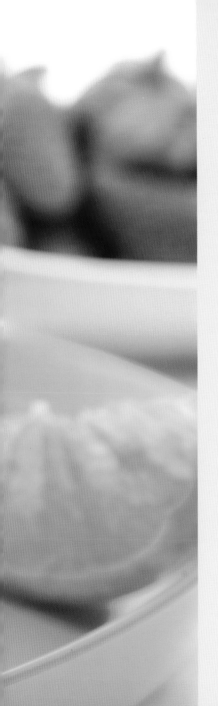

038 pink grapefruit

2 grapefruits

1 handful raspberries

1 handful strawberries

Just the colour of this makes you want to schlurp it up, not to mention how great it is for your body's defences.

NUTRIENTS

Beta-carotene, biotin, folic acid, vitamin C; calcium, magnesium, manganese, phosphorus, potassium, sodium, sulphur

ENERGY	★★★★☆
DETOX	★☆☆☆☆
IMMUNITY	★★★★★
DIGESTION	☆☆☆☆☆
SKIN	★★★★☆

039   greatfruit c

2 grapefruits

1 guava

1 kiwi fruit

Not just for colds, high doses of vitamin C such as are found in this tasty drink can ward off all sorts of other illnesses and aging.

NUTRIENTS
Beta-carotene, folic acid, vitamin C; calcium, magnesium, phosphorus, potassium, sodium, sulphur

ENERGY	★★★★☆
DETOX	★★★☆☆
IMMUNITY	★★★★★
DIGESTION	☆☆☆☆☆
SKIN	★★★★☆

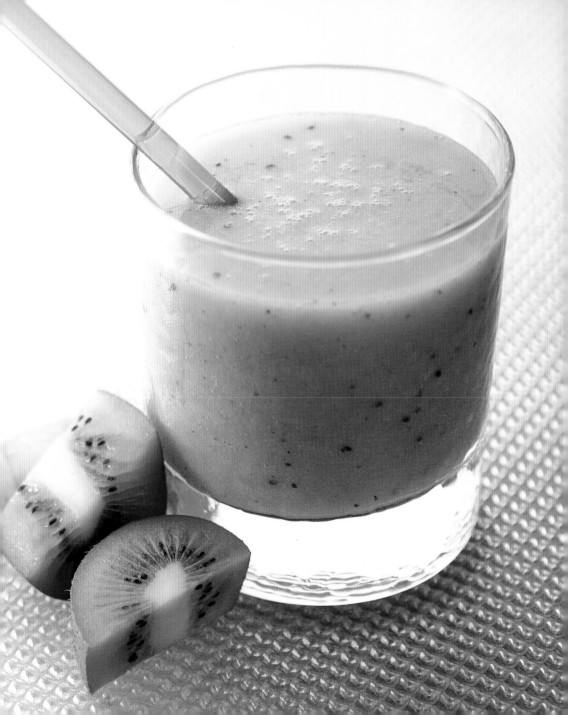

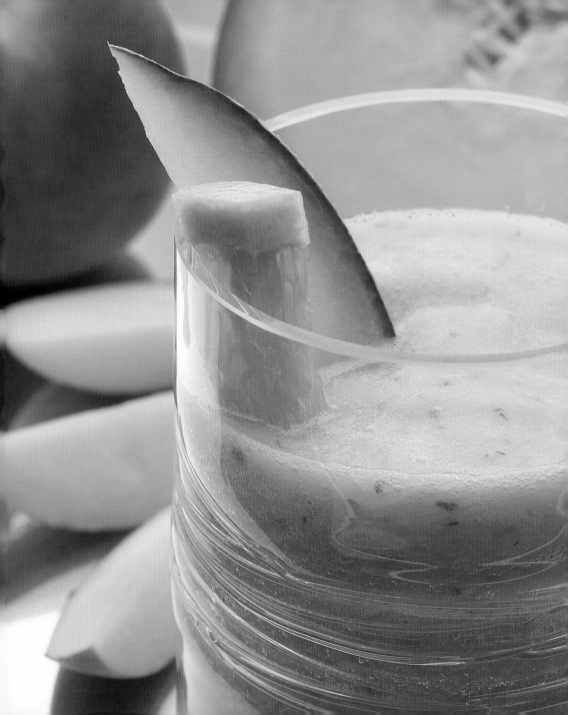

040 surprising sweetie

2 grapefruits

1 thick slice melon

1 peach

You would never imagine that anything with grapefruit could be so sweet, let alone pack such an immune-boosting punch.

NUTRIENTS
Beta-carotene, folic acid, vitamin B3, vitamin C; calcium, magnesium, phosphorus, potassium, sodium, sulphur

ENERGY	★★★★☆
DETOX	★★☆☆☆
IMMUNITY	★★★★☆
DIGESTION	★★☆☆☆
SKIN	★★★★★

041 pale faced

2 grapefruits

1 apple

½ fennel bulb

1 small bunch fresh mint

A blend of three distinctly strong flavours makes a delicious whole, with the more subtle undertones of the apple.

NUTRIENTS
Beta-carotene, folic acid, vitamin C; calcium, magnesium, phosphorus, potassium, sodium, sulphur

ENERGY	★★★★☆
DETOX	★☆☆☆☆
IMMUNITY	★★☆☆☆
DIGESTION	★★★☆☆
SKIN	★★☆☆☆

042 grapefruit tonic

3 grapefruits

1 teaspoon spirulina

Simple but strong, the earthy taste of spirulina goes well with grapefruit. Best shaken in a jar with the juice to avoid lumps of spirulina powder.

NUTRIENTS
Beta-carotene, folic acid, vitamins B1, B3,
B5, B6 and C; calcium, iron, magnesium,
phosphorus, potassium, sodium, sulphur;
protein; essential fatty acids

ENERGY ★★★★☆
DETOX ★★★★☆
IMMUNITY ★★★☆☆
DIGESTION ★☆☆☆☆
SKIN ★★★★☆

043   peppery grapefruit

2 grapefruits

¼ red cabbage

It's the strong red cabbage here that gives this juice its distinctive, peppery taste and vibrant colour.

NUTRIENTS
Beta-carotene, folic acid, vitamin C,
vitamin E; calcium, magnesium,
phosphorus, potassium, sodium,
sulphur

ENERGY ★★★☆☆
DETOX ★☆☆☆☆
IMMUNITY ★★★★☆
DIGESTION ★★★☆☆
SKIN ★★☆☆☆

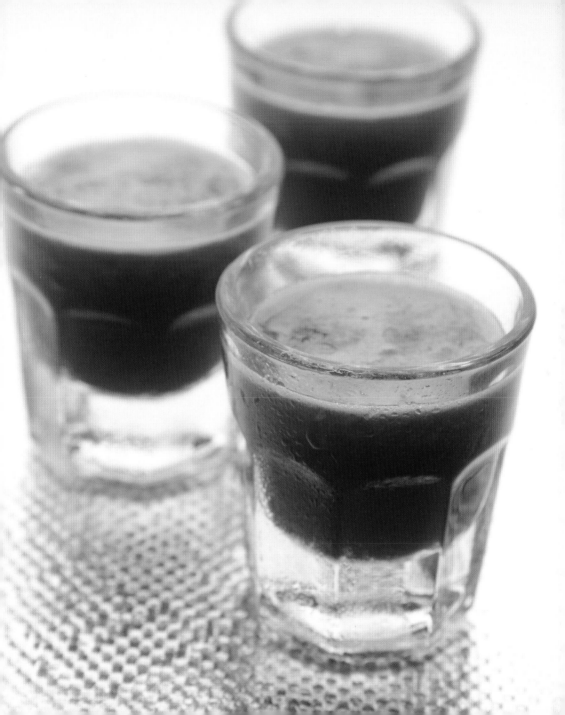

044 orange morning

2 grapefruits

3 carrots

½ inch (1 cm) ginger root

Another great morning staple but one where the sharp,
awakening grapefruit tang is tempered by the sweet,
rich carrot.

NUTRIENTS
Beta-carotene, folic acid, vitamin C;
calcium, magnesium, phosphorus,
potassium, sodium, sulphur

ENERGY	★★★★☆
DETOX	★★★☆☆
IMMUNITY	★★★★☆
DIGESTION	★★★☆☆
SKIN	★★★☆☆

045 grapefruit greens

2 grapefruits

1 handful watercress

1 bunch parsley

You can certainly taste the cleansing goodness in this one, and the strong flavour of the grapefruit can carry the greens' taste very well.

NUTRIENTS
Beta-carotene, folic acid, vitamins B3,
C and E; calcium, iron, magnesium,
phosphorus, potassium, sodium,
sulphur

ENERGY	★★★☆☆
DETOX	★★★☆☆
IMMUNITY	★★☆☆☆
DIGESTION	★☆☆☆☆
SKIN	★★★☆☆

046   cloudy day

2 grapefruits

½ long cucumber

2 sticks celery

1 small bunch fresh mint

The sweet tang of the grapefruit contrasts wonderfully with the
almost melon-like cucumber and salty celery, all lifted by the mint.

NUTRIENTS
Beta-carotene, folic acid, vitamin C;
calcium, magnesium, phosphorus,
potassium, sodium, sulphur

ENERGY	★★★☆☆
DETOX	★★☆☆☆
IMMUNITY	★★☆☆☆
DIGESTION	★★☆☆☆
SKIN	★★☆☆☆

047 black grapefruit

2 grapefruits

1 handful blackberries

1 handful blackcurrants

A fabulous contrast of the colours as they blend in the jug…
and then a fantastic boost to immunity. Best made in summer
with fresh berries.

NUTRIENTS
Beta-carotene, folic acid, vitamins B5,
C and E; calcium, iron, magnesium,
manganese, phosphorus, potassium,
sodium, sulphur

ENERGY	★★★★☆
DETOX	★☆☆☆☆
IMMUNITY	★★★★★
DIGESTION	☆☆☆☆☆
SKIN	★★★★☆

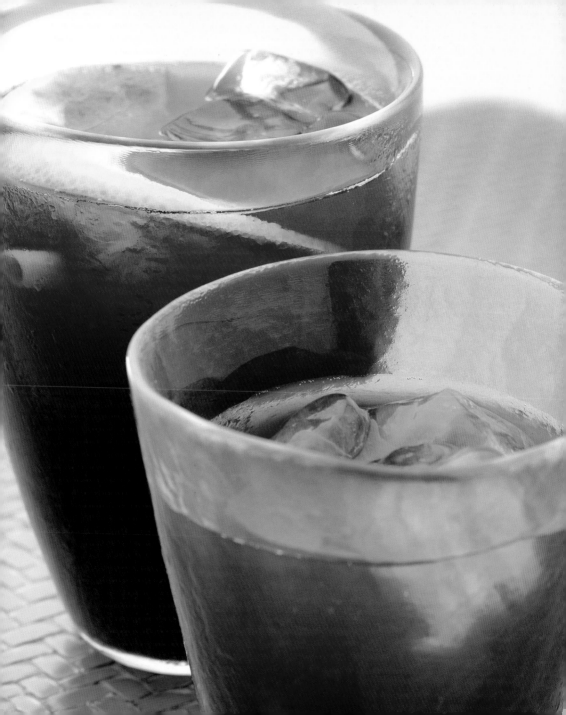

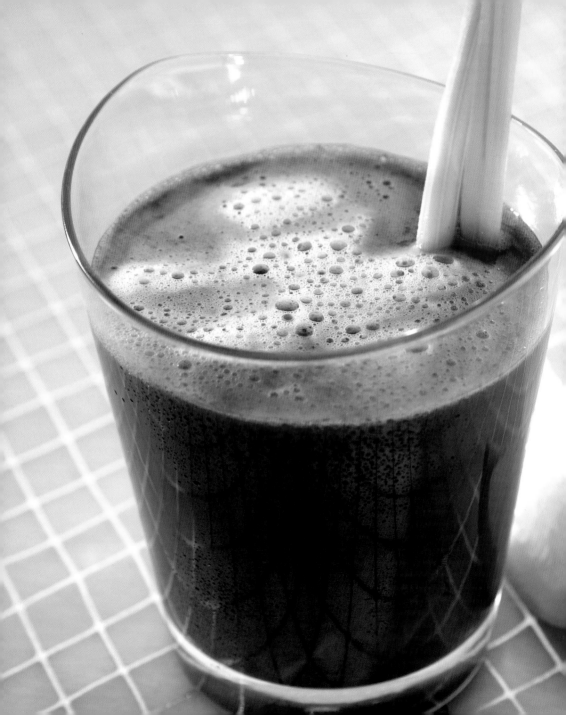

048 bleeding grapefruit

2 grapefruits

2 sticks celery

½ beet (beetroot)

The earthy sweetness of the beet nicely balances the sharpness of white grapefruit, while the salty celery brings out all the flavours.

NUTRIENTS

Beta-carotene, folic acid, vitamin C; calcium, magnesium, manganese, phosphorus, potassium, sodium, sulphur

ENERGY	★★★☆☆
DETOX	★★★★☆
IMMUNITY	★★☆☆☆
DIGESTION	★☆☆☆☆
SKIN	★★★☆☆

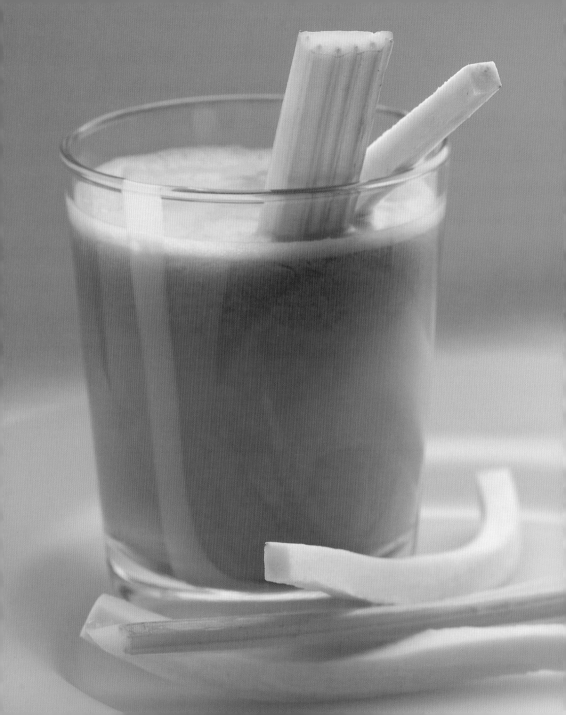

049 tangy veggie

2 grapefruits

2 inches (5 cm) sweet potato

1 parsnip

1 stick celery

Another great combination of sweet, earthy root vegetables and sharp, white grapefruit, or pink if you prefer. The celery serves to magnify the flavours.

NUTRIENTS
Beta-carotene, folic acid, vitamin C, vitamin E; calcium, magnesium, manganese, phosphorus, potassium, sodium, sulphur

ENERGY	★★★☆☆
DETOX	★★★☆☆
IMMUNITY	★★☆☆☆
DIGESTION	★☆☆☆☆
SKIN	★★☆☆☆

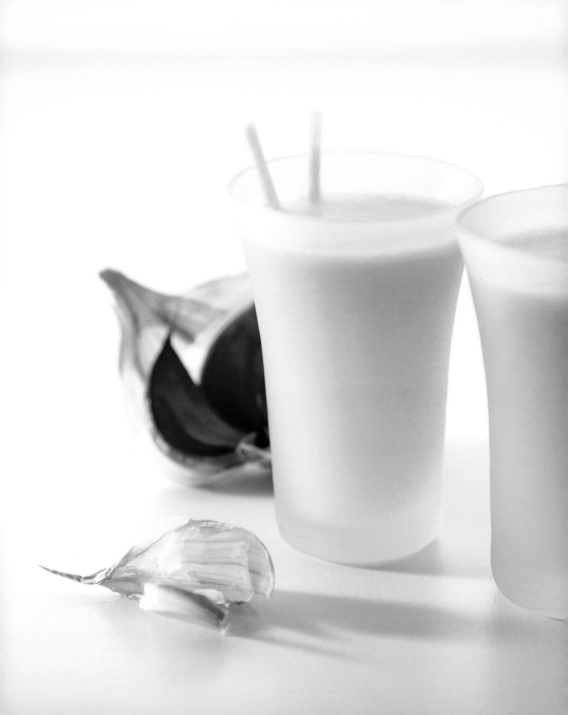

050 grapefruit cold zap

2 grapefruits

1 lemon

1 inch (2.5 cm) ginger root

1 clove garlic

You'd only really want this one if you were full of cold, unless you're trying to keep vampires away.

NUTRIENTS
Beta-carotene, folic acid, vitamin C; calcium, magnesium, phosphorus, potassium, sulphur

ENERGY	★★★☆☆
DETOX	★★☆☆☆
IMMUNITY	★★★★★
DIGESTION	★★☆☆☆
SKIN	★★★☆☆

051 creamy grapefruit

2 grapefruits

1 large beet (beetroot)

2 carrots

½ inch (1 cm) ginger root

This juice takes on a very velvety texture.

NUTRIENTS
Beta-carotene, folic acid, vitamin C;
calcium, magnesium, phosphorus,
potassium, sodium, sulphur

ENERGY ★★★★☆

DETOX ★★★☆☆

IMMUNITY ★★★☆☆

DIGESTION ★★☆☆☆

SKIN ★★★☆☆

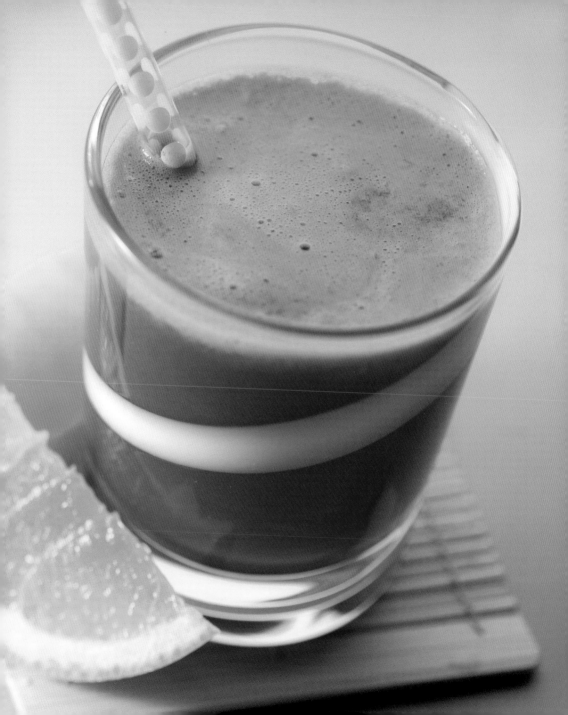

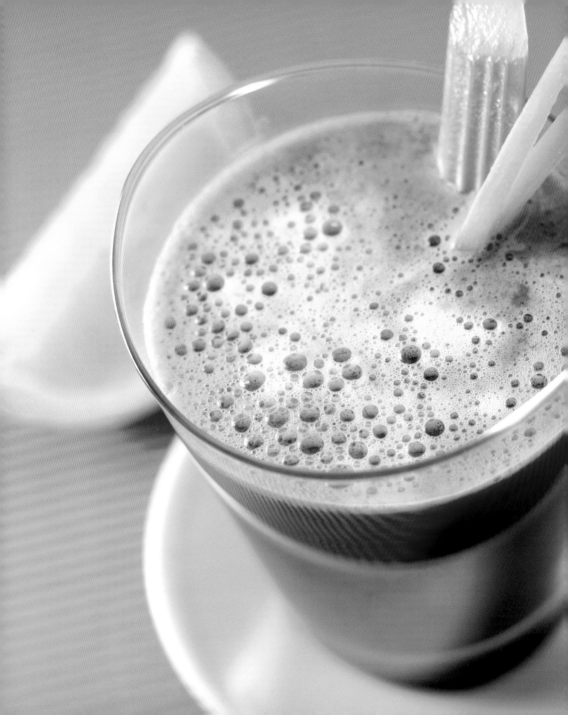

052 delicious darkness

2 grapefruits

1 carrot

1 large beet (beetroot)

1 stick celery

1 handful spinach

This weird combo is surprisingly delicious and creamy. Don't be put off by the spinach!

NUTRIENTS
Beta-carotene, folic acid, vitamin B3, vitamin C; calcium, iron, magnesium, phosphorus, potassium, sodium, sulphur

ENERGY	★★★★☆
DETOX	★★★★☆
IMMUNITY	★★★★☆
DIGESTION	★★☆☆☆
SKIN	★★★★☆

053 the original juice

4 oranges

Pure OJ is certainly the number one juice in the West, but not even the so-called "freshly squeezed" juices come close to making your own and drinking it immediately.

NUTRIENTS
Beta-carotene, vitamin C; calcium,
magnesium, phosphorus, potassium

ENERGY ★★★★☆
DETOX ★☆☆☆☆
IMMUNITY ★★★★☆
DIGESTION ☆☆☆☆☆
SKIN ★★☆☆☆

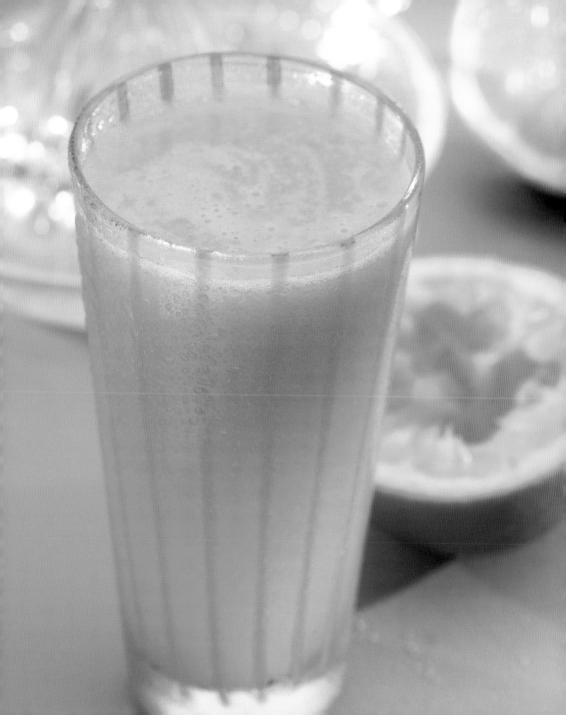

054 bloodthirst

6 blood oranges

A winter speciality, sweet, red blood oranges remind me of rare trips to my family home in Malta in the winter. You can often find them in supermarkets – particularly small, juicy organic ones. Best left unadulterated by other fruits.

NUTRIENTS
Beta-carotene, vitamin C; calcium,
magnesium, phosphorus, potassium

ENERGY ★★★★☆
DETOX ★☆☆☆☆
IMMUNITY ★★★★☆
DIGESTION ☆☆☆☆☆
SKIN ★★☆☆☆

055 orange basic

2 oranges

1 apple

3 carrots

1 stick celery

1 inch (2.5 cm) ginger root

One of my everyday staples – it doesn't require too much imagination as most refrigerators and fruit bowls will have the ingredients.

NUTRIENTS
Beta-carotene, folic acid, vitamin C; calcium, magnesium, manganese, phosphorus, potassium, sodium, sulphur

ENERGY	★★★★☆
DETOX	★★★★☆
IMMUNITY	★★★★☆
DIGESTION	★★☆☆☆
SKIN	★★★☆☆

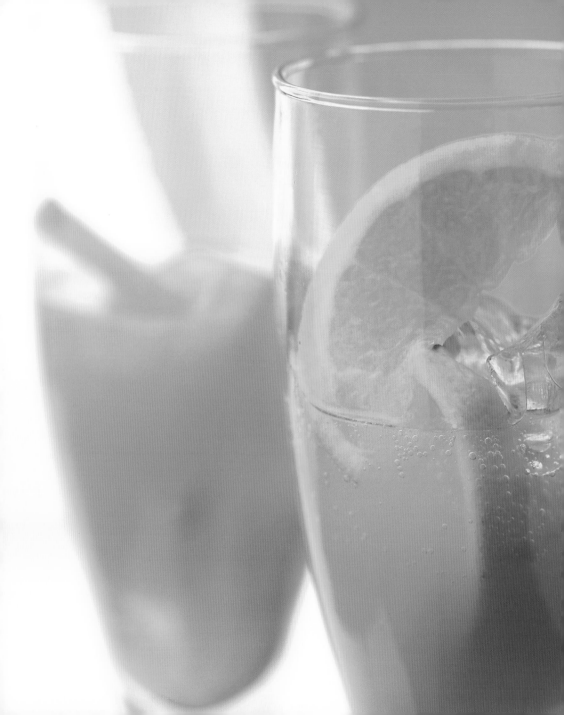

056 bright orange

2 oranges

4 carrots

The incredible colour of this simple combination, even easier to make than basic OJ, heralds an equally amazing taste.

NUTRIENTS
Beta-carotene, folic acid, vitamin C; calcium, magnesium, phosphorus, potassium, sodium, sulphur

ENERGY	★★★★☆
DETOX	★★★☆☆
IMMUNITY	★★★★☆
DIGESTION	★☆☆☆☆
SKIN	★★★☆☆

057 florida blue

2 oranges

1 pink grapefruit

1 handful blueberries

If you use a sweet pink grapefruit, rather than a sharper white one, this blend is divine.

NUTRIENTS
Beta-carotene, biotin, folic acid,
vitamins B1, B2, B6, C and E; calcium,
magnesium, phosphorus, potassium,
sodium, sulphur

ENERGY	★★★★☆
DETOX	★☆☆☆☆
IMMUNITY	★★★★★
DIGESTION	★★☆☆☆
SKIN	★★★☆☆

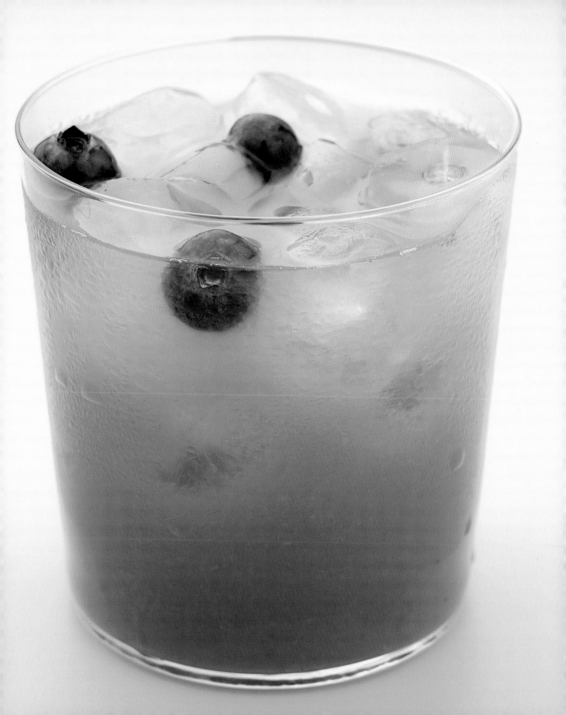

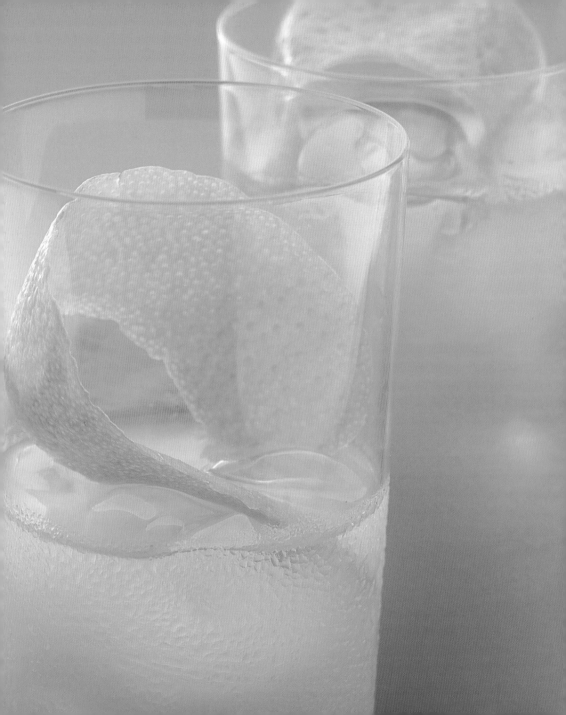

058 orange crudités

2 oranges

½ long cucumber

2 carrots

1 stick celery

The three vegetables in this juice gently dilute the sweet, sharp taste of the oranges, and make it a lighter, more refreshing drink.

NUTRIENTS
Beta-carotene, folic acid, vitamin C;
calcium, magnesium, manganese,
phosphorus, potassium, sodium,
sulphur

ENERGY ★★★☆☆
DETOX ★★☆☆☆
IMMUNITY ★★★☆☆
DIGESTION ★★☆☆☆
SKIN ★★★☆☆

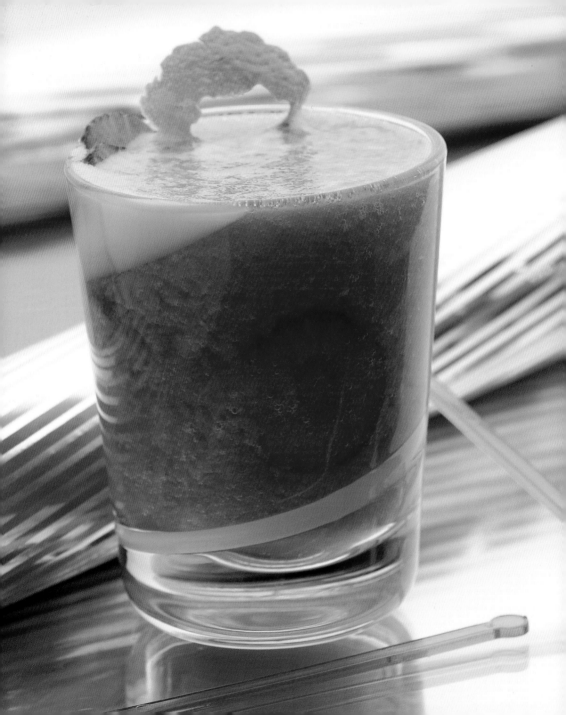

059 power-packed c

3 oranges

1 guava

1 handful strawberries

Combining three of the richest sources of vitamin C, this is not only a delicious drink but also a strong immunity booster that helps keep illnesses at bay.

NUTRIENTS

Beta-carotene, biotin, folic acid, vitamin B3, vitamin C; calcium, magnesium, phosphorus, potassium, sodium, sulphur

ENERGY	★★★★★
DETOX	★☆☆☆☆
IMMUNITY	★★★★★
DIGESTION	☆☆☆☆☆
SKIN	★★★★☆

060 william's orange

2 oranges

2 pears

You'd think the pears would get swamped by the oranges in this juice, but, in fact, they just tone down the tang beautifully. It's best to use a sweet variety of pear such as Williams.

NUTRIENTS
Beta-carotene, folic acid, vitamin C; calcium, magnesium, phosphorus, potassium, sulphur

ENERGY	★★★★☆
DETOX	★☆☆☆☆
IMMUNITY	★★★☆☆
DIGESTION	★★☆☆☆
SKIN	★☆☆☆☆

061 orange medley

2 oranges

½ melon

1 nectarine

Use a cantaloupe melon to make this a wonderful blend of orange-coloured fruits.

NUTRIENTS
Beta-carotene, folic acid, vitamin C;
calcium, magnesium, phosphorus,
potassium, sodium

ENERGY	★★★★★
DETOX	★☆☆☆☆
IMMUNITY	★★★★★
DIGESTION	★★☆☆☆
SKIN	★★★★☆

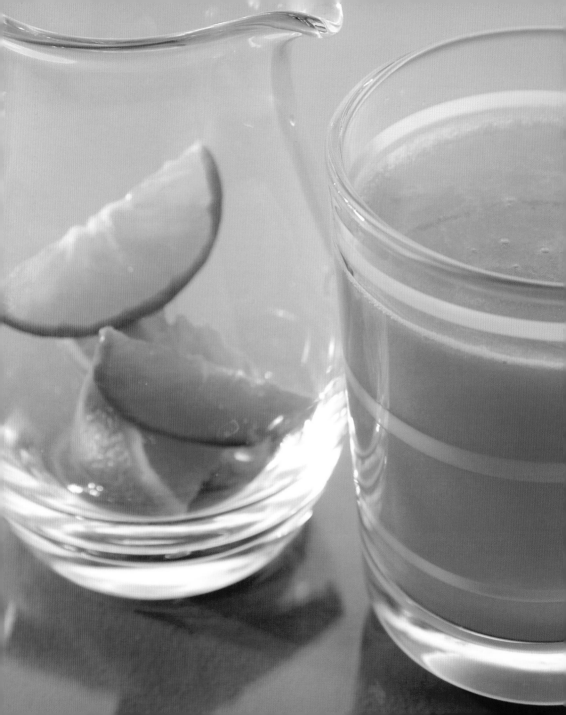

062 citrus sweet

2 oranges

3 tangerines

This juice really highlights the differences between the tastes of oranges and the smaller tangerines or other similar fruits. Clementines or any small, easily peeled orange citrus fruits may be used.

NUTRIENTS
Beta-carotene, folic acid, vitamin C; calcium, magnesium, phosphorus, potassium, sodium

ENERGY	★★★★☆
DETOX	★☆☆☆☆
IMMUNITY	★★★★☆
DIGESTION	☆☆☆☆☆
SKIN	☆☆☆☆☆

063 biting orange

4 oranges

½ inch (1 cm) ginger root

Almost any juice goes well with ginger in my book, but this sweet orange with a ginger bite – giving it a festive winter flavour – is a particular favourite.

NUTRIENTS
Beta-carotene, vitamin C; calcium, magnesium, phosphorus, potassium

ENERGY ★★★★☆
DETOX ☆☆☆☆☆
IMMUNITY ★★★★☆
DIGESTION ★★☆☆☆
SKIN ★☆☆☆☆

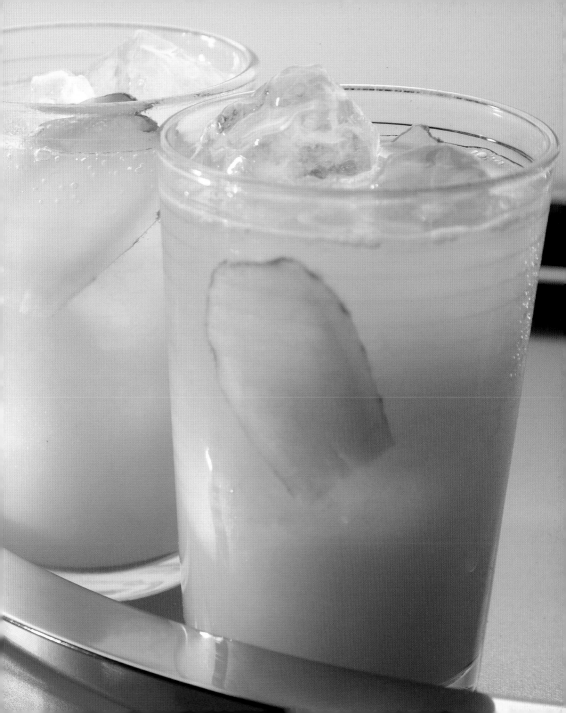

064 bitter melon

2 oranges

2 thick slices melon

Bitter Melon is actually the name of an Indian vegetable (and a '90s American rock band), but also sums up this juice's tangy twist on sweet melon. Use a cantaloupe or honeydew melon.

NUTRIENTS
Beta-carotene, folic acid, vitamin C; calcium, magnesium, phosphorus, potassium, sodium, sulphur

ENERGY	★★★★★
DETOX	★☆☆☆☆
IMMUNITY	★★★★★
DIGESTION	☆☆☆☆☆
SKIN	★★★★☆

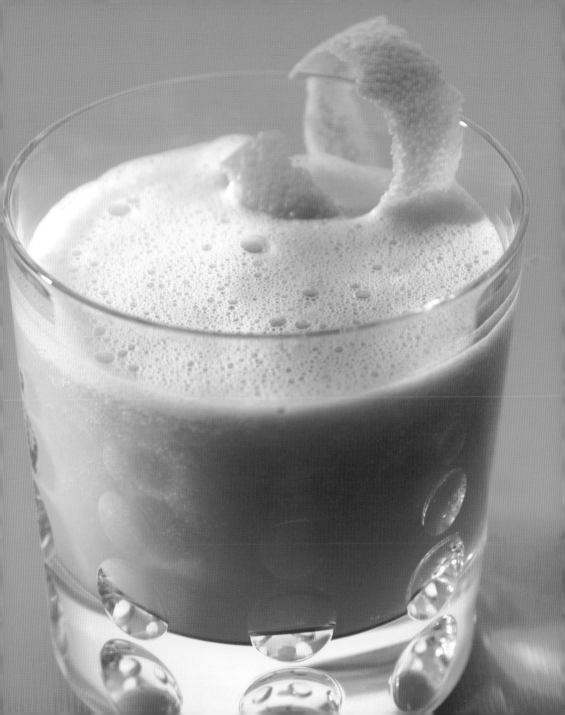

065 orange winter crumble

2 oranges

2 apples

1 handful blackberries

I love the blend of orange juice with the traditional winter mixture of apple and blackberry used in pies and crumbles.

NUTRIENTS
Beta-carotene, folic acid, vitamin C,
vitamin E; calcium, iron, magnesium,
manganese, phosphorus, potassium,
sodium, sulphur

ENERGY	★★★★★
DETOX	★★☆☆☆
IMMUNITY	★★★★★
DIGESTION	★☆☆☆☆
SKIN	★★★★☆

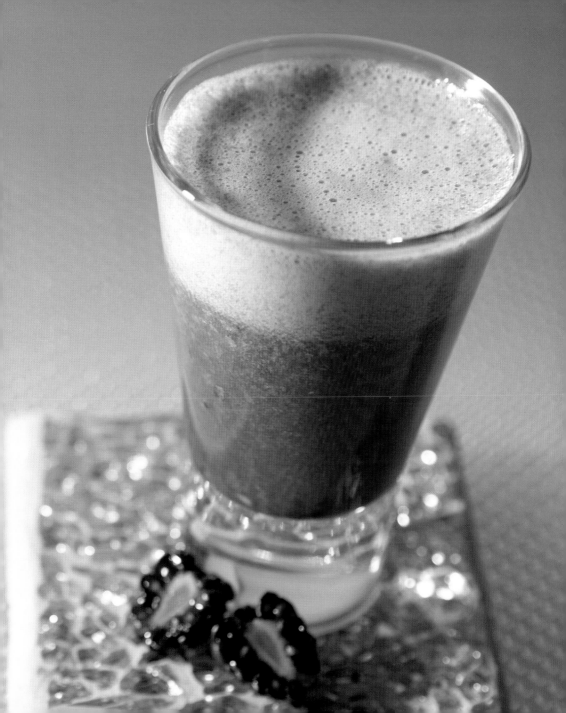

066 muddy puddle

3 oranges

1 handful spinach

1 handful watercress

2 broccoli spears

The name of this originates from a drink a friend of mine used to have at college – orange juice and cola. But it's a far cry from that in terms of sweetness and health properties. The strength of flavour of the oranges carries the earthy, strong taste of the greens.

NUTRIENTS
Beta-carotene, vitamin B5, vitamin C; calcium, magnesium, phosphorus, potassium, sodium

ENERGY	★★★☆☆
DETOX	★★★★☆
IMMUNITY	★★★☆☆
DIGESTION	★☆☆☆☆
SKIN	★★★☆☆

067 blackcurrant twist

3 oranges

1 handful blackcurrants

¼ fennel bulb

This always reminds me of a tangy version of the blackcurrant and aniseed sweets I would buy as a child.

NUTRIENTS
Beta-carotene, biotin, vitamins B5,
C and E; calcium, magnesium,
phosphorus, potassium, sodium,
sulphur

ENERGY	★★★☆☆
DETOX	☆☆☆☆☆
IMMUNITY	★★★☆☆
DIGESTION	☆☆☆☆☆
SKIN	★★☆☆☆

068 citrus sharp

3 oranges

1 lemon

1 lime

The colour of this refreshing juice hails a tart tickling of the tastebuds, and all that citrus fruit gives you a great immunity boost.

NUTRIENTS
Beta-carotene, folic acid, vitamin C;
calcium, magnesium, phosphorus,
potassium, sodium, sulphur

ENERGY	★★★★☆
DETOX	★☆☆☆☆
IMMUNITY	★★★★★
DIGESTION	☆☆☆☆☆
SKIN	★★☆☆☆

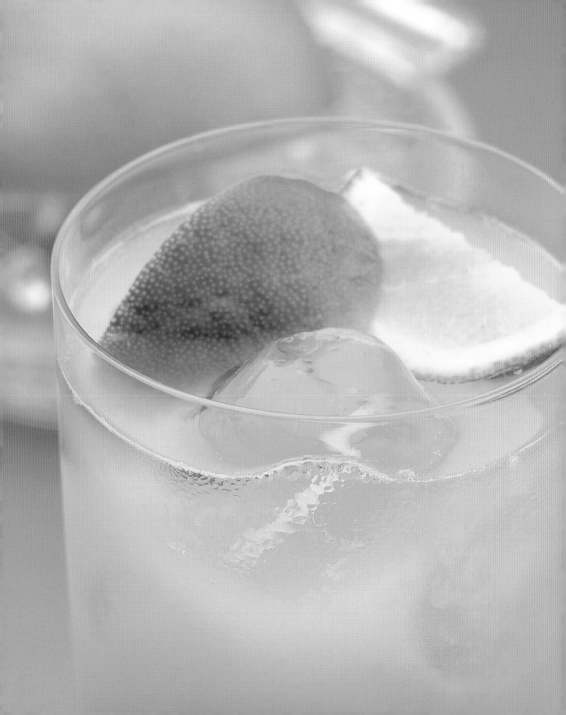

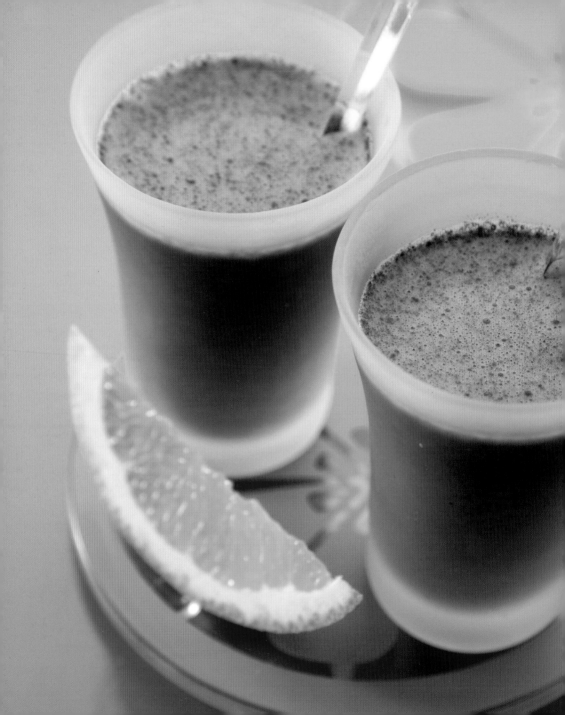

069 muddy tonic

4 oranges

1 teaspoon spirulina

I love the earthy green taste mixed with orange, although the brown colour isn't the most appealing. It's best to shake the juice (or a portion of it) with the spirulina in a jar so it doesn't go lumpy.

NUTRIENTS
Beta-carotene, vitamins B1, B3, B5, B6 and C; calcium, iron, magnesium, phosphorus, potassium, sodium; protein; essential fatty acids

ENERGY	★★★☆☆
DETOX	★★★☆☆
IMMUNITY	★★☆☆☆
DIGESTION	☆☆☆☆☆
SKIN	★★☆☆☆

070 bloody orange

3 oranges

1 beet (beetroot)

The name is a reference to this juice's thick red colour and not to blood oranges which are, unfortunately, all too rare – the earthy taste of beet cuts through the sharpness of good oranges well.

NUTRIENTS
Beta-carotene, folic acid, vitamin C; calcium, magnesium, phosphorus, potassium, sodium

ENERGY	★★★☆☆
DETOX	★★☆☆☆
IMMUNITY	★★★☆☆
DIGESTION	☆☆☆☆☆
SKIN	★★★☆☆

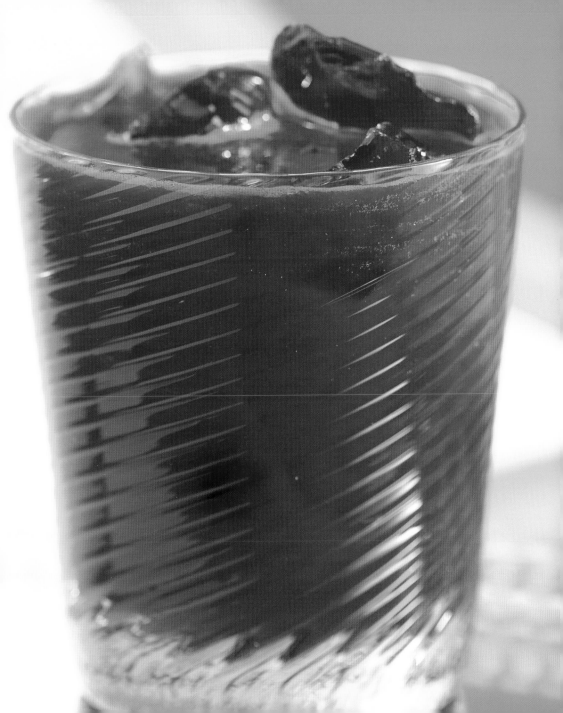

071 orange aniseed twist

3 oranges

2 sticks celery

¼ fennel bulb

The fennel gives a great turn to this recipe, while the saltiness of the celery brings out the flavours. All in all, very refreshing.

NUTRIENTS
Beta-carotene, folic acid, vitamin C;
calcium, magnesium, manganese,
phosphorus, potassium, sodium,
sulphur

ENERGY	★★★☆☆
DETOX	★☆☆☆☆
IMMUNITY	★☆☆☆☆
DIGESTION	★★★☆☆
SKIN	★☆☆☆☆

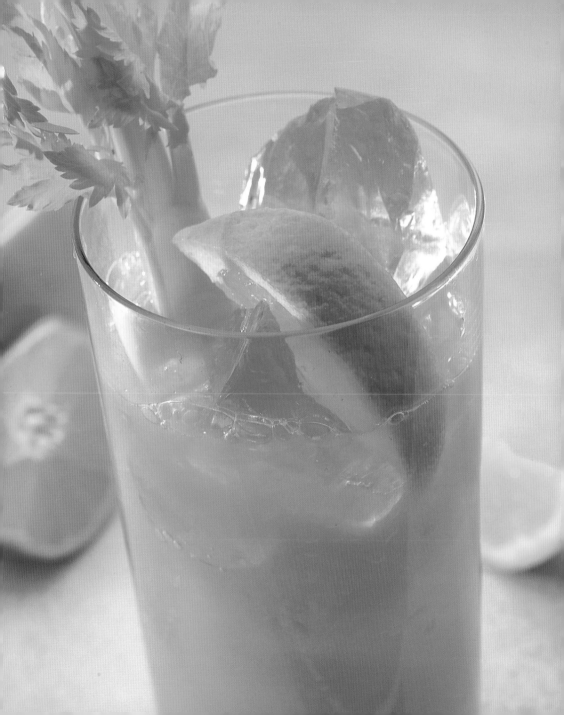

072   water cooler II

3 oranges

1 thick slice watermelon

Unbelievably light and refreshing, the watermelon takes the edge off the tangy orange.

NUTRIENTS
Beta-carotene, vitamin C; calcium, iron, magnesium, phosphorus, potassium, sodium, sulphur

ENERGY	★★★★☆
DETOX	★★☆☆☆
IMMUNITY	★★★☆☆
DIGESTION	☆☆☆☆☆
SKIN	★★★★☆

073   orange pepper

3 oranges

½ red or yellow bell pepper

1 kale leaf

1 handful watercress

The strong taste of oranges carries the more subtle flavours of the vegetables in this juice. Don't be put off by the muddy colour.

NUTRIENTS
Beta-carotene, folic acid, vitamins B3,
C and E; calcium, iron, magnesium,
manganese, phosphorus, potassium,
sodium, sulphur

ENERGY	★★☆☆☆
DETOX	★★★☆☆
IMMUNITY	★★★☆☆
DIGESTION	★★☆☆☆
SKIN	★★★★☆

074 orange blush

3 oranges

1 apple

1 handful raspberries

A tangy pink juice which blends three fantastic fruits perfectly
– definitely greater than the sum of its parts.

NUTRIENTS
Beta-carotene, biotin, folic acid,
vitamin C; calcium, magnesium,
manganese, phosphorus,
potassium, sodium, sulphur

ENERGY	★★★★★
DETOX	★☆☆☆☆
IMMUNITY	★★★☆☆
DIGESTION	★☆☆☆☆
SKIN	★★★☆☆

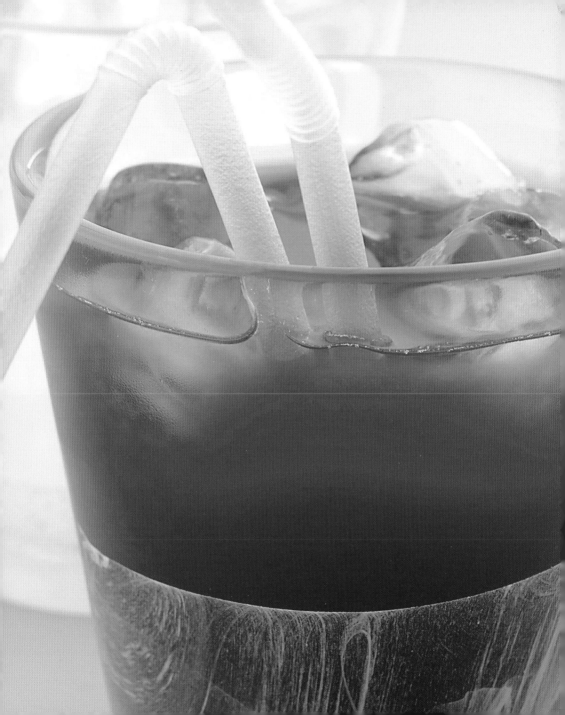

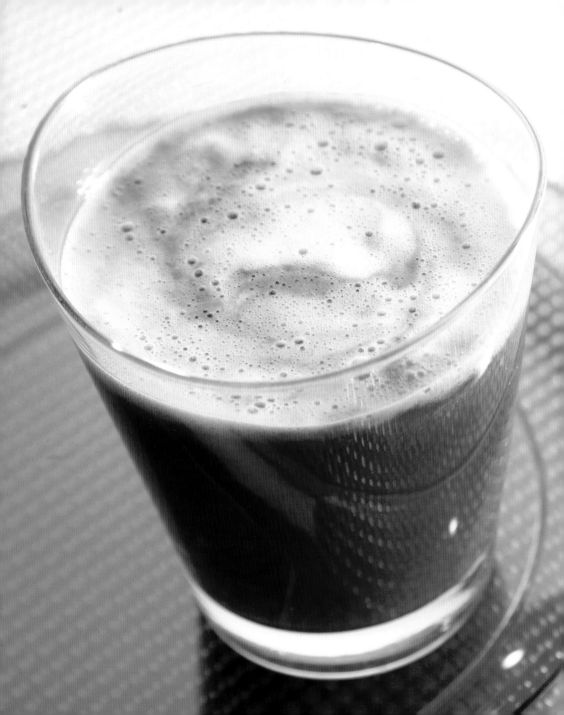

075   counteractor

3 oranges

¼ red cabbage

¼ inch (0.5 cm) ginger root

Some people find oranges too
acidic on their digestion – here
the soothing cabbage and ginger
provide the perfect balance.

NUTRIENTS
Beta-carotene, folic acid, vitamin C,
vitamin E; calcium, magnesium,
phosphorus, potassium, sodium

ENERGY	★★★☆☆
DETOX	★☆☆☆☆
IMMUNITY	★★☆☆☆
DIGESTION	★★★☆☆
SKIN	★★☆☆☆

076   pure raspberry

2 large handfuls raspberries

For the vast majority of us this juice is an absurd luxury, so make just a small glassful and savour every drop.

NUTRIENTS
Beta-carotene, biotin, vitamin C;
calcium, magnesium, manganese,
phosphorus, potassium, sodium,
sulphur

ENERGY	★★★★★
DETOX	★☆☆☆☆
IMMUNITY	★★★☆☆
DIGESTION	☆☆☆☆☆
SKIN	★★★☆☆

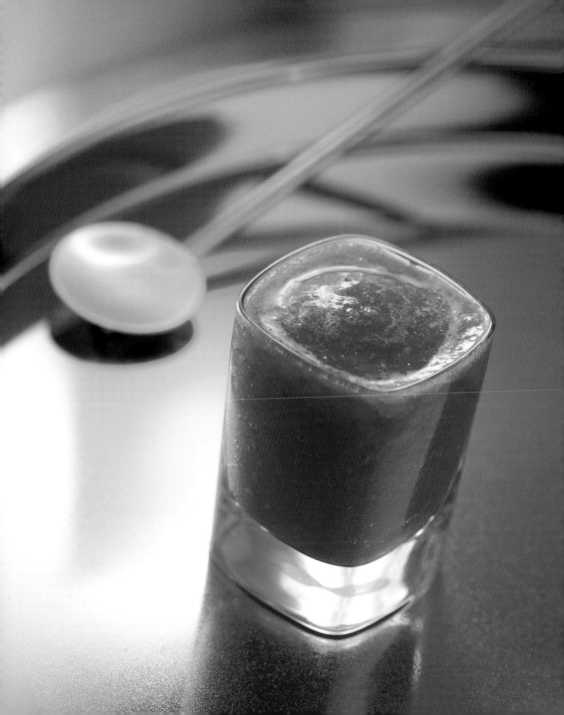

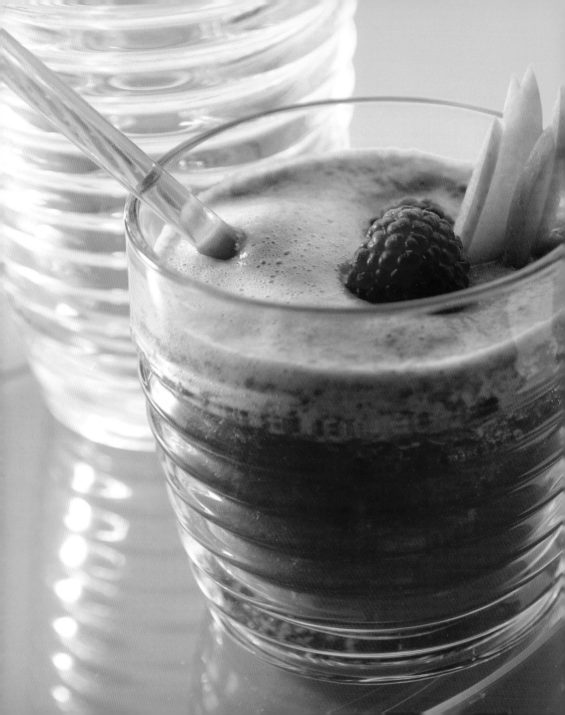

077   raspapple

2 large handfuls raspberries

2 large apples

A simple but splendid blend of juices.

NUTRIENTS
Beta-carotene, biotin, folic acid,
vitamin C; calcium, magnesium,
manganese, phosphorus, potassium,
sodium, sulphur

ENERGY ★★★★★

DETOX ★☆☆☆☆

IMMUNITY ★★☆☆☆

DIGESTION ★☆☆☆☆

SKIN ★★★☆☆

078 raspapple tang

2 large handfuls raspberries

2 large apples

1 lime

Remarkably different from Raspapple (blend 077) with just
the addition of a little lime.

NUTRIENTS
Beta-carotene, biotin, folic acid,
vitamin C; calcium, magnesium,
manganese, phosphorus, potassium,
sodium, sulphur

ENERGY	★★★★☆
DETOX	★☆☆☆☆
IMMUNITY	★★★★☆
DIGESTION	★☆☆☆☆
SKIN	★★☆☆☆

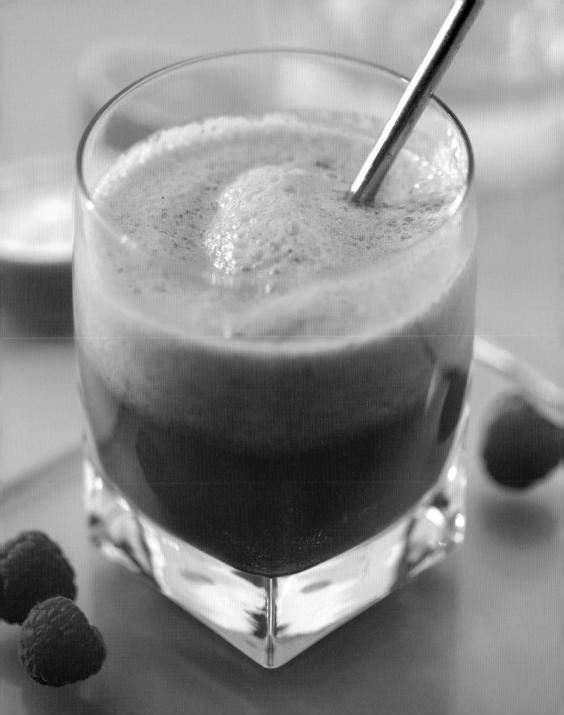

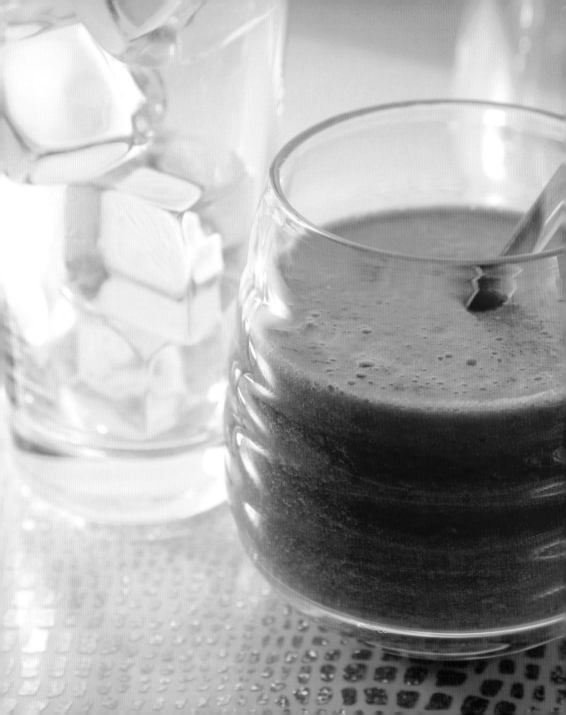

079   citrusberry

2 large handfuls raspberries

2 large oranges

1 tangerine

This is such a classic, delicious blend, they even sell it in supermarkets without the tangerine, which I find just tones it down a nice touch.

NUTRIENTS

Beta-carotene, biotin, vitamin C; calcium, magnesium, manganese, phosphorus, potassium, sodium, sulphur

ENERGY	★★★★★
DETOX	★☆☆☆☆
IMMUNITY	★★★★☆
DIGESTION	☆☆☆☆☆
SKIN	★★★☆☆

080 creamy raspberry

2 large handfuls raspberries

½ melon

1 stick celery

With the creaminess of the melon, you'd think you were drinking more than just fruit juice, while the salty celery lifts all the flavours.

NUTRIENTS
Beta-carotene, biotin, folic acid,
vitamin C; calcium, magnesium,
manganese, phosphorus, potassium,
sodium, sulphur

ENERGY	★★★★★
DETOX	★☆☆☆☆
IMMUNITY	★★★☆☆
DIGESTION	☆☆☆☆☆
SKIN	★★★★☆

081   gently raspberry

2 large handfuls raspberries

2 pears

¼ cucumber

Not quite as strange a combination as you may initially think – the cucumber in this appears to save the pears from being drowned out by the raspberries.

NUTRIENTS
Beta-carotene, biotin, folic acid,
vitamin C; calcium, magnesium,
manganese, phosphorus, potassium,
sodium, sulphur

ENERGY	★★★☆☆
DETOX	★☆☆☆☆
IMMUNITY	★★☆☆☆
DIGESTION	★☆☆☆☆
SKIN	★★☆☆☆

082 raspberry sensation

2 large handfuls raspberries

½ pineapple

A truly sensational combination – go on, spoil yourself with two independently rich fruits laden with goodness.

NUTRIENTS		
Beta-carotene, biotin, folic acid,	ENERGY	★★★★★
vitamin C; calcium, magnesium,	DETOX	★☆☆☆☆
manganese, phosphorus,	IMMUNITY	★★☆☆☆
potassium, sodium, sulphur	DIGESTION	★★★★☆
	SKIN	★★★☆☆

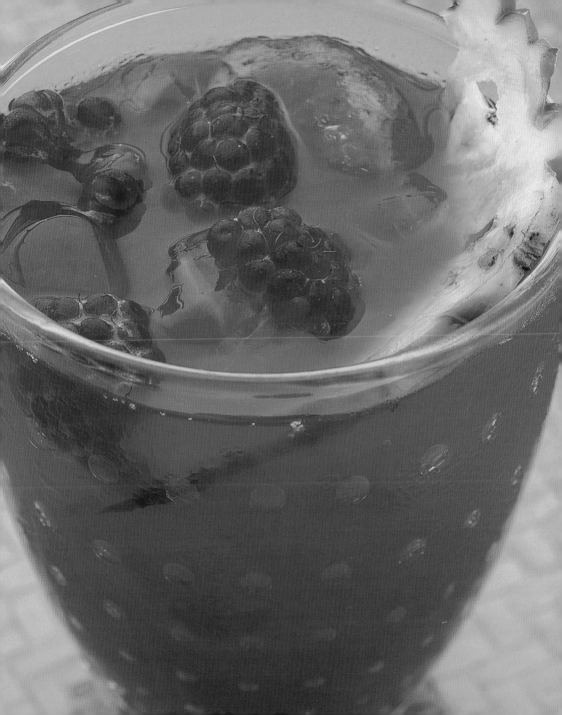

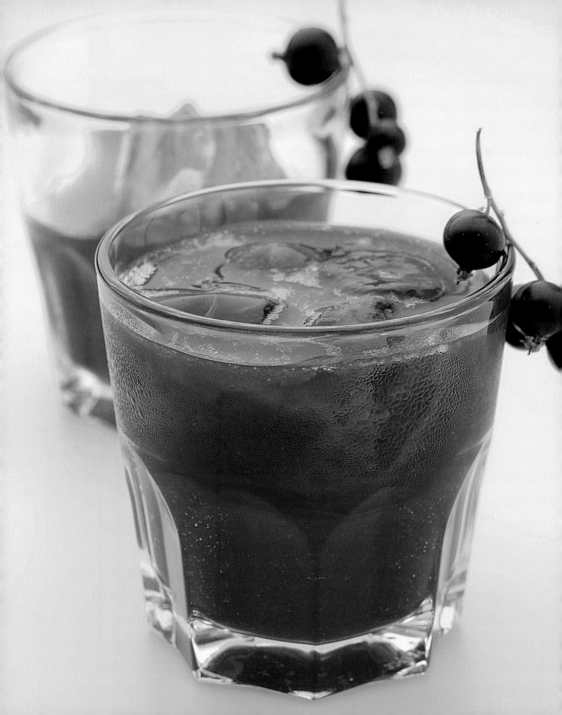

083   berry bonanza

2 large handfuls raspberries

1 handful blackcurrants

1 handful blueberries

Taking the luxury even further… this berry combination is a
blessing to your tastebuds and your body.

NUTRIENTS
Beta-carotene, biotin, folic acid,
vitamins B1, B2, B5, B6, C and E;
calcium, chromium, magnesium,
phosphorus, potassium, sodium, sulphur

ENERGY	★★★★★
DETOX	★☆☆☆☆
IMMUNITY	★★★★★
DIGESTION	☆☆☆☆☆
SKIN	★★★★☆

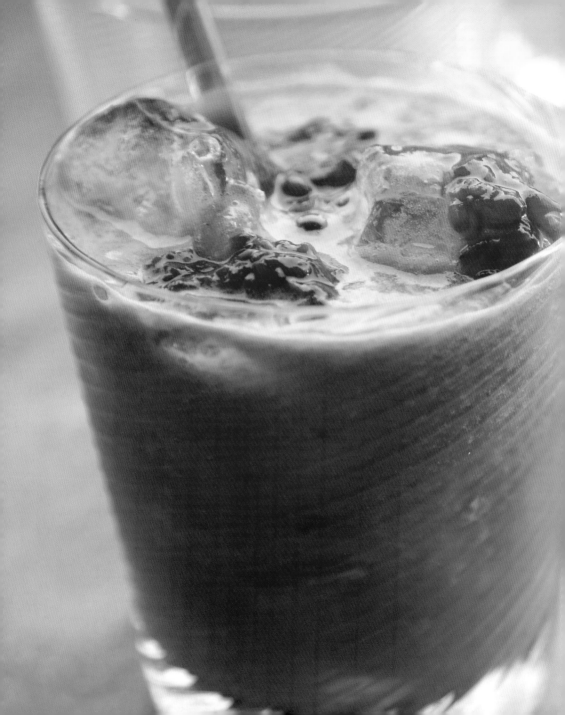

084 sharp citrusberry

2 large handfuls raspberries

1 grapefruit

½ lemon

I almost prefer this one to the orange blend of Citrusberry (see blend 079), with the bite of the grapefruit and the nose-curling lemon.

NUTRIENTS
Beta-carotene, biotin, folic acid, vitamin C; calcium, magnesium, manganese, phosphorus, potassium, sodium, sulphur

ENERGY ★★★★☆
DETOX ★☆☆☆☆
IMMUNITY ★★★☆☆
DIGESTION ☆☆☆☆☆
SKIN ★★★☆☆

085 morning berry basic

2 large handfuls raspberries

2 apples

1 orange

1 teaspoon spirulina

Fruit-bowl classics with the raspberries and some spirulina for an extra health kick. To avoid green lumps, shake the spirulina in a jar with a little of the juice before mixing it in with the rest.

NUTRIENTS
Beta-carotene, vitamins B1, B3, B5, B6 and C; calcium, iron, magnesium, manganese, phosphorus, potassium, sodium, sulphur; protein; essential fatty acids

ENERGY	★★★★☆
DETOX	★★★★☆
IMMUNITY	★★★☆☆
DIGESTION	★☆☆☆☆
SKIN	★★★★☆

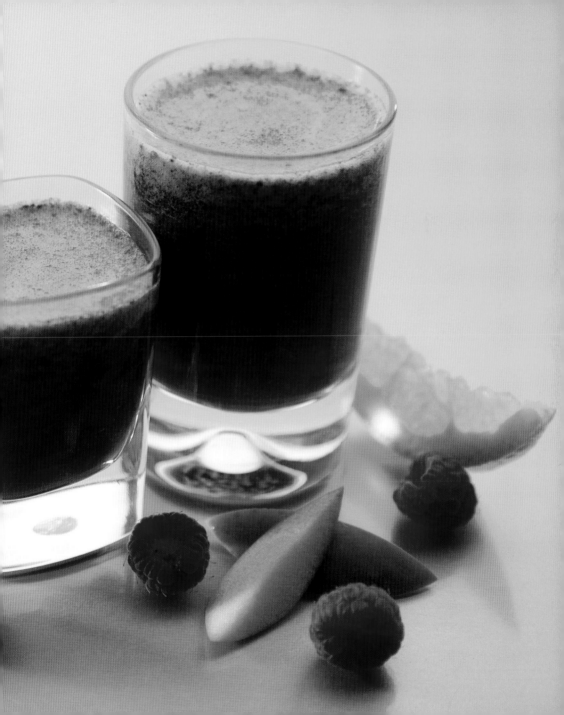

086   pure peach

4 peaches or nectarines

Pure heaven for anyone with the slightest penchant for fruit
of any sort.

NUTRIENTS
Beta-carotene, folic acid, vitamin B3,
vitamin C; calcium, magnesium,
phosphorus, potassium, sodium,
sulphur

ENERGY	★★★★★
DETOX	★☆☆☆☆
IMMUNITY	★★★★☆
DIGESTION	★★☆☆☆
SKIN	★★★★☆

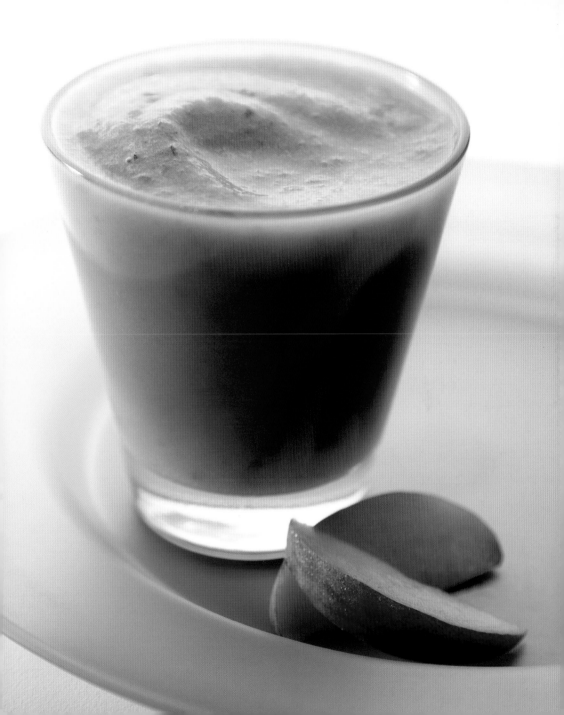

087 eve's peach

2 peaches or nectarines

2 apples

I'm sure the serpent would not have had to do much persuading
with this one!

NUTRIENTS
Beta-carotene, folic acid, vitamin B3,
vitamin C; calcium, magnesium,
phosphorus, potassium, sodium,
sulphur

ENERGY	★★★★★
DETOX	★☆☆☆☆
IMMUNITY	★★★★☆
DIGESTION	★★☆☆☆
SKIN	★★★★☆

088   peach 'n' pine

2 peaches or nectarines

½ pineapple

Tropical and temperate, tangy and delicate.

NUTRIENTS
Beta-carotene, folic acid, vitamin B3,
vitamin C; calcium, magnesium,
manganese, phosphorus, potassium,
sodium, sulphur

ENERGY	★★★★★
DETOX	★☆☆☆☆
IMMUNITY	★★★☆☆
DIGESTION	★★★☆☆
SKIN	★★★☆☆

089 black peach

2 peaches or nectarines

2 handfuls blueberries, blackberries
and/or blackcurrants

A summer delight – each drop to be savoured. Play with
the different berry combinations to change the flavour
and the sweetness.

NUTRIENTS
Beta-carotene, biotin, folic acid, vitamins
B1, B2, B3, B6, C and E; calcium, chromium,
iron, magnesium, manganese, phosphorus,
potassium, sodium, sulphur

ENERGY	★★★★★
DETOX	★★☆☆☆
IMMUNITY	★★★★☆
DIGESTION	★☆☆☆☆
SKIN	★★★★★

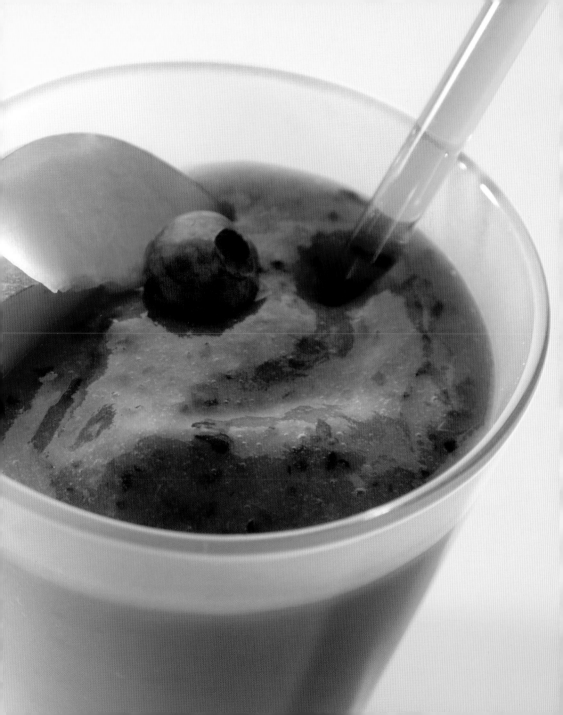

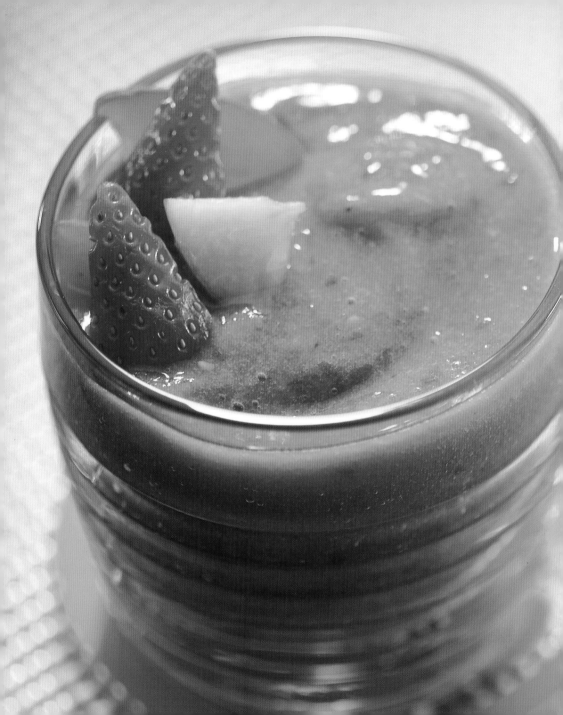

090 pink peach

2 peaches or nectarines

2 handfuls strawberries and raspberries

Another exquisite summer luxury – choose
your favourite combination.

NUTRIENTS
Beta-carotene, biotin, folic acid,
vitamin B3, vitamin C; calcium,
magnesium, phosphorus, potassium,
sodium, sulphur

ENERGY	★★★★★
DETOX	★★☆☆☆
IMMUNITY	★★★★☆
DIGESTION	★☆☆☆☆
SKIN	★★★★★

091 peaches and cream

2 peaches or nectarines

½ melon

If any creamless drink comes close to peaches and cream this delicious concoction is it.

NUTRIENTS
Beta-carotene, folic acid, vitamin B3, vitamin C; calcium, magnesium, phosphorus, potassium, sodium, sulphur

ENERGY ★★★★★
DETOX ★☆☆☆☆
IMMUNITY ★★★★☆
DIGESTION ★☆☆☆☆
SKIN ★★★★☆

092 peaches and green

3 peaches or nectarines

2 sticks celery

1 teaspoon spirulina

Even the less inviting earthiness of the celery and spirulina are forgotten in this super-healthy blend. To avoid green lumps, shake the spirulina in a jar with a little of the juice before mixing it in with the rest.

NUTRIENTS
Beta-carotene, folic acid, vitamin B3, vitamin C; calcium, magnesium, manganese, phosphorus, potassium, sodium, sulphur; protein; essential fatty acids

ENERGY	★★★☆☆
DETOX	★★★★☆
IMMUNITY	★★☆☆☆
DIGESTION	★☆☆☆☆
SKIN	★★★★☆

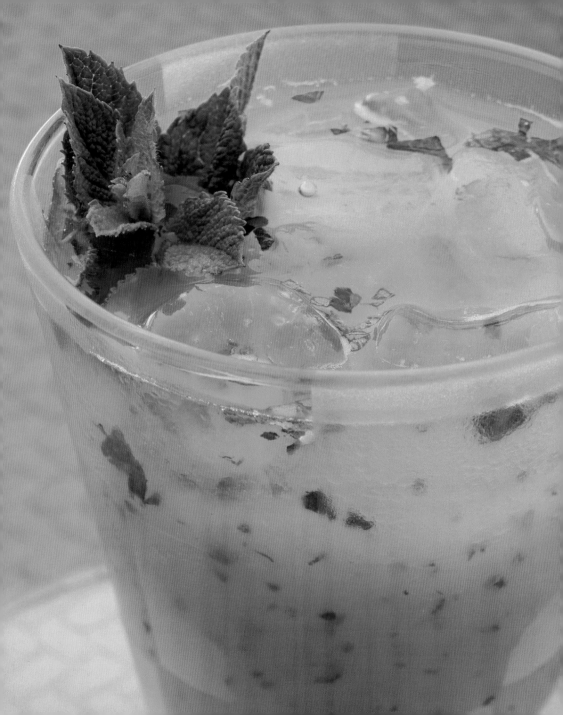

093 minty peach

3 peaches or nectarines

1 apple

1 lime

1 small bunch fresh mint

One of the most refreshing combinations possible, blended with the nectar of peaches.

NUTRIENTS
Beta-carotene, folic acid, vitamin B3,
vitamin C; calcium, magnesium,
phosphorus, potassium, sodium,
sulphur

ENERGY	★★★★☆
DETOX	★☆☆☆☆
IMMUNITY	★★☆☆☆
DIGESTION	★★☆☆☆
SKIN	★★★★☆

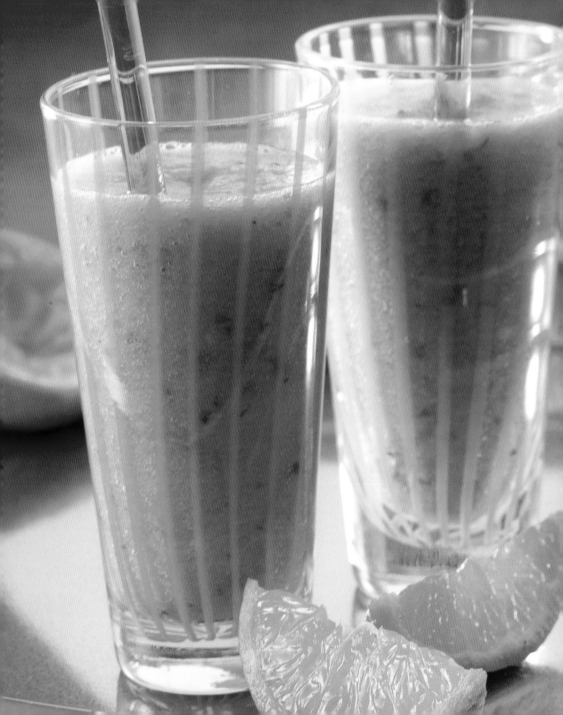

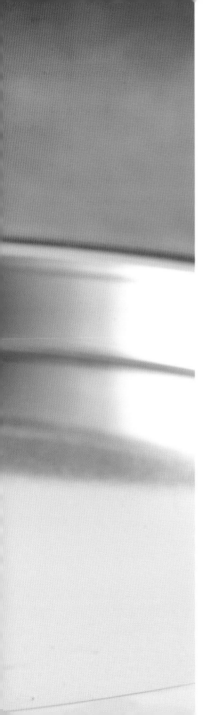

094 tangerine cream

3 peaches or nectarines

2 tangerines or clementines

When oranges simply won't do – only the delicate taste of tangerine or any similar citrus fruit. Combine with peach or nectarine and you get a creamy, sweet blend.

NUTRIENTS

Beta-carotene, folic acid, vitamin B3, vitamin C; calcium, magnesium, phosphorus, potassium, sodium, sulphur

ENERGY	★★★★★
DETOX	★☆☆☆☆
IMMUNITY	★★★★★
DIGESTION	★☆☆☆☆
SKIN	★★★★☆

095 sunset peach

2 peaches or nectarines

1 apple

2 carrots

1 handful raspberries

The carrots add a surprising creamy sweetness to this one and can even make up for getting a dud batch of raspberries that aren't that sweet.

NUTRIENTS

Beta-carotene, biotin, folic acid, vitamin B3, vitamin C; calcium, magnesium, manganese, phosphorus, potassium, sodium, sulphur

ENERGY	★★★★★
DETOX	★★☆☆☆
IMMUNITY	★★★★★
DIGESTION	★★☆☆☆
SKIN	★★★★☆

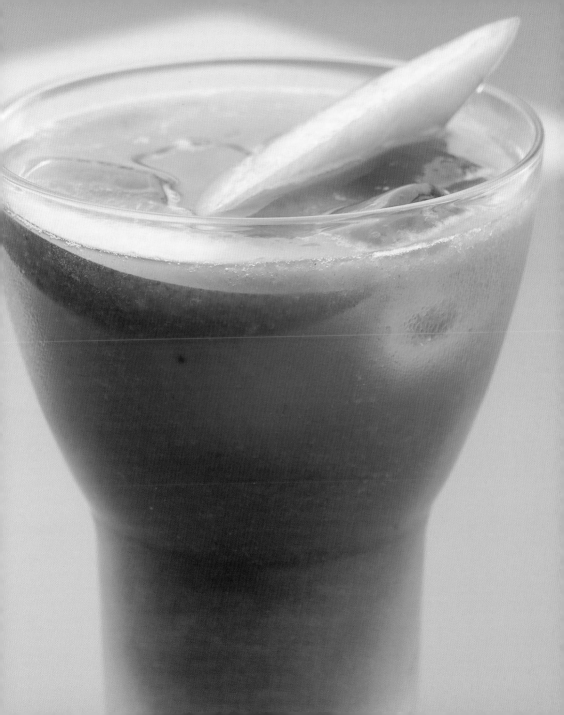

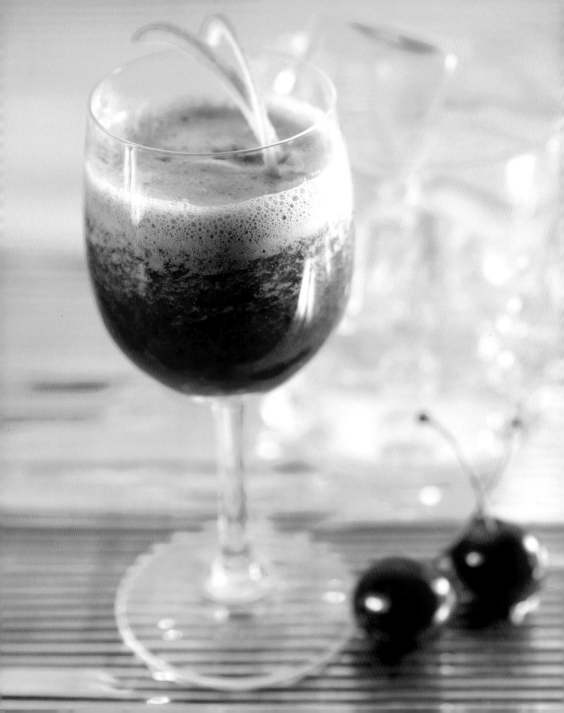

096 cherry pie

2 large handfuls cherries

2 apples

Nothing to do with pies at all, but the sweetness of apples blends beautifully with the cherries.

NUTRIENTS
Beta-carotene, folic acid, vitamin C; calcium, magnesium, phosphorus, potassium, sodium, sulphur

ENERGY	★★★★★
DETOX	★★★☆☆
IMMUNITY	★★★★☆
DIGESTION	★★☆☆☆
SKIN	★★★☆☆

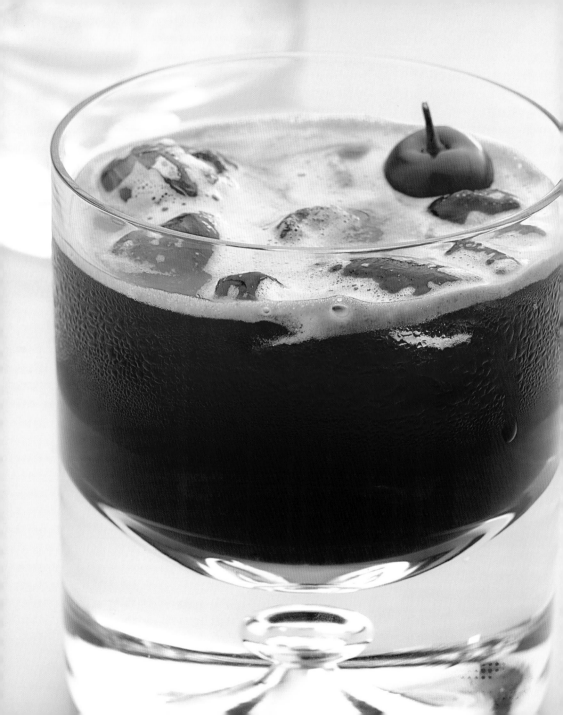

097   thicker than water

2 large handfuls cherries

2 apples

½ beet (beetroot)

The colour of this smooth, sumptuous juice almost makes you
want to hold it as though it were soft, pink velvet.

NUTRIENTS
Beta-carotene, folic acid, vitamin C;
calcium, magnesium, phosphorus,
potassium, sodium, sulphur

ENERGY	★★★★★
DETOX	★★★☆☆
IMMUNITY	★★★★☆
DIGESTION	★★★☆☆
SKIN	★★★★☆

098 citrus cherry

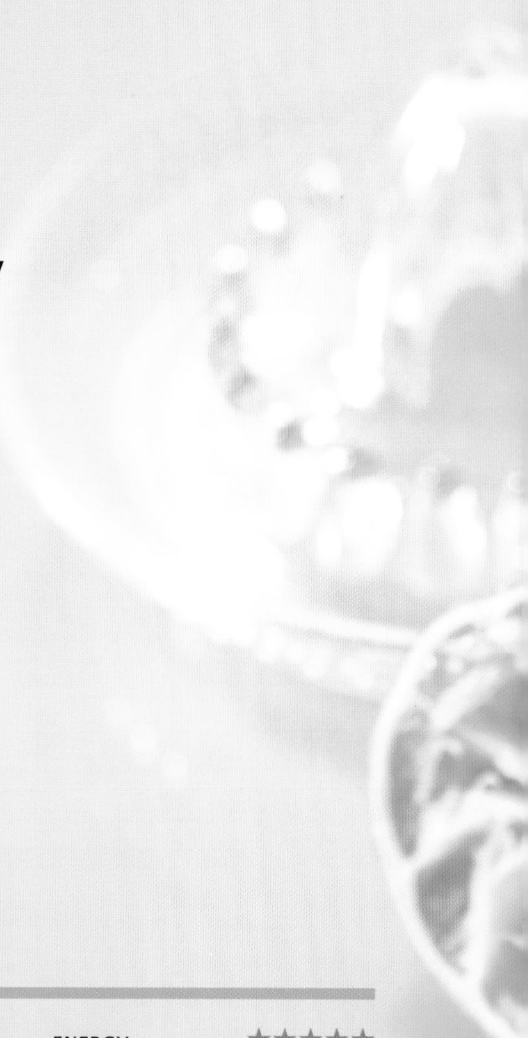

2 large handfuls cherries

2 oranges

½ lime

You'll be hard pressed to enjoy a better combination with orange juice than this.

NUTRIENTS
Beta-carotene, folic acid, vitamin C; calcium, magnesium, phosphorus, potassium, sodium, sulphur

ENERGY	★★★★★
DETOX	★☆☆☆☆
IMMUNITY	★★★★☆
DIGESTION	★☆☆☆☆
SKIN	★★★★☆

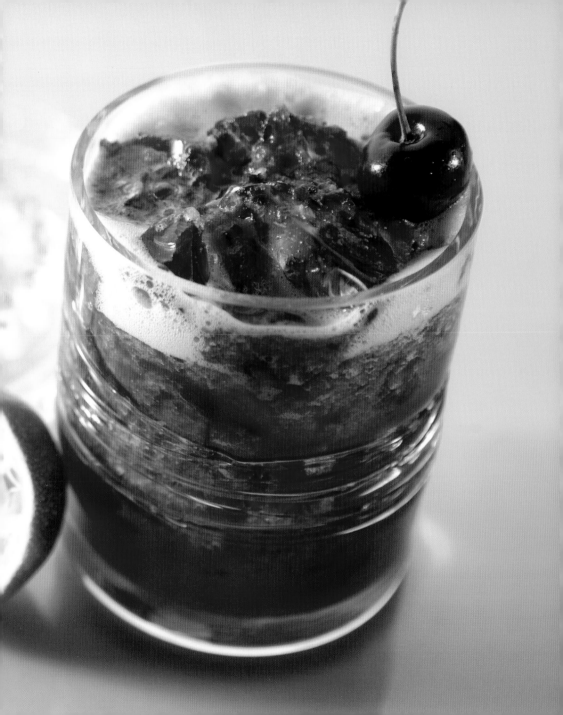

099 sweet cherry pine

2 large handfuls cherries

½ pineapple

The combination of these two fruits produces an unbelievable sensation of intense taste and texture with the rich sweetness of the cherries and the pineapple's tang.

NUTRIENTS
Beta-carotene, folic acid, vitamin C; calcium, magnesium, manganese, phosphorus, potassium, sodium, sulphur

ENERGY	★★★★☆
DETOX	★★☆☆☆
IMMUNITY	★★★★☆
DIGESTION	★★★☆☆
SKIN	★★★★☆

100 cherry cooler

2 large handfuls cherries

½ long cucumber

2 sticks celery

This may seem like a peculiar combination but the cucumber and celery provide delicious light relief from the density of the cherry juice.

NUTRIENTS
Beta-carotene, folic acid, vitamin C;
calcium, magnesium, manganese,
phosphorus, potassium, sodium,
sulphur

ENERGY	★★★☆☆
DETOX	★★☆☆☆
IMMUNITY	★★★☆☆
DIGESTION	★★☆☆☆
SKIN	★★☆☆☆

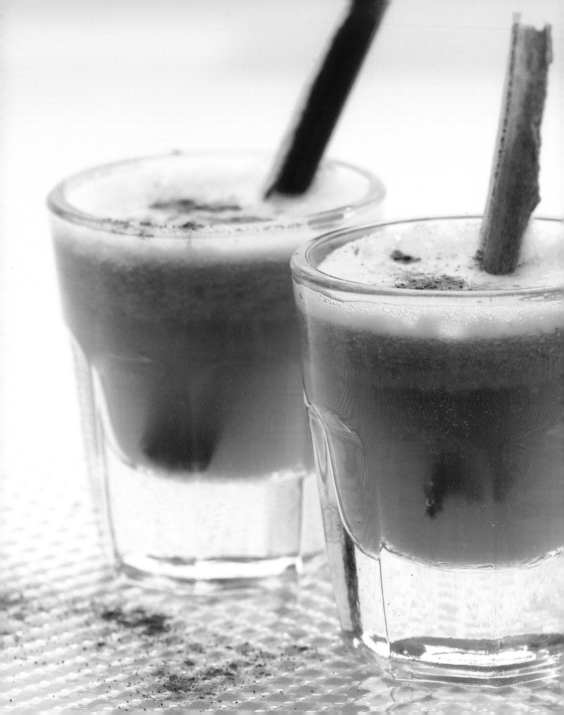

101 pear tart

4 pears

½ inch (1 cm) ginger root

¼ teaspoon ground cinnamon

Pears go so well with a gentle hint of spices.
The cinnamon is best shaken up with the juice
in a jar after it's made.

NUTRIENTS
Beta-carotene, folic acid, vitamin C;
calcium, magnesium, phosphorus,
potassium, sulphur

ENERGY	★★★★☆
DETOX	★☆☆☆☆
IMMUNITY	★★★☆☆
DIGESTION	★★★☆☆
SKIN	★☆☆☆☆

102 pure pear

4 pears

In addition to some of the tropical fruits, I think a ripe Williams pear
ranks right up there as one of my favourites.

NUTRIENTS
Beta-carotene, folic acid, vitamin C;
calcium, magnesium, phosphorus,
potassium, sulphur

ENERGY	★★★★☆
DETOX	★★☆☆☆
IMMUNITY	★☆☆☆☆
DIGESTION	★★★☆☆
SKIN	★★☆☆☆

103   pear basic

2 pears

1 apple

2 carrots

½ inch (1 cm) ginger root

A good, standard morning blend to set you up for the day ahead.

NUTRIENTS
Beta-carotene, folic acid, vitamin C;
calcium, magnesium, phosphorus,
potassium, sodium, sulphur

ENERGY	★★★★☆
DETOX	★★★☆☆
IMMUNITY	★★★☆☆
DIGESTION	★★☆☆☆
SKIN	★★★☆☆

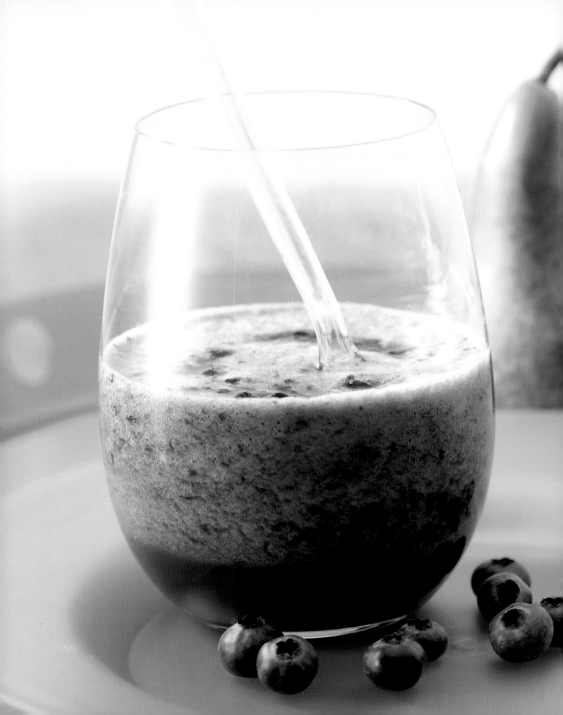

104 blue pear

2 pears

1 handful blueberries

1 handful blackberries

The sweetness of all three of these fruits is divine.

NUTRIENTS
Beta-carotene, biotin, folic acid, vitamins B1, B2, B6, C and E; calcium, chromium, iron, magnesium, manganese, phosphorus, potassium, sodium, sulphur

ENERGY	★★★★☆
DETOX	★★★☆☆
IMMUNITY	★★★★☆
DIGESTION	★☆☆☆☆
SKIN	★★★☆☆

105   pink pear

2 pears

1 handful raspberries

1 handful strawberries

In my view, raspberries and strawberries go well with pretty much any fruit, and this is certainly no exception.

NUTRIENTS
Beta-carotene, biotin, folic acid,
vitamin C; calcium, magnesium,
manganese, phosphorus, potassium,
sodium, sulphur

ENERGY	★★★★★
DETOX	★★☆☆☆
IMMUNITY	★★★★☆
DIGESTION	★☆☆☆☆
SKIN	★★★☆☆

106 pink pear II

3 pears

1 handful cranberries

Another bright pink juice, this one is fantastic for the immune system, particularly for urinary-tract infections. Unless you want a very sharp taste, make sure you use nearly ripe Williams pears.

NUTRIENTS

Beta-carotene, folic acid, vitamin C;
calcium, iron, magnesium, phosphorus,
potassium, sodium, sulphur

ENERGY	★★★☆☆
DETOX	★★☆☆☆
IMMUNITY	★★★★☆
DIGESTION	★☆☆☆☆
SKIN	★★★☆☆

107 black pear

3 pears

1 handful blackcurrants

Quite distinct from Blue Pear (see blend 104) –
the sweet sharpness of the blackcurrants blends
wonderfully with pears.

NUTRIENTS
Beta-carotene, biotin, folic acid,
vitamins B5, C and E; calcium,
magnesium, phosphorus, potassium,
sodium, sulphur

ENERGY	★★★★☆
DETOX	★★★☆☆
IMMUNITY	★★★★☆
DIGESTION	★☆☆☆☆
SKIN	★★★☆☆

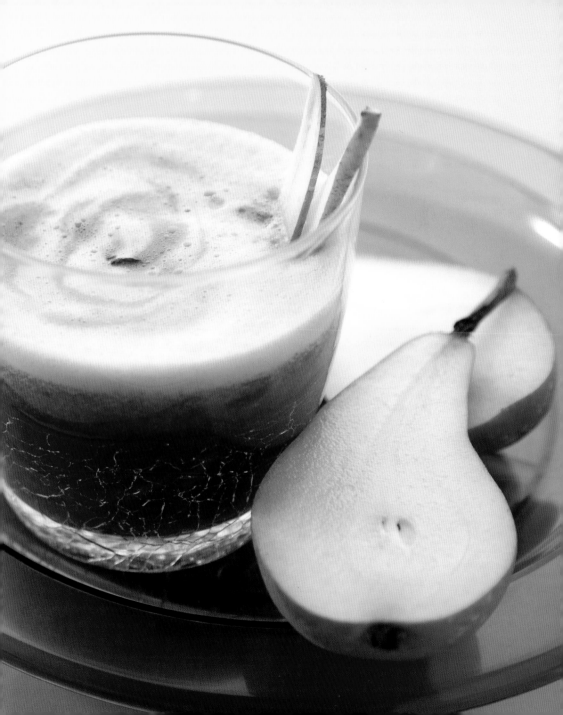

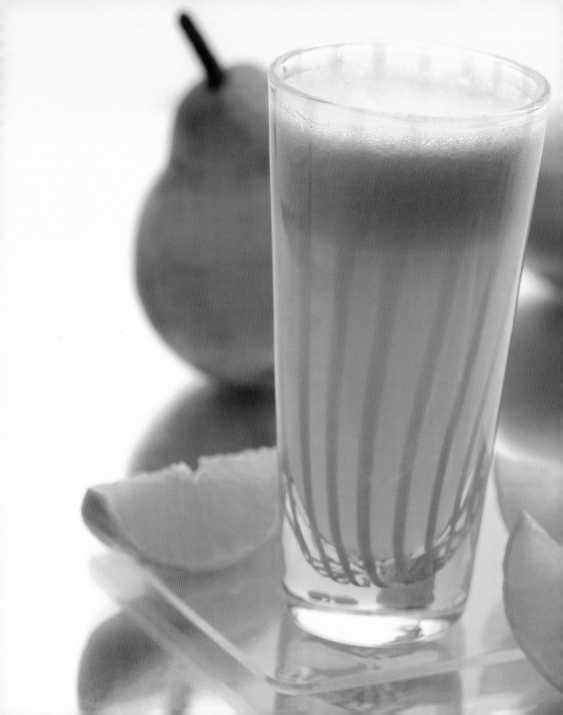

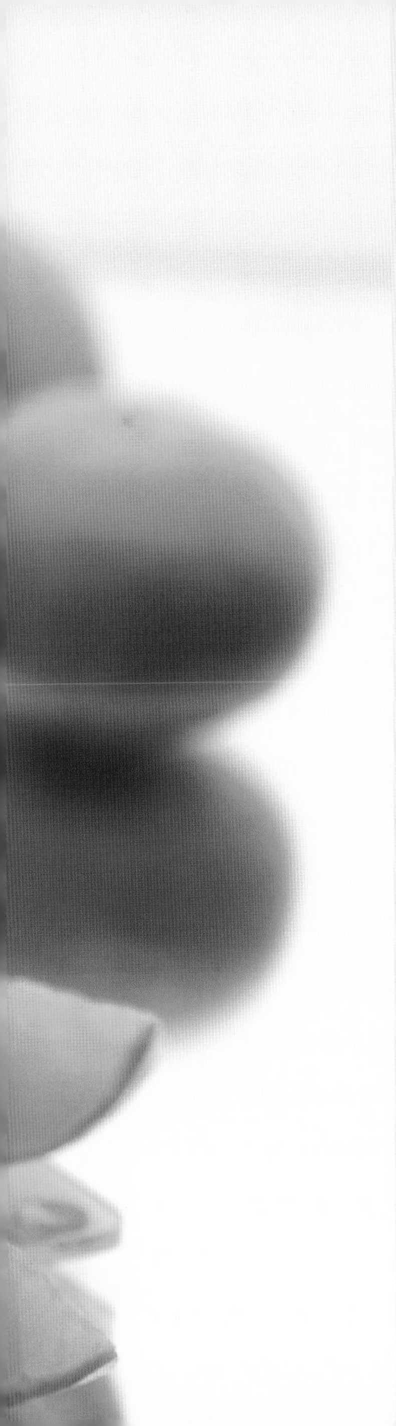

108 tangerine dream

3 pears

2 tangerines

Although pears go well with any citrus fruit, the slightly more delicate flavour of tangerine (or clementine) really draws out the taste of the pear.

NUTRIENTS
Beta-carotene, folic acid, vitamin C; calcium, magnesium, phosphorus, potassium, sodium, sulphur

ENERGY ★★★★☆
DETOX ★★☆☆☆
IMMUNITY ★★★☆☆
DIGESTION ★☆☆☆☆
SKIN ★★★☆☆

109 big c pear

2 pears

2 kiwi fruits

2 guavas

These two vitamin C-packed fruits create a divine taste with pear.

NUTRIENTS
Beta-carotene, folic acid, vitamin B3,
vitamin C; calcium, magnesium,
phosphorus, potassium, sodium,
sulphur

ENERGY ★★★★★
DETOX ★★☆☆☆
IMMUNITY ★★★★★
DIGESTION ★★☆☆☆
SKIN ★★★★☆

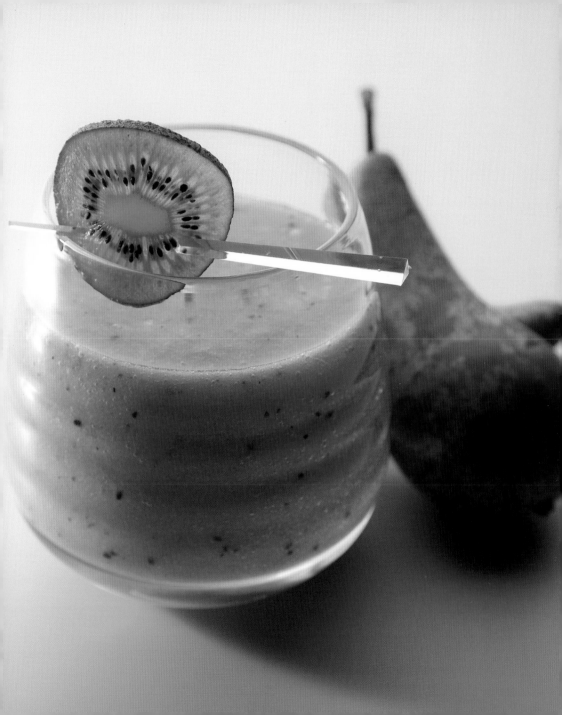

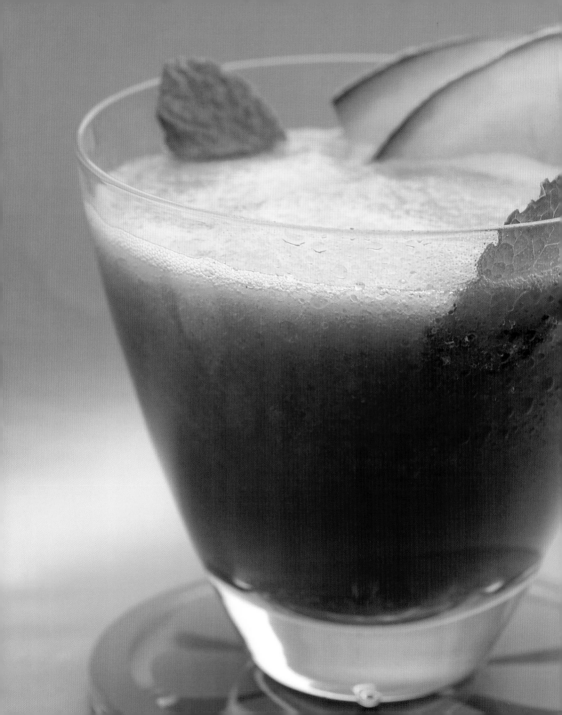

110   creamy pear

3 pears

1 thick slice melon

1 small bunch fresh mint

The taste and texture of melon juice somehow conjures up the sensation of creaminess.

NUTRIENTS
Beta-carotene, folic acid, vitamin C;
calcium, magnesium, phosphorus,
potassium, sodium, sulphur

ENERGY ★★★★☆
DETOX ★☆☆☆☆
IMMUNITY ★★★★☆
DIGESTION ★★☆☆☆
SKIN ★★★☆☆

111 tropical pear

3 pears

¼ pineapple

½ lime

Perhaps two of my favourite fruits with a hint of tangy lime.

NUTRIENTS
Beta-carotene, folic acid, vitamin C;
calcium, magnesium, manganese,
phosphorus, potassium, sodium,
sulphur

ENERGY	★★★★☆
DETOX	★★☆☆☆
IMMUNITY	★★★★☆
DIGESTION	★★★☆☆
SKIN	★★☆☆☆

112   pear dream

3 pears

4 apricots

Two delicate, gentle flavours bound to create a dreamy combination.

NUTRIENTS
Beta-carotene, folic acid, vitamin C;
calcium, magnesium, phosphorus,
potassium, sulphur

ENERGY	★★★★☆
DETOX	★★☆☆☆
IMMUNITY	★★★★☆
DIGESTION	★★☆☆☆
SKIN	★★★★☆

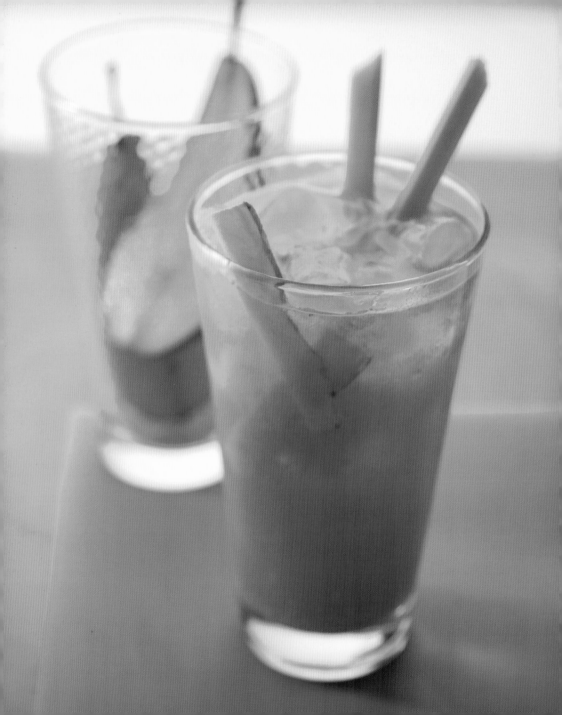

113 breakfast pear

3 pears

2 sticks celery

½ inch (1 cm) ginger root

The saltiness of celery and the hot bite of the ginger make this a great morning recipe for awakening the tastebuds.

NUTRIENTS
Beta-carotene, folic acid, vitamin C;
calcium, magnesium, phosphorus,
potassium, sodium, sulphur

ENERGY	★★★☆☆
DETOX	★★★★☆
IMMUNITY	★★★☆☆
DIGESTION	★★☆☆☆
SKIN	★☆☆☆☆

114 fresh pear

3 pears

½ long cucumber

1 small bunch fresh mint

There aren't many juices like that of a cucumber to
quench your thirst, and combined with pear and
then the mint too… mmm.

NUTRIENTS
Beta-carotene, folic acid, vitamin C;
calcium, magnesium, phosphorus,
potassium, sodium, sulphur

ENERGY ★★★☆☆
DETOX ★★★★☆
IMMUNITY ★☆☆☆☆
DIGESTION ★★☆☆☆
SKIN ★★☆☆☆

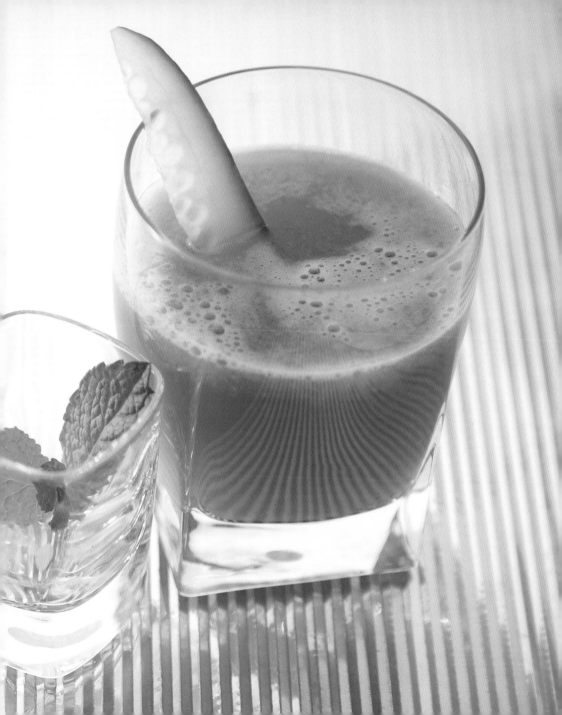

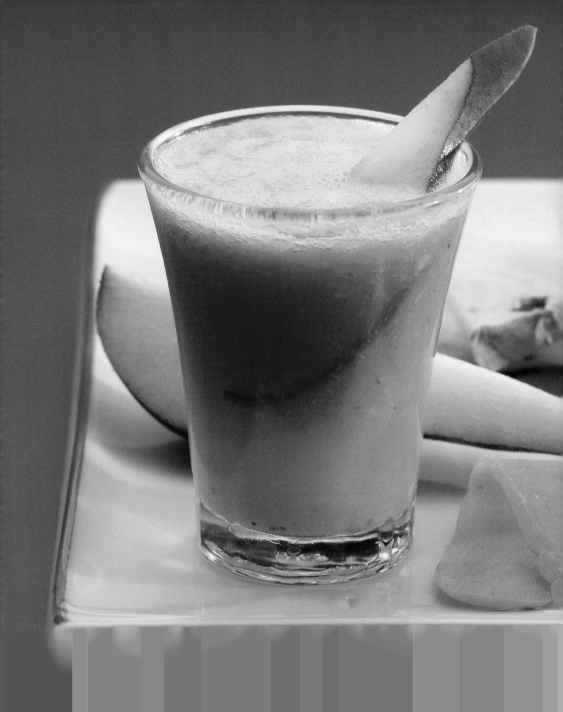

115 gut soother

2 pears

2 carrots

½ pineapple

½ inch (1 cm) ginger root

The blend of these three along
with the ginger not only make
a great taste, but they're good for
the digestive tract too.

NUTRIENTS

Beta-carotene, folic acid, vitamin C;
calcium, magnesium, manganese,
phosphorus, potassium, sodium,
sulphur

ENERGY	★★★☆☆
DETOX	★★☆☆☆
IMMUNITY	★★★☆☆
DIGESTION	★★★★★
SKIN	★★★☆☆

116 pink pineapple

½ pineapple

1 handful raspberries

1 handful strawberries

This rich yet fresh juice is a beautiful shade of pink created by a blend of fruits from tropical and temperate climes.

NUTRIENTS
Beta-carotene, biotin, folic acid,
vitamin C; calcium, magnesium,
manganese, phosphorus, potassium,
sodium, sulphur

ENERGY ★★★★★
DETOX ★☆☆☆☆
IMMUNITY ★★★★☆
DIGESTION ★★★☆☆
SKIN ★★★☆☆

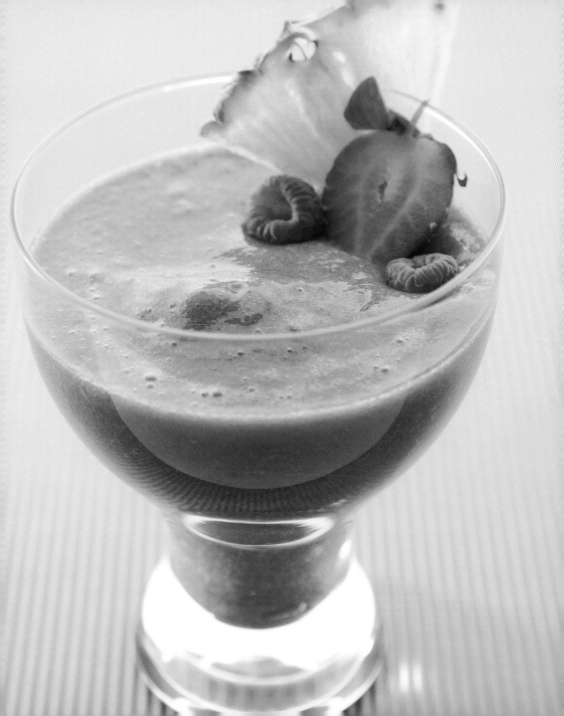

117 pure pineapple

1 pineapple

It was always my favourite juice in a can, bottle or carton…
until I discovered the real thing.

NUTRIENTS
Beta-carotene, folic acid, vitamin C;
calcium, magnesium, manganese,
phosphorus, potassium, sodium

ENERGY	★★★★★
DETOX	★★★☆☆
IMMUNITY	★★★☆☆
DIGESTION	★★★★★
SKIN	★★★☆☆

118 pineapple tang

1 pineapple

1 lime

Mixed with lime, pineapple takes me straight to the streets of Bangkok.

NUTRIENTS
Beta-carotene, folic acid, vitamin C;
calcium, magnesium, manganese,
phosphorus, potassium, sodium,
sulphur

ENERGY	★★★★★
DETOX	★★★☆☆
IMMUNITY	★★★☆☆
DIGESTION	★★★★★
SKIN	★★★☆☆

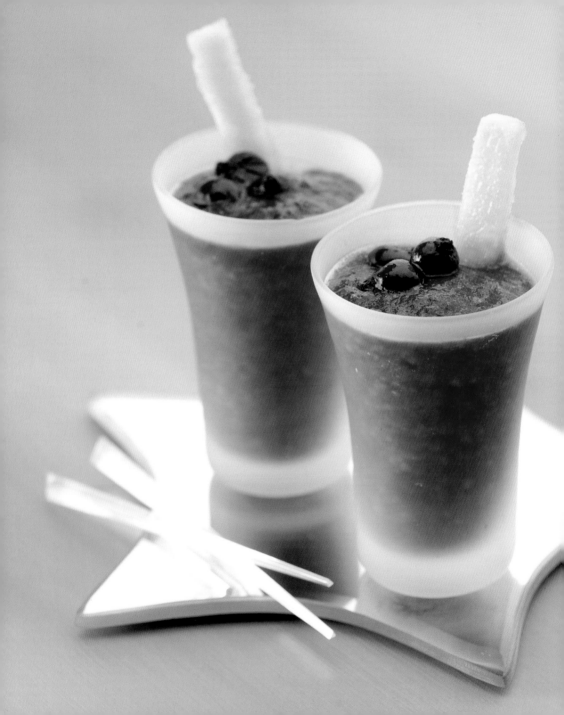

119 black pineapple

½ pineapple

1 handful blackcurrants

1 handful blackberries

Another tropic-temperate blend of fruits which goes down perfectly.

NUTRIENTS
Beta-carotene, biotin, folic acid,
vitamins B5, C and E; calcium, iron,
magnesium, manganese, phosphorus,
potassium, sodium, sulphur

ENERGY	★★★★★
DETOX	★★☆☆☆
IMMUNITY	★★★★☆
DIGESTION	★★★☆☆
SKIN	★★★★☆

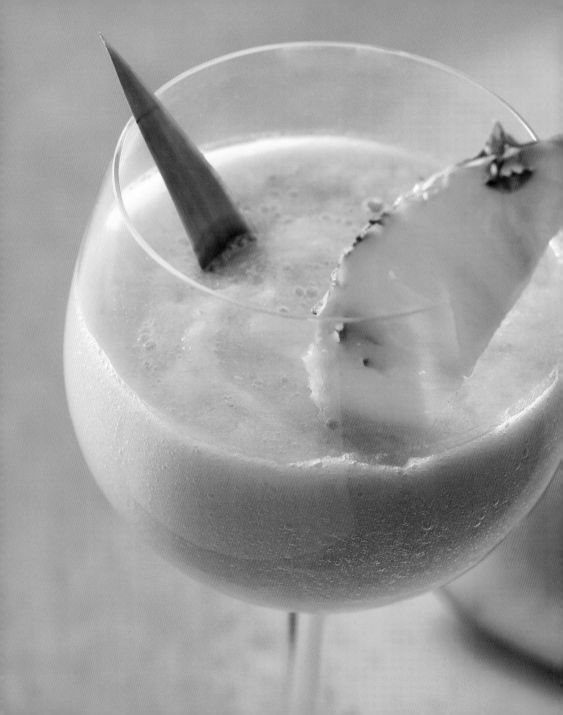

120 sweet sunset

½ pineapple

1 thick slice watermelon

The watery sweetness of the melon contrasts ideally with the rich tang of pineapple in this all-round health-affirming, thirst-quenching drink.

NUTRIENTS
Beta-carotene, folic acid, vitamin B5, vitamin C; calcium, magnesium, manganese, phosphorus, potassium, sodium

ENERGY	★★★★★
DETOX	★★★☆☆
IMMUNITY	★★★★☆
DIGESTION	★★☆☆☆
SKIN	★★★★☆

121 aniseed black

½ pineapple

1 large handful blackcurrants

½ fennel bulb

A nostalgic reminder of blackcurrant-and-aniseed
boiled candy but with a tangy difference.

NUTRIENTS
Beta-carotene, biotin, folic acid,
vitamins B5, C and E; calcium,
magnesium, manganese, phosphorus,
potassium, sodium, sulphur

ENERGY	★★★★☆
DETOX	★☆☆☆☆
IMMUNITY	★★★☆☆
DIGESTION	★★★★☆
SKIN	★★★★☆

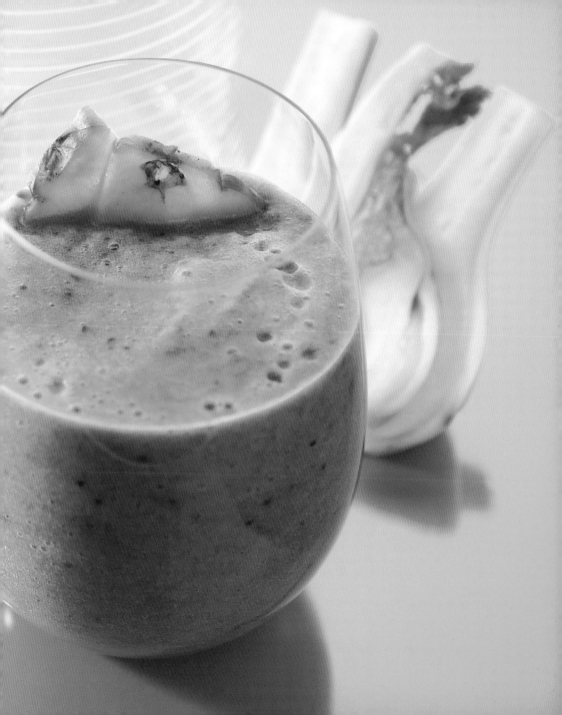

122 ginger zinger

½ pineapple

2 oranges

1 inch (2.5 cm) ginger root

One of the most refreshing, flavourful combinations there is. You could add more ginger if you're a real fan and get an even greater boost from this all-round wonderfood.

NUTRIENTS
Beta-carotene, folic acid, vitamin C; calcium, magnesium, manganese, phosphorus, potassium, sodium

ENERGY   ★★★★☆
DETOX   ★☆☆☆☆
IMMUNITY   ★★★★☆
DIGESTION   ★★★☆☆
SKIN   ★★☆☆☆

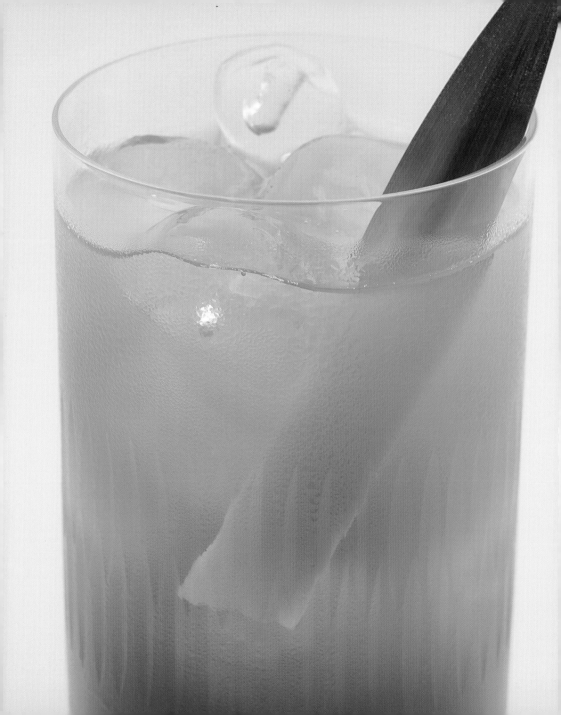

123 muddy pine

1 pineapple

1 teaspoon spirulina

The tangy, strong taste of the pineapple easily carries the earthy goodness of the spirulina. Best to shake a bit of the juice with the spirulina in a jar and then mix it all up to avoid getting lumps of green powder.

NUTRIENTS
Beta-carotene, folic acid, vitamins B1, B3, B5, B6 and C; calcium, iron, magnesium, manganese, phosphorus, potassium, sodium; protein; essential fatty acids

ENERGY	★★★★★
DETOX	★★★★★
IMMUNITY	★★★☆☆
DIGESTION	★★★★☆
SKIN	★★★★☆

124 pineapple basic

½ pineapple

1 apple

3 carrots

1 stick celery

Apart from the essential pineapple, this is a simple mixture of ingredients you're likely to have in your fruit bowl and refrigerator, and one which turns out a delicious morning juice.

NUTRIENTS
Beta-carotene, folic acid, vitamin C; calcium, magnesium, manganese, phosphorus, potassium, sodium, sulphur

ENERGY	★★★★☆
DETOX	★★★★☆
IMMUNITY	★★★★☆
DIGESTION	★★★★☆
SKIN	★★★☆☆

125 aniseed twist

½ pineapple

2 apples

½ fennel bulb

The fennel comes as an unexpected twist against the pineapple and apple. A delicious afternoon pick-me-up.

NUTRIENTS
Beta-carotene, folic acid, vitamin C; calcium, magnesium, manganese, phosphorus, potassium, sodium, sulphur

ENERGY	★★★★☆
DETOX	★★★☆☆
IMMUNITY	★★★☆☆
DIGESTION	★★★★☆
SKIN	★★★☆☆

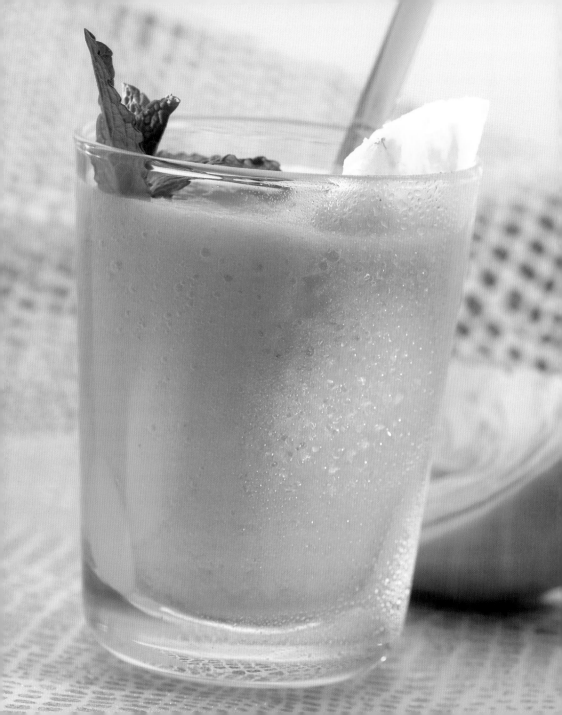

126 digestaid

½ pineapple

1 thick slice white cabbage

1 inch (2.5 cm) ginger root

1 small bunch fresh mint

Pineapple contains bromelain (a natural substance that helps digestion), cabbage soothes the stomach lining and ginger calms the digestive tract – an all-round gut tonic.

NUTRIENTS
Beta-carotene, folic acid, vitamin C, vitamin E; calcium, magnesium, manganese, phosphorus, potassium, sodium

ENERGY ★★★☆☆
DETOX ★★★☆☆
IMMUNITY ★★☆☆☆
DIGESTION ★★★★★
SKIN ★★★☆☆

127 bloody pineapple

½ pineapple

1 beet (beetroot)

Another mixture where the powerful taste of pineapple carries
a flavour that some people find too earthy in other combinations.

NUTRIENTS
Beta-carotene, folic acid, vitamin C;
calcium, magnesium, manganese,
phosphorus, potassium, sodium

ENERGY   ★★★★☆
DETOX   ★★★★☆
IMMUNITY   ★★★☆☆
DIGESTION ★★★★☆
SKIN   ★★★★☆

128 green pines

½ pineapple

3 sticks celery

1 large handful watercress

This is a very cleansing juice with rich, peppery undertones supplied by the watercress.

NUTRIENTS
Beta-carotene, folic acid, vitamin C, vitamin E; calcium, iron, magnesium, manganese, phosphorus, potassium, sodium, sulphur

ENERGY	★★★☆☆
DETOX	★★★★☆
IMMUNITY	★★★☆☆
DIGESTION	★★★☆☆
SKIN	★★★★☆

129 pineapple magic

½ pineapple

1 thick slice melon

2 guavas

This exquisite combination of three flavoursome fruits creates a creamy, magical taste which is also very rich in immunity-boosting nutrients.

NUTRIENTS
Beta-carotene, folic acid, vitamin
B3, vitamin C; calcium, magnesium,
manganese, phosphorus, potassium,
sodium, sulphur

ENERGY	★★★★★
DETOX	★★☆☆☆
IMMUNITY	★★★★★
DIGESTION	★★★☆☆
SKIN	★★★☆☆

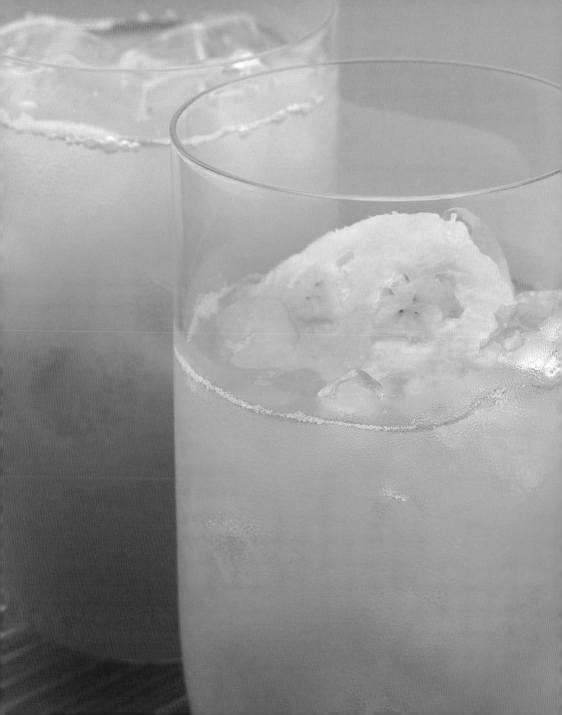

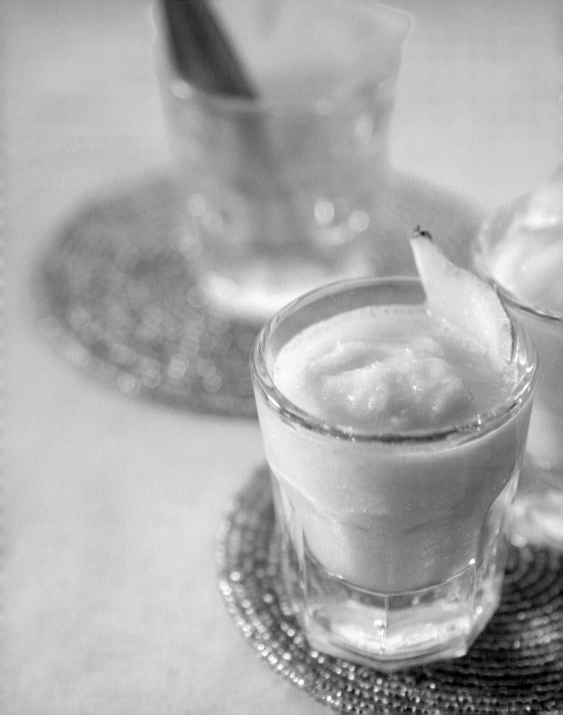

130 joint aid

1 pineapple

2 inches (5 cm) ginger root

1 tablespoon (15 ml) flaxseed (linseed) oil

The bromelain in pineapple can help reduce inflammation, as can ginger and the essential fatty acids in flaxseed oil. Two inches of ginger is a pretty hefty dose, so reduce it if you find it too strong.

NUTRIENTS
Beta-carotene, folic acid, vitamin C; calcium, magnesium, manganese, phosphorus, potassium, sodium; essential fatty acids

ENERGY	★★★★★
DETOX	★★★☆☆
IMMUNITY	★★★★★
DIGESTION	★★★★☆
SKIN	★★★★☆

131 pixie pine

½ pineapple

2 beets (beetroot)

1 inch (2.5 cm) ginger root

This is named in honour of Dr Pixie, the fabulous Irish TV celebrity GP, because there's something Guinness-like about it!

NUTRIENTS
Beta-carotene, folic acid, vitamin C;
calcium, magnesium, phosphorus,
potassium, sodium

ENERGY	★★★★☆
DETOX	★★☆☆☆
IMMUNITY	★☆☆☆☆
DIGESTION	★★★★☆
SKIN	★★★☆☆

132 clear cleanser

½ pineapple

1 large handful spinach

½ fennel bulb

The worthy, earthy taste of the spinach is offset well by the pineapple and fennel.

NUTRIENTS
Beta-carotene, folic acid, vitamin B3,
vitamin C; calcium, iron, magnesium,
phosphorus, potassium, sodium

ENERGY	★★★★☆
DETOX	★★★★☆
IMMUNITY	☆☆☆☆☆
DIGESTION	★★★☆☆
SKIN	★★☆☆☆

133　what's up, doc?

5 carrots

The original basic vegetable juice, this is pure orange, creamy and vibrant, and probably the most popular and palatable of all the solo vegetable juices.

NUTRIENTS
Beta-carotene, folic acid, vitamin C; calcium, magnesium, phosphorus, potassium, sodium, sulphur

ENERGY	★★★★☆
DETOX	★★★★☆
IMMUNITY	★★★★☆
DIGESTION	★★☆☆☆
SKIN	★★★★★

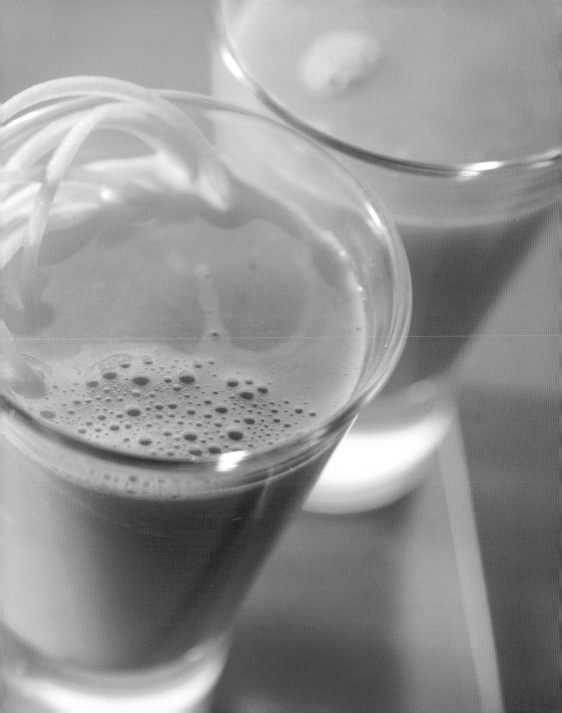

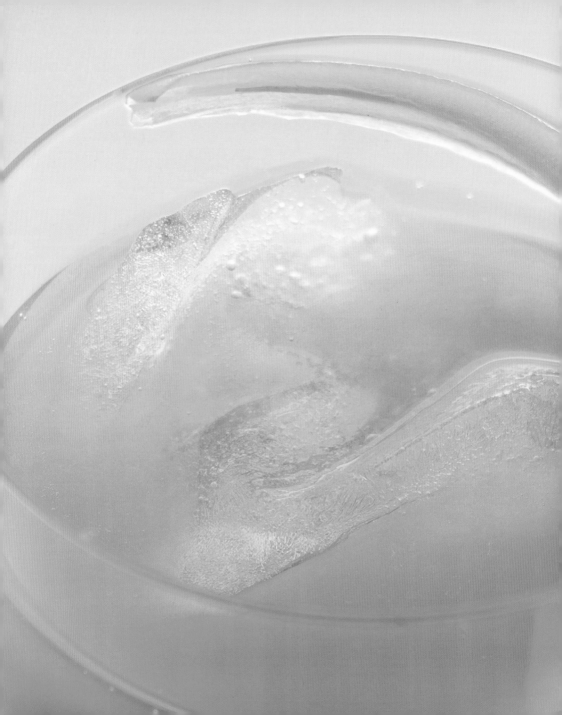

134 easy morning

3 carrots

1 apple

½ orange

1 stick celery

½ inch (1 cm) ginger root

This is my absolute staple – when I'm not feeling any more adventurous, this is what pours daily from my juicer. It makes an invigorating start to any day.

NUTRIENTS

Beta-carotene, folic acid, vitamin C; calcium, magnesium, manganese, phosphorus, potassium, sodium, sulphur

ENERGY	★★★★☆
DETOX	★★★☆☆
IMMUNITY	★★★☆☆
DIGESTION	★★☆☆☆
SKIN	★★★☆☆

135 apple basic

4 carrots

1 apple

Most refrigerators house a couple of carrots and most fruit bowls an apple, so this is a good, basic standby for any morning.

NUTRIENTS
Beta-carotene, folic acid, vitamin C; calcium, magnesium, phosphorus, potassium, sodium, sulphur

ENERGY	★★★★★
DETOX	★★★☆☆
IMMUNITY	★★☆☆☆
DIGESTION	★★★☆☆
SKIN	★★★☆☆

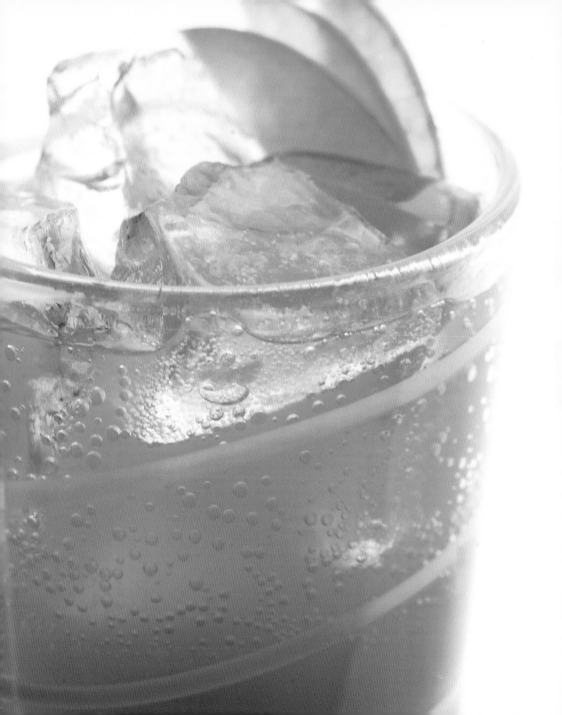

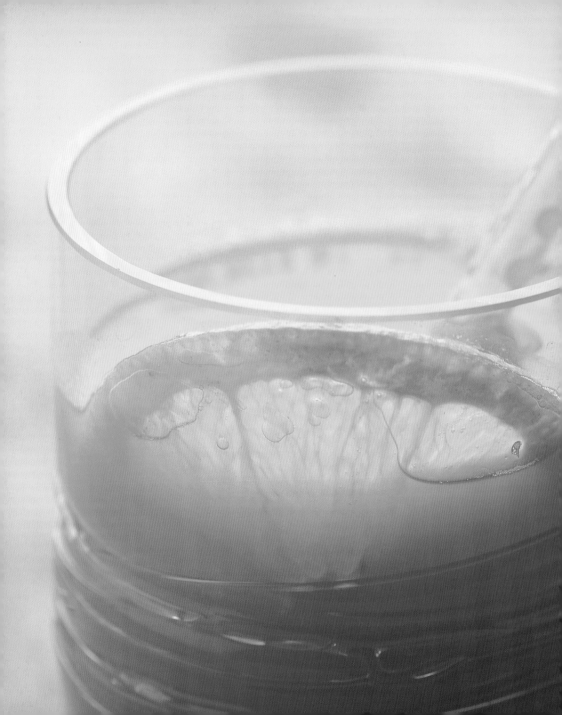

136 orange carrot

4 carrots

1 orange

Double-orange blast of colour and goodness
– a great, basic blend for any morning.

NUTRIENTS
Beta-carotene, folic acid, vitamin C;
calcium, magnesium, phosphorus,
potassium, sodium, sulphur

ENERGY ★★★☆☆

DETOX ★★★☆☆

IMMUNITY ★★★☆☆

DIGESTION ★☆☆☆☆

SKIN ★★☆☆☆

137 carrot cleanser

3 carrots

½ apple

½ orange

¼ beet (beetroot)

1 stick celery

2 large kale leaves

Any juice using beet or kale can take some getting used to for the vegetable-juice initiate, but once you've had it, you can fully appreciate its cleansing properties.

NUTRIENTS
Beta-carotene, folic acid, vitamins B3, B6 and C; calcium, iron, magnesium, manganese, phosphorus, potassium, sodium, sulphur

ENERGY	★★★☆☆
DETOX	★★★★★
IMMUNITY	★★★★☆
DIGESTION	★★★☆☆
SKIN	★★★☆☆

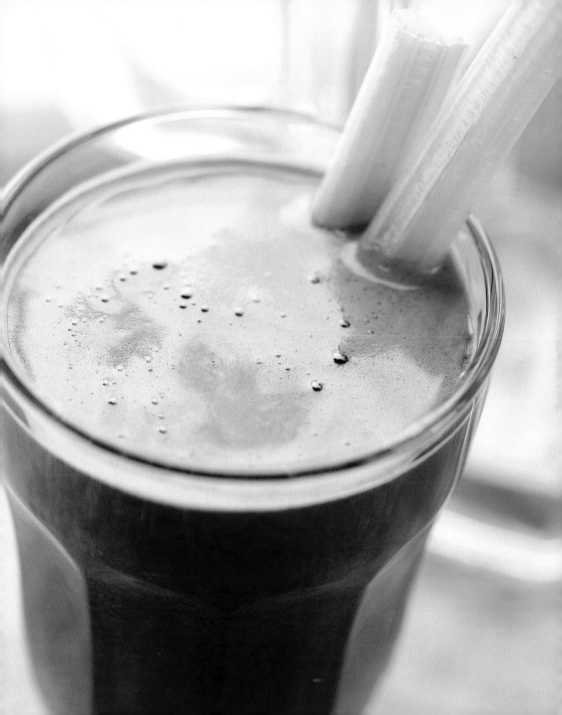

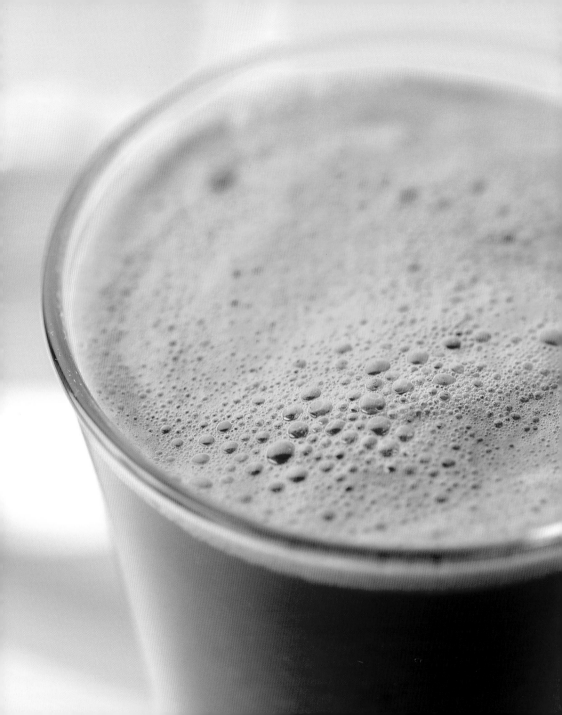

138 carrot deep cleanser

3 carrots

½ apple

½ beet (beetroot)

1 stick celery

3 large kale leaves

If you are at all wary of having beet or kale juice, start with the Carrot Cleanser (blend 137) before you graduate to this.

NUTRIENTS
Beta-carotene, folic acid, vitamins B3, B6 and C; calcium, iron, magnesium, manganese, phosphorus, potassium, sodium, sulphur

ENERGY	★★★☆☆
DETOX	★★★★★
IMMUNITY	★★★★☆
DIGESTION	★★★☆☆
SKIN	★★★☆☆

139 carrot crunch

4 carrots

2 sticks celery

½ inch (1 cm) ginger root

Well, of course this isn't crunchy, but if it weren't a juice it would certainly get your jaw moving. An excellent contrasting blend of flavours.

NUTRIENTS
Beta-carotene, folic acid, vitamin C; calcium, magnesium, phosphorus, potassium, sodium, sulphur

ENERGY ★★★☆☆

DETOX ★★★☆☆

IMMUNITY ★★★★☆

DIGESTION ★★★☆☆

SKIN ★★★☆☆

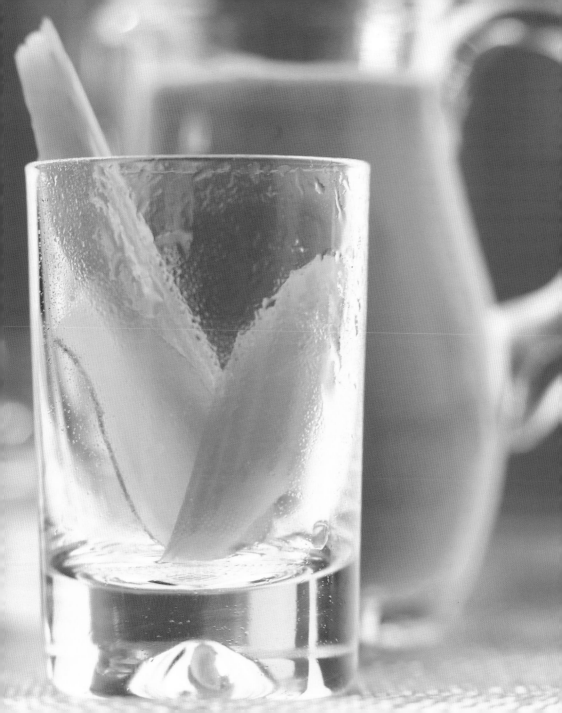

140 carrot digestif

4 carrots

¼ pineapple

2 large white cabbage leaves

The beta-carotene in the carrots, combined with the particularly soothing constituents of the other ingredients, makes this a great juice for helping ease digestive problems.

NUTRIENTS
Beta-carotene, folic acid, vitamin C;
calcium, magnesium, manganese,
phosphorus, potassium, sodium,
sulphur

ENERGY	★★★☆☆
DETOX	★★★☆☆
IMMUNITY	★☆☆☆☆
DIGESTION	★★★★★
SKIN	★★★☆☆

141   carotene catapult

3 carrots

½ melon

1 slice watermelon

1 teaspoon spirulina

Beta-carotene is a crucial vitamin, which the body can convert to vitamin A. It's needed for healthy immunity, skin, digestive tract, lungs and much more. All of the ingredients in this tasty juice are excellent beta-carotene sources.

NUTRIENTS
Beta-carotene, folic acid, vitamins B1, B3, B5, B6 and C; calcium, iron, magnesium, phosphorus, potassium, sodium, sulphur; protein; essential fatty acids

ENERGY	★★★★☆
DETOX	★★★☆☆
IMMUNITY	★★★★★
DIGESTION	★★★☆☆
SKIN	★★★★★

142 sweet pepper

3 carrots

1 red bell pepper

1 yellow bell pepper

The sweetness of the carrots with bell peppers is remarkable and makes this fresh drink a great introduction to vegetable-based juicing.

NUTRIENTS
Beta-carotene, folic acid, vitamin C; calcium, magnesium, phosphorus, potassium, sodium, sulphur

ENERGY	★★★☆☆
DETOX	★★☆☆☆
IMMUNITY	★★★★★
DIGESTION	★★☆☆☆
SKIN	★★★★☆

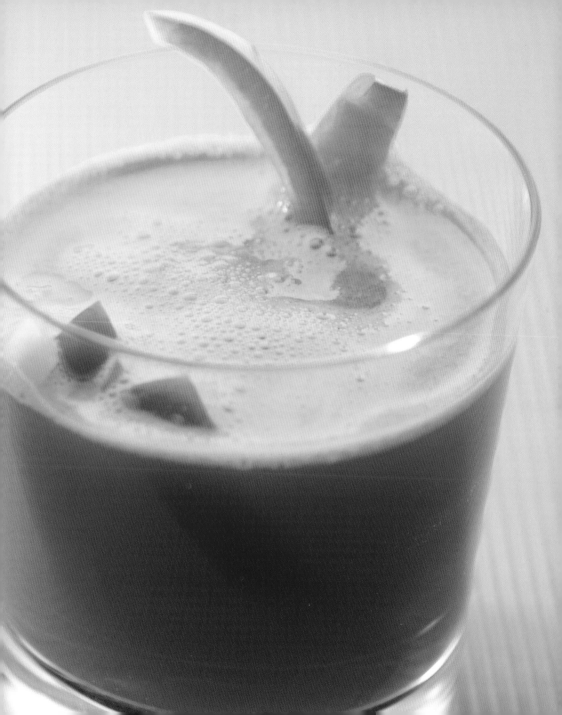

143 breath freshener

4 carrots

1 handful fresh parsley

This juice helps work on your breath from the inside, rather than just washing out your mouth.

NUTRIENTS
Beta-carotene, folic acid, vitamin B3, vitamin C; calcium, iron, magnesium, phosphorus, potassium, sodium, sulphur

ENERGY ★★★★☆
DETOX ★★★☆☆
IMMUNITY ★★★★☆
DIGESTION ★★★★☆
SKIN ★★★★☆

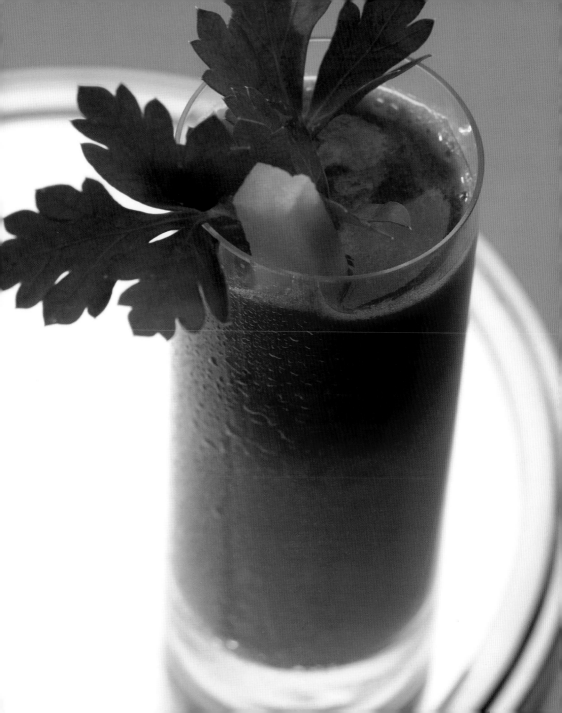

144 veggie carotene catapult

3 carrots

1 red bell pepper

1 broccoli spear

½ sweet potato

Superbly rich in anti-aging and cancer-protective carotenes – and it tastes good.

NUTRIENTS

Beta-carotene, folic acid, vitamins C, B5 and E; calcium, magnesium, phosphorus, potassium, sodium, sulphur

ENERGY	★★★★☆
DETOX	★★★☆☆
IMMUNITY	★★★★★
DIGESTION	★★★☆☆
SKIN	★★★★★

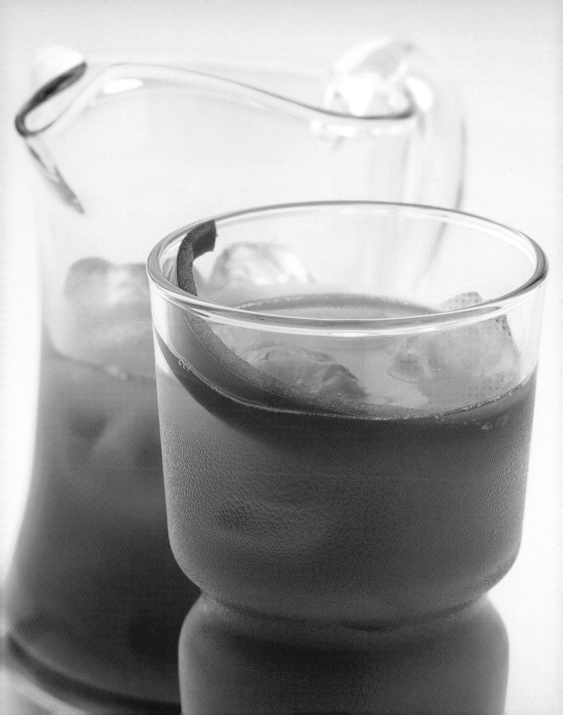

145 cold war

4 carrots

1 orange

½ inch (1 cm) ginger root

2 cloves garlic

The garlic in here is purely for therapeutic use – to give your immune system a powerful punch in the face of a cold or any other infection. It's a brave person who can stomach it on any normal morning, let alone the breath you're likely to have afterwards. If your chest is feeling congested, you could add half an onion.

NUTRIENTS
Beta-carotene, folic acid, vitamin C; calcium, magnesium, phosphorus, potassium, sodium, sulphur

ENERGY	★★★☆☆
DETOX	★★☆☆☆
IMMUNITY	★★★★★
DIGESTION	★★☆☆☆
SKIN	★★★★☆

146 sharp carrot

4 carrots

2 sticks celery

1 lime

1 small bunch fresh mint

This one has a fantastic bite from the lime, nicely lifted by the salty celery and hint of mint.

NUTRIENTS	ENERGY	★★★★☆
Beta-carotene, folic acid, vitamin C;	DETOX	★★★☆☆
calcium, magnesium, phosphorus,	IMMUNITY	★★★☆☆
potassium, sodium, sulphur	DIGESTION	★★★☆☆
	SKIN	★★★☆☆

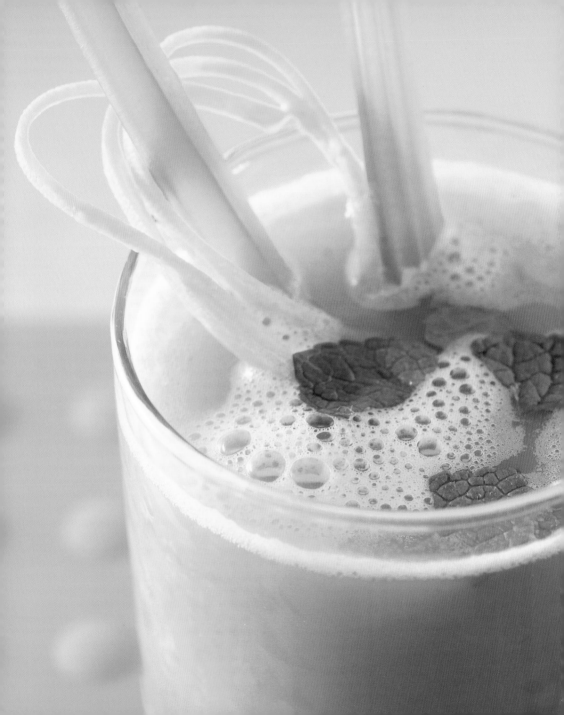

147 minty carrot

3 carrots

1 apple

1 stick celery

1 small bunch fresh mint

A creamy, orange-coloured juice that could almost be pure fruit, it's so sweet, but the celery gives it a different turn.

NUTRIENTS
Beta-carotene, folic acid, vitamin C; calcium, magnesium, manganese, phosphorus, potassium, sodium, sulphur

ENERGY	★★★☆☆
DETOX	★★★☆☆
IMMUNITY	★★★★☆
DIGESTION	★★☆☆☆
SKIN	★★★☆☆

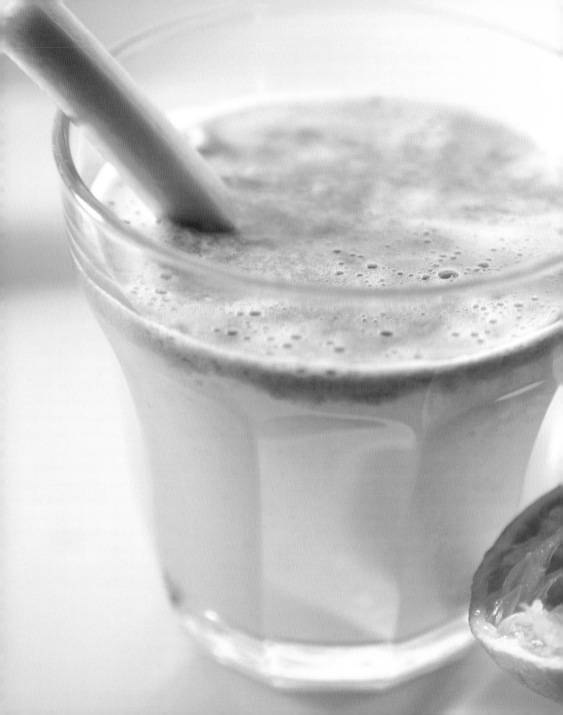

148 carrot salad

3 carrots

2 tomatoes

2 sticks celery

½ lime

A fantastic blend of vegetable juices – makes you wonder why you would ever buy juice in a carton.

NUTRIENTS

Beta-carotene, biotin, folic acid, vitamin C; calcium, magnesium, phosphorus, potassium, sodium, sulphur

ENERGY	★★★☆☆
DETOX	★★☆☆☆
IMMUNITY	★★★☆☆
DIGESTION	★☆☆☆☆
SKIN	★★★★☆

149 green hit

3 carrots

2 sticks celery

1 bunch watercress

1 large handful spinach

This is another very cleansing combination with earthy, grassy undertones.

NUTRIENTS
Beta-carotene, folic acid, vitamins B3, C and E; calcium, iron, magnesium, manganese, phosphorus, potassium, sodium, sulphur

ENERGY	★★☆☆☆
DETOX	★★★☆☆
IMMUNITY	★★★☆☆
DIGESTION	★☆☆☆☆
SKIN	★★★☆☆

150 carrot cooler

3 carrots

½ long cucumber

½ lime

Just the idea of cucumber is refreshing, let alone when you're drinking the juice, and it contrasts wonderfully well with the carrot.

NUTRIENTS
Beta-carotene, folic acid, vitamin C;
calcium, magnesium, phosphorus,
potassium, sodium, sulphur

ENERGY	★★★★☆
DETOX	★★★☆☆
IMMUNITY	★★★☆☆
DIGESTION	★☆☆☆☆
SKIN	★★★★☆

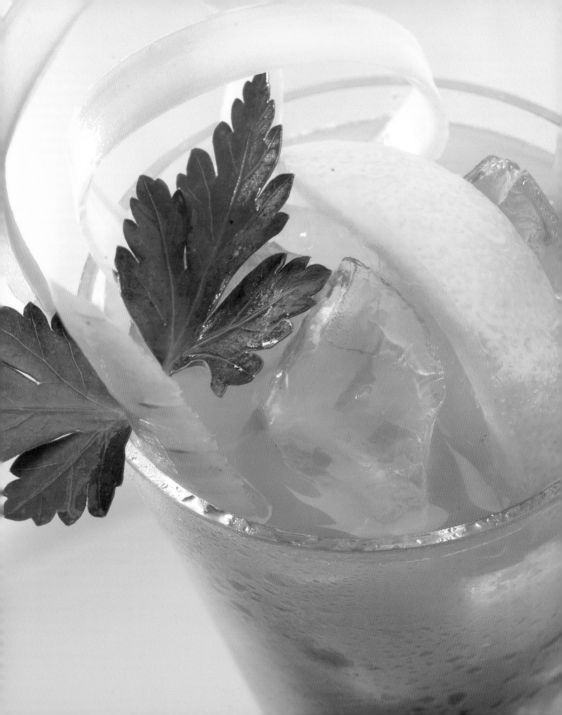

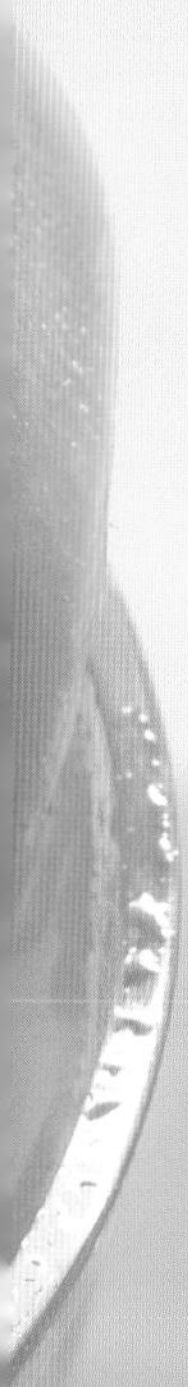

151 carrot lift

4 carrots

2 sticks celery

1 small bunch fresh parsley

½ lemon

A very refreshing combination – the creamy, sweet carrot is offset by the other ingredients.

NUTRIENTS
Beta-carotene, folic acid, vitamin B3, vitamin C; calcium, iron, magnesium, phosphorus, potassium, sodium, sulphur

ENERGY ★★★★☆
DETOX ★★★☆☆
IMMUNITY ★★★☆☆
DIGESTION ★★★☆☆
SKIN ★★★☆☆

152 bloody carrot

3 carrots

1 beet (beetroot)

2 sticks celery

½ lime

A doubly rooty mix of sweetness lifted by the celery and
lime – wonderfully cleansing and fortifying.

NUTRIENTS
Beta-carotene, folic acid, vitamin C;
calcium, magnesium, manganese,
phosphorus, potassium, sodium,
sulphur

ENERGY	★★★☆☆
DETOX	★★★★☆
IMMUNITY	★★★★☆
DIGESTION	★★☆☆☆
SKIN	★★★★☆

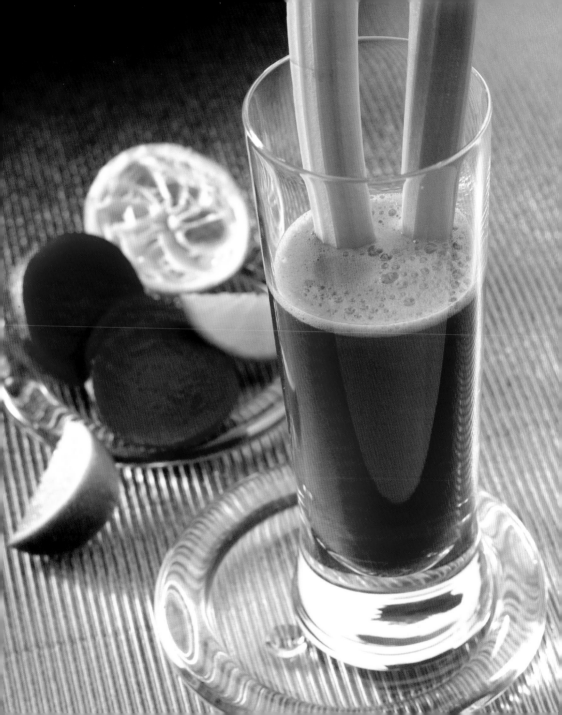

153 carrot tang

3 carrots

1 grapefruit

½ inch (1 cm) ginger root

I love the tang of the grapefruit tempered by the creamy carrot and then lifted by the zing of ginger – altogether an uplifting combination.

NUTRIENTS
Beta-carotene, folic acid, vitamin C; calcium, magnesium, phosphorus, potassium, sodium, sulphur

ENERGY ★★★★☆
DETOX ★★☆☆☆
IMMUNITY ★★★★☆
DIGESTION ★☆☆☆☆
SKIN ★★★☆☆

154 triple orange

3 carrots

1 orange

½ melon

If you use the orange-fleshed variety of melon, you get a threesome of orange, an explosion of tastes plus a powerful beta-carotene hit.

NUTRIENTS
Beta-carotene, folic acid, vitamin C; calcium, magnesium, phosphorus, potassium, sodium, sulphur

ENERGY	★★★★★
DETOX	★★☆☆☆
IMMUNITY	★★★★★
DIGESTION	★☆☆☆☆
SKIN	★★★★☆

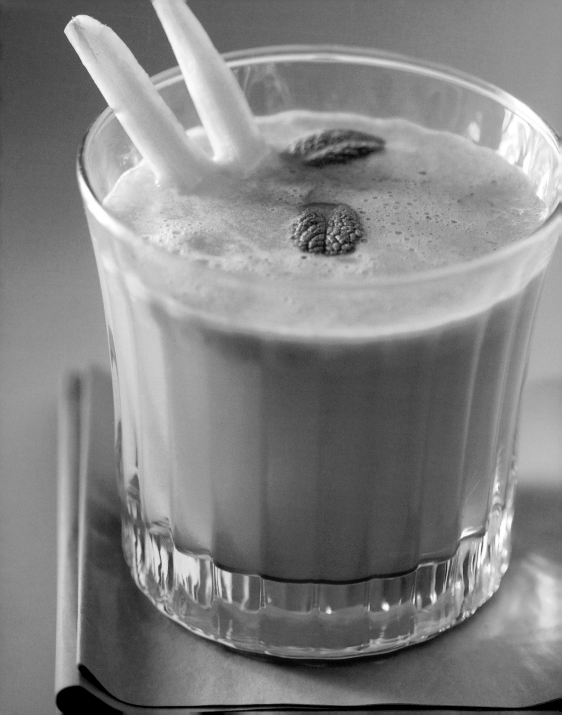

155 florida carrot

3 carrots

½ grapefruit

1 orange

1 small handful fresh mint leaves

The tang of the citrus complements the sweetness of the carrots perfectly.

NUTRIENTS
Beta-carotene, folic acid, vitamin C; calcium, magnesium, phosphorus, potassium, sodium, sulphur

ENERGY	★★★★☆
DETOX	★★☆☆☆
IMMUNITY	★★★★★
DIGESTION	★☆☆☆☆
SKIN	★★★☆☆

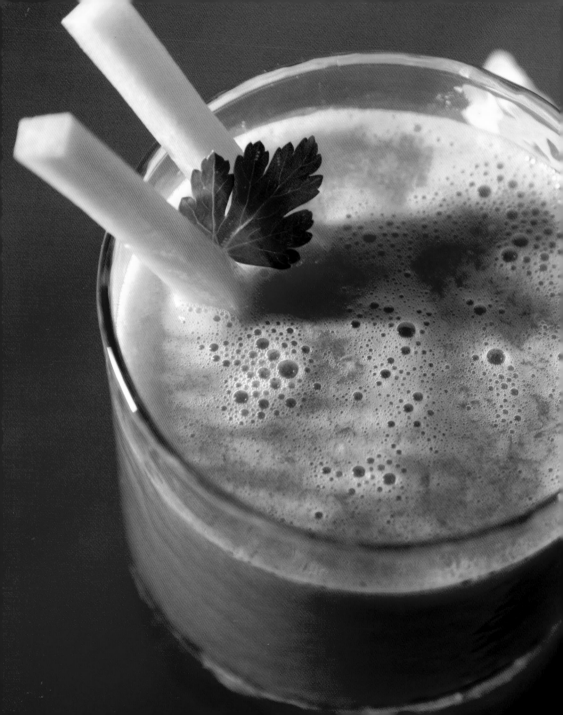

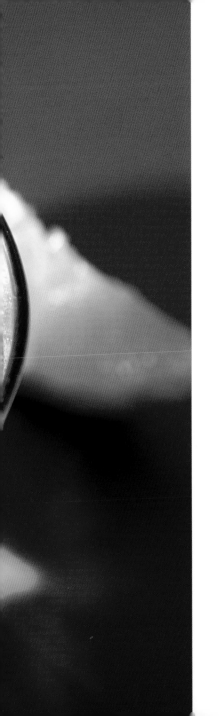

156 chlorophyll carrot

4 carrots

1 orange

1 bunch fresh parsley

A surprisingly good combination and the high chlorophyll content of the parsley is wonderfully cleansing.

NUTRIENTS

Beta-carotene, folic acid, vitamin B3, vitamin C; calcium, iron, magnesium, phosphorus, potassium, sodium, sulphur

ENERGY ★★★★☆
DETOX ★★★★☆
IMMUNITY ★★★★☆
DIGESTION ★☆☆☆☆
SKIN ★★★★☆

157 capple zing

4 carrots

1 apple

½ inch (1 cm) ginger root

½ lime

Uplifting and fresh on the palate. This is a wonderful morning combination – very refreshing to awaken your tastebuds for the day.

NUTRIENTS
Beta-carotene, folic acid, vitamin C; calcium, magnesium, phosphorus, potassium, sodium, sulphur

ENERGY	★★★☆☆
DETOX	★★☆☆☆
IMMUNITY	★★★☆☆
DIGESTION	★☆☆☆☆
SKIN	★★☆☆☆

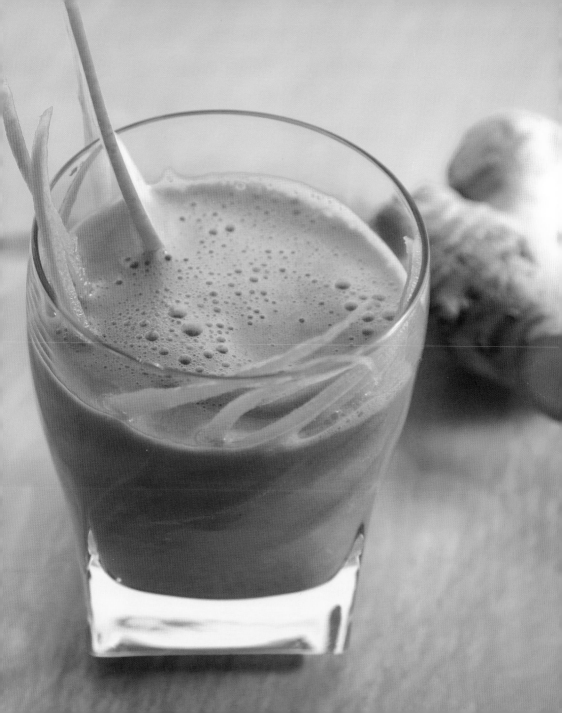

158　capple kiwi

3 carrots

1 apple

2 kiwi fruits

Kiwis can often be a bit soft to juice – choose firm ones and you'll get a delicious green juice. A crisp apple such as Discovery goes particularly well here.

NUTRIENTS
Beta-carotene, folic acid, vitamin C;
calcium, magnesium, phosphorus,
potassium, sodium, sulphur

ENERGY	★★★★★
DETOX	★★★☆☆
IMMUNITY	★★★★☆
DIGESTION	★★☆☆☆
SKIN	★★★★☆

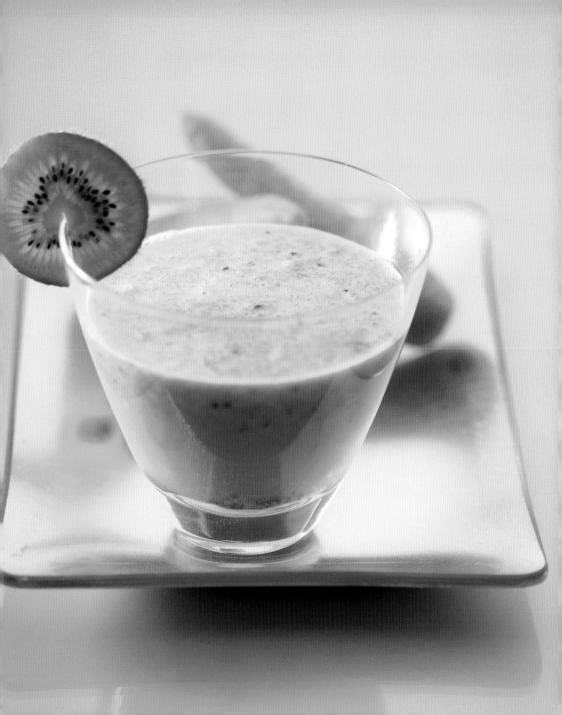

159 capple and black

4 carrots

1 apple

1 handful blackcurrants

The traditional favourite mix of apple and blackcurrant blended with creamy, sweet carrots makes a great combination.

NUTRIENTS
Beta-carotene, biotin, folic acid, vitamin C, vitamin E; calcium, magnesium, manganese, phosphorus, potassium, sodium, sulphur

ENERGY	★★★☆☆
DETOX	★★☆☆☆
IMMUNITY	★★★★☆
DIGESTION	★☆☆☆☆
SKIN	★★★☆☆

160   carrot jointaid

3 carrots

½ pineapple

1 inch (2.5 cm) ginger root

1 tablespoon (15 ml) flaxseed (linseed) oil

A fine marriage of antioxidants and essential fats to help soothe joints, plus pineapple and ginger which have been shown to be anti-inflammatory and are good for problems such as asthma.

NUTRIENTS		
Beta-carotene, folic acid, vitamin C;	ENERGY	★★★☆☆
calcium, magnesium, manganese,	DETOX	★★★☆☆
phosphorus, potassium, sodium,	IMMUNITY	★★★☆☆
	DIGESTION	★★★☆☆
sulphur; essential fatty acids	SKIN	★★☆☆☆

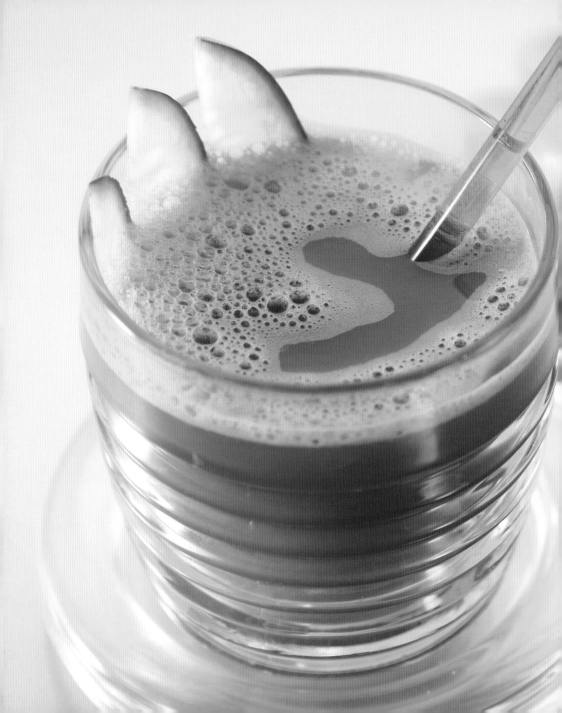

161 cool 'n' creamy

1 cucumber

4 carrots

Each of these juices brings out the best in the other.
You'll be surprised at just how much flavour you
can extract from a cucumber by juicing it, and how
delicious it is.

NUTRIENTS
Beta-carotene, folic acid, vitamin C;
calcium, magnesium, phosphorus,
potassium, sodium, sulphur

ENERGY	★★☆☆☆
DETOX	★★★☆☆
IMMUNITY	★★☆☆☆
DIGESTION	★☆☆☆☆
SKIN	★★☆☆☆

162 cool 'n' pale

1 cucumber

2 apples

A dreamy shade of green, with a taste to match – this refreshing combination of two highly juicy ingredients is very cleansing on the palate.

NUTRIENTS
Beta-carotene, folic acid,
vitamin C; calcium, magnesium,
phosphorus, potassium, sulphur

ENERGY	★★★☆☆
DETOX	★★★★☆
IMMUNITY	★★☆☆☆
DIGESTION	★★★☆☆
SKIN	★★★☆☆

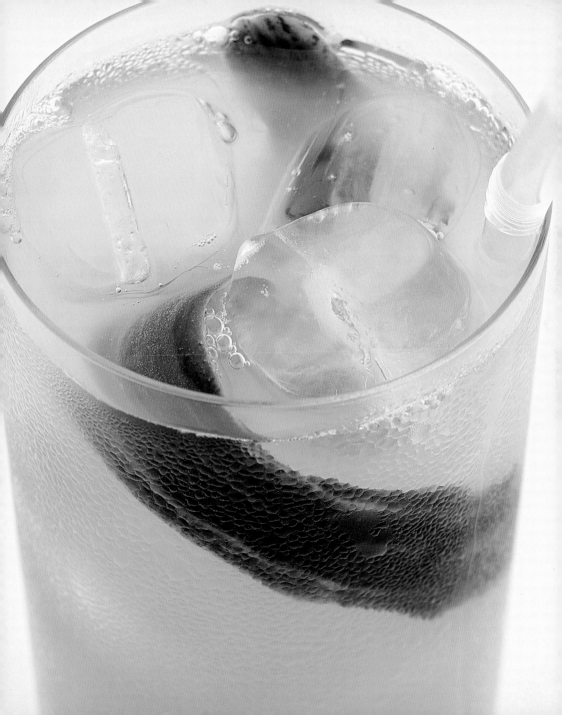

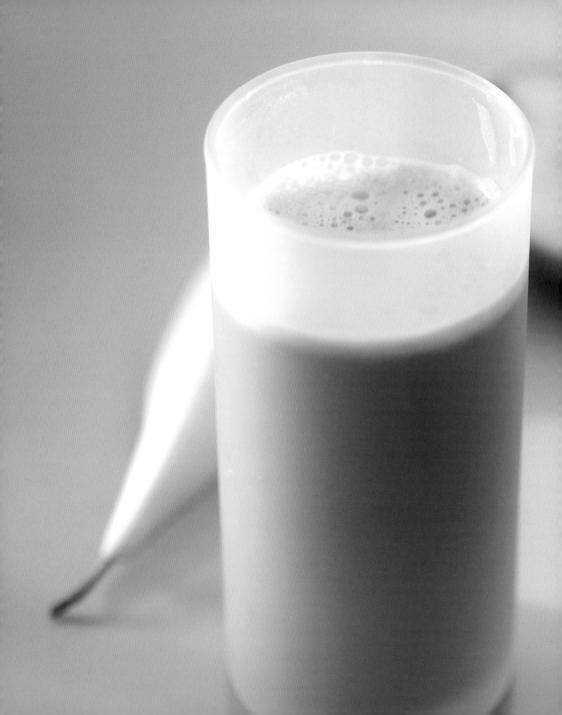

163 cucumber refresher

1 cucumber

2 pears

Another delicate mix of pale green with two subtly flavoured ingredients blending to form a refreshing, cleansing juice.

NUTRIENTS
Beta-carotene, folic acid, vitamin C; calcium, magnesium, phosphorus, potassium, sulphur

ENERGY	★★★☆☆
DETOX	★★★★☆
IMMUNITY	★★☆☆☆
DIGESTION	★★★☆☆
SKIN	★★★☆☆

164 apple cooler

1 cucumber

2 apples

4 sprigs fresh mint

½ inch (1 cm) ginger root

A wonderful summer drink. You could even add a splash of ginger ale or fizzy mineral water for a non-alcoholic cocktail.

NUTRIENTS
Beta-carotene, folic acid, vitamin C;
calcium, magnesium, phosphorus,
potassium, sulphur

ENERGY	★★★☆☆
DETOX	★★★★☆
IMMUNITY	★★☆☆☆
DIGESTION	★★★☆☆
SKIN	★★★☆☆

165　mellow melon

¾ cucumber

½ melon

1 pear

2 sprigs fresh mint

From the same family, cucumber and melon combine beautifully.
You can leave out the mint if you prefer.

NUTRIENTS
Beta-carotene, folic acid, vitamin C;
calcium, magnesium, phosphorus,
potassium, sodium, sulphur

ENERGY	★★★★☆
DETOX	★★★★☆
IMMUNITY	★★★☆☆
DIGESTION	★★★☆☆
SKIN	★★★☆☆

166 water, water everywhere

1 cucumber

1 thick slice watermelon

Two of the juiciest of nature's pickings blend to create a rich but subtle flavour. A perfect summer thirst-quencher.

NUTRIENTS
Beta-carotene, folic acid, vitamin B5, vitamin C; calcium, magnesium, phosphorus, potassium, sodium

ENERGY	★★★★☆
DETOX	★★★★☆
IMMUNITY	★★★★☆
DIGESTION	★★☆☆☆
SKIN	★★★☆☆

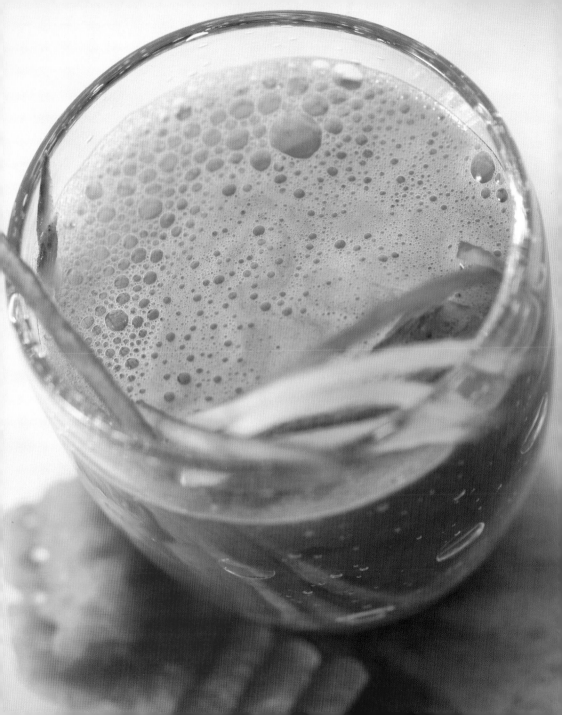

167   citrus cuke

1 cucumber

1 orange

1 grapefruit

Although the actual flavour of the cucumber gets a bit lost, its watery freshness transforms the orange and grapefruit to a more refreshing drink.

NUTRIENTS
Beta-carotene, folic acid, vitamin C; calcium, magnesium, phosphorus, potassium, sulphur

ENERGY	★★★★☆
DETOX	★★☆☆☆
IMMUNITY	★★★★☆
DIGESTION	☆☆☆☆☆
SKIN	★★★☆☆

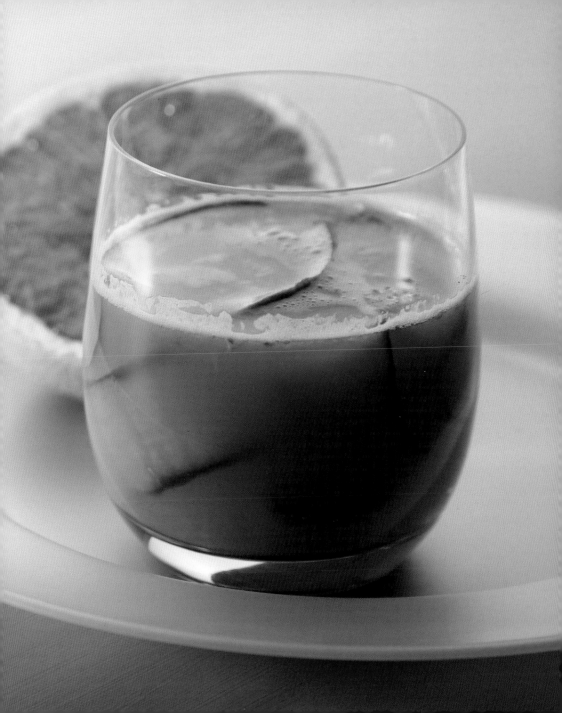

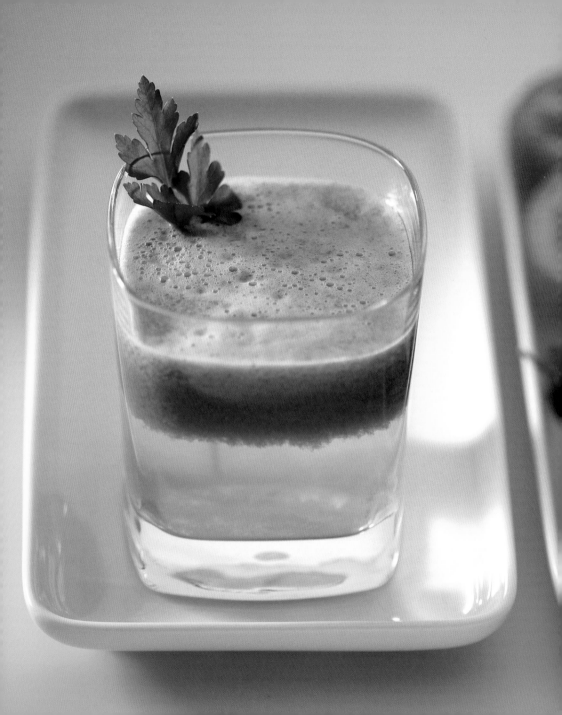

168 salad cooler

1 cucumber

3 tomatoes

1 small bunch fresh parsley

½ lemon

A great veggie cocktail which always reminds me of a fresh, tasty Middle Eastern salad.

NUTRIENTS

Beta-carotene, biotin, folic acid, vitamin B3, vitamin C; calcium, iron, magnesium, phosphorus, potassium, sodium, sulphur

ENERGY	★★☆☆☆
DETOX	★★★★☆
IMMUNITY	★★★☆☆
DIGESTION	★☆☆☆☆
SKIN	★★★★☆

169 tropical cucumber

1 cucumber

2 guavas

1 apple

The rich, tangy, tropical taste of guavas is toned down by the cucumber to form an unusual, cooling juice.

NUTRIENTS		
Beta-carotene, folic acid, vitamin B3,	ENERGY	★★★★☆
vitamin C; calcium, magnesium,	DETOX	★★★★☆
	IMMUNITY	★★★★☆
phosphorus, potassium, sodium,	DIGESTION	★★☆☆☆
sulphur	SKIN	★★★★☆

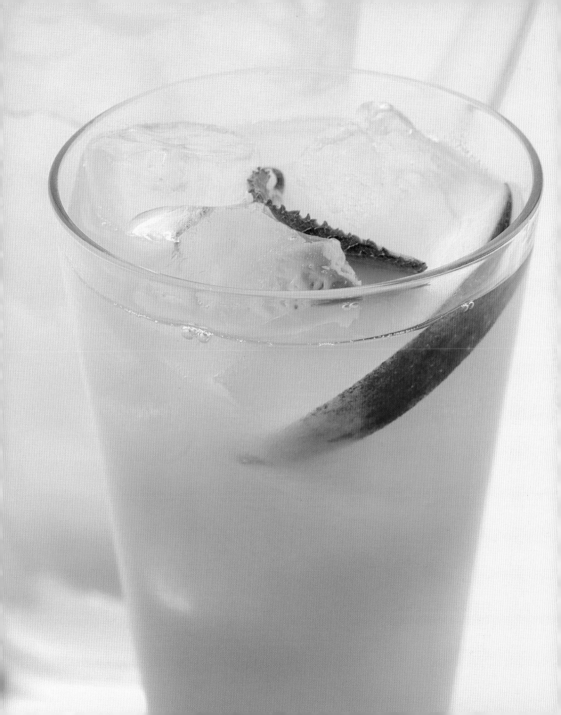

170 bloody cuke

1 cucumber

2 apples

1 beet (beetroot)

The richness of the beet is perfectly tempered by the cucumber and sweetened by the apple in this colourful magenta juice.

NUTRIENTS
Beta-carotene, folic acid, vitamin C; calcium, magnesium, phosphorus, potassium, sodium, sulphur

ENERGY	★★★☆☆
DETOX	★★★★★
IMMUNITY	★★★☆☆
DIGESTION	★★★★☆
SKIN	★★★★☆

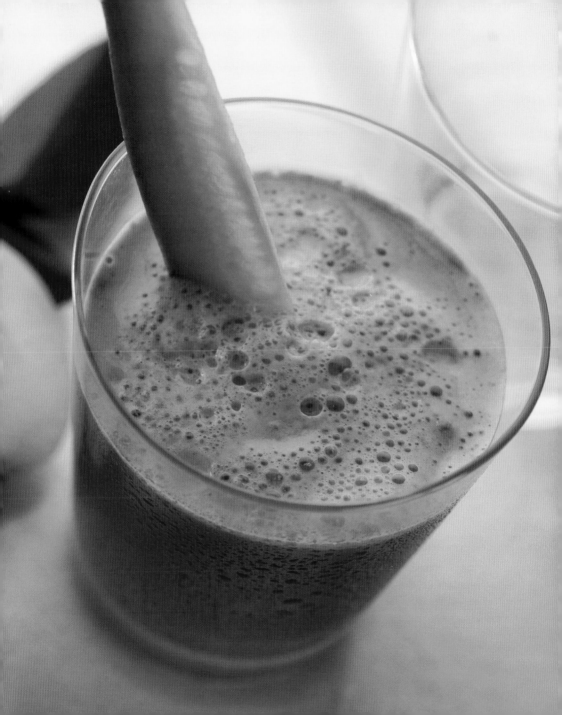

171 clear green

1 cucumber

1 apple

1 stick celery

1 lime

This delicate-coloured juice is a wonderfully refreshing palate-cleanser.

NUTRIENTS
Beta-carotene, folic acid, vitamin C;
calcium, magnesium, phosphorus,
potassium, sodium, sulphur

ENERGY	★★☆☆☆
DETOX	★★☆☆☆
IMMUNITY	★★☆☆☆
DIGESTION	☆☆☆☆☆
SKIN	★★☆☆☆

172 red cucumber

1 cucumber

1 beet (beetroot)

½ pineapple

The watery, light cucumber blends well with the rich, earthy beetroot in this nutritious juice.

NUTRIENTS
Beta-carotene, folic acid, vitamin C;
calcium, magnesium, phosphorus,
potassium, sodium, sulphur

ENERGY ★★☆☆☆
DETOX ★★★☆☆
IMMUNITY ★☆☆☆☆
DIGESTION ★★★★☆
SKIN ★★☆☆☆

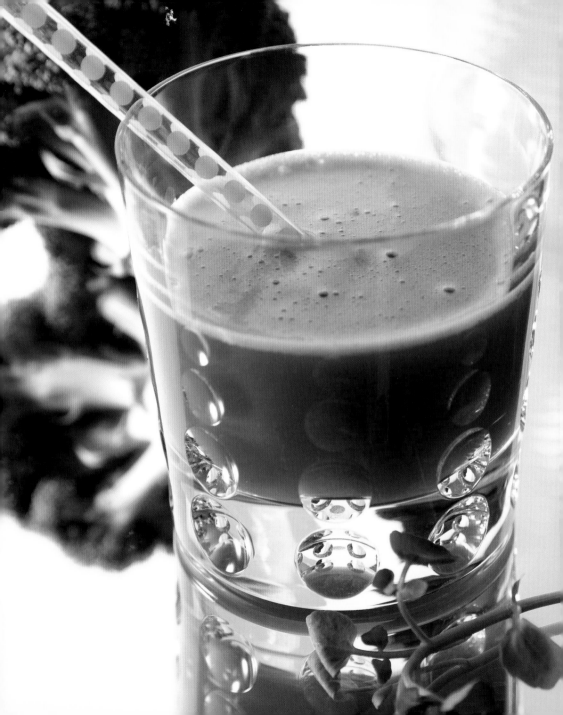

173 green goddess

1 bunch fresh parsley

1 handful watercress

4 broccoli spears

½ pineapple

There had to be one juice with this name and this is it – anything with pineapple is good in my book.

NUTRIENTS
Beta-carotene, folic acid, vitamins B3, B5, C and E; calcium, iron, magnesium, phosphorus, potassium, sodium, sulphur

ENERGY	★★★☆☆
DETOX	★★★★★
IMMUNITY	★★☆☆☆
DIGESTION	★★★★☆
SKIN	★★★★☆

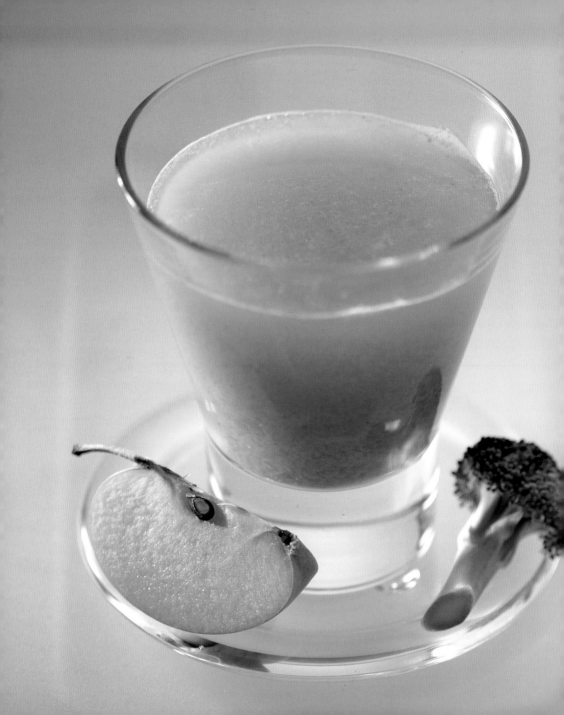

174 green apple

8 broccoli spears

1 bunch fresh parsley

3 apples

To counteract the strong-tasting green vegetables, it's best to use an apple variety with a powerful flavour, such as Granny Smith, for this one.

NUTRIENTS
Beta-carotene, folic acid, vitamins B3, B5 and C; calcium, iron, magnesium, phosphorus, potassium, sodium, sulphur

ENERGY	★★☆☆☆
DETOX	★★★★★
IMMUNITY	★★★★☆
DIGESTION	★★★★☆
SKIN	★★★★☆

175 green 'n' pear it

8 broccoli spears

3 sticks celery

2 pears

You may not wish to adulterate your pear with broccoli juice, but believe me, it's a surprising winner.

NUTRIENTS
Beta-carotene, folic acid, vitamin B5, vitamin C; calcium, magnesium, phosphorus, potassium, sodium, sulphur

ENERGY ★★★☆☆
DETOX ★★★★★
IMMUNITY ★★★★☆
DIGESTION ★★★★☆
SKIN ★★★★☆

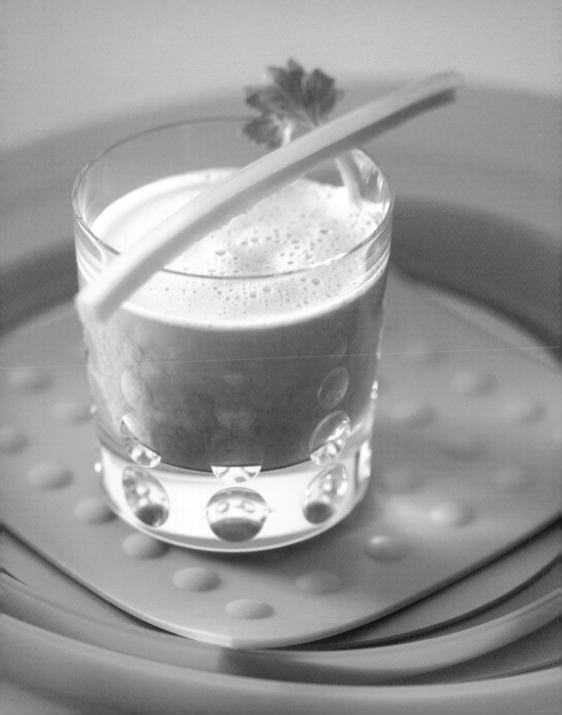

176 green citrus

2 handfuls spinach

2 sticks celery

2 oranges

Fresh orange juice is so flavourful that it can carry
pretty much anything, even the powerful taste of
iron-rich spinach.

NUTRIENTS
Beta-carotene, folic acid, vitamin B3,
vitamin C; calcium, iron, magnesium,
phosphorus, potassium, sodium,
sulphur

ENERGY	★★★☆☆
DETOX	★★★☆☆
IMMUNITY	★★★★☆
DIGESTION	★☆☆☆☆
SKIN	★★★☆☆

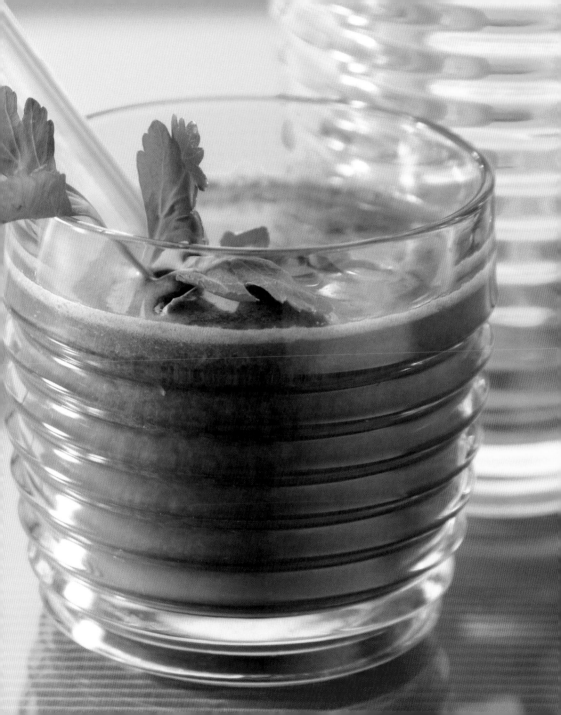

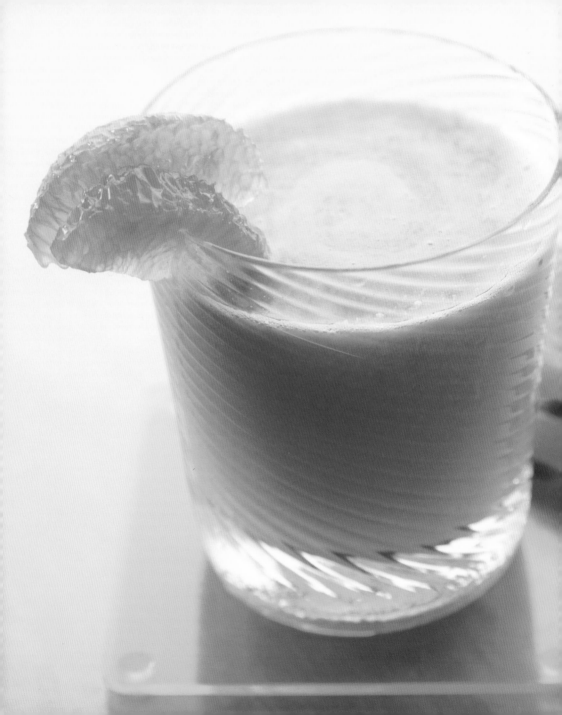

177 green grapefruit

8 broccoli spears

2 grapefruits

If anything is going to temper the strong, earthy taste of broccoli juice and make it more palatable, it's going to be grapefruit.

NUTRIENTS

Beta-carotene, folic acid, vitamin B5, vitamin C; calcium, magnesium, phosphorus, potassium, sodium, sulphur

ENERGY	★★★☆☆
DETOX	★★★★★
IMMUNITY	★★★★☆
DIGESTION	★☆☆☆☆
SKIN	★★★★☆

178 green waldorf

5 large kale leaves

2 apples

2 sticks celery

1 tablespoon (15 ml) flaxseed (linseed) oil

Well, not quite a Waldorf, but it tastes good and is super-healthy. The flaxseed brings an unusual dimension in taste, texture and health properties to this cleansing juice.

NUTRIENTS
Beta-carotene, folic acid, vitamin B3, vitamin C; calcium, iron, magnesium, manganese, phosphorus, potassium, sodium, sulphur

ENERGY	★★★☆☆
DETOX	★★★★☆
IMMUNITY	★★★☆☆
DIGESTION	★★★★☆
SKIN	★★★★☆

179 sweet green melon

1 bunch fresh parsley

¼ white cabbage

½ long cucumber

½ melon

The green in this doesn't just belong to the melon – it's a cleansing
punch, tempered by cucumber.

NUTRIENTS

Beta-carotene, folic acid, vitamins B3,
C and E; calcium, iron, magnesium,
phosphorus, potassium, sodium,
sulphur

ENERGY	★★★☆☆
DETOX	★★★★☆
IMMUNITY	★★★☆☆
DIGESTION	★★★★★
SKIN	★★★★☆

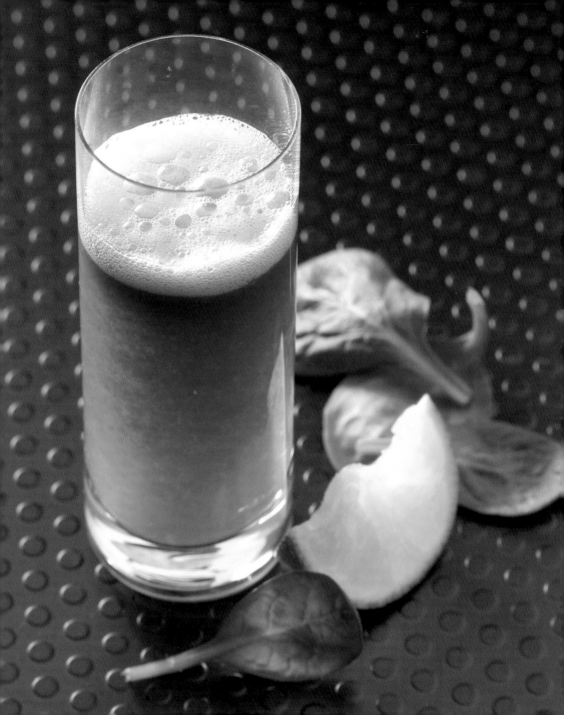

180 green lullaby

½ lettuce

2 apples

½ lime

1 small handful spinach

Lettuce contains substances which act as mild sedatives, so this one should help send you into the land of nod.

NUTRIENTS
Beta-carotene, folic acid, vitamin B3, vitamin C; calcium, iron, magnesium, phosphorus, potassium, sodium, sulphur

ENERGY	★☆☆☆☆
DETOX	★★★☆☆
IMMUNITY	★★★☆☆
DIGESTION	☆☆☆☆☆
SKIN	★★☆☆☆

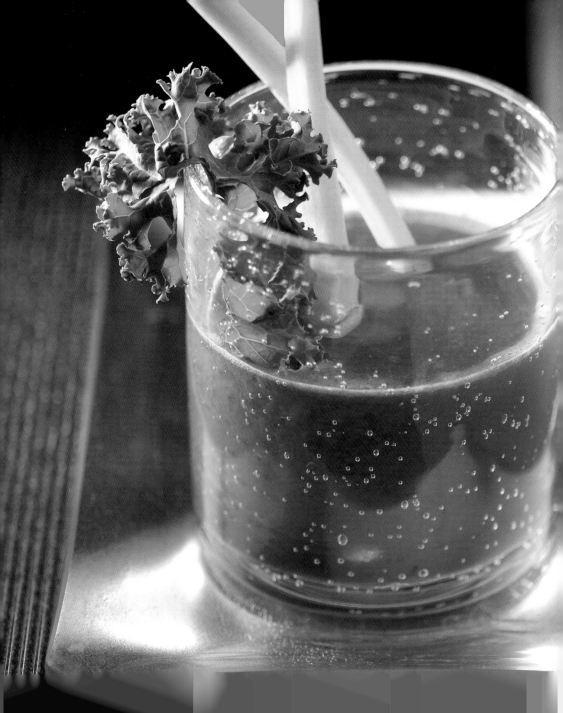

181 super defender

5 large kale leaves

3 carrots

1 orange

Kale, orange and carrot — muddy to look at, magnificent to taste.

NUTRIENTS
Beta-carotene, folic acid, vitamin B3, vitamin C; calcium, iron, magnesium, manganese, phosphorus, potassium, sodium, sulphur

ENERGY	★★★☆☆
DETOX	★★★★☆
IMMUNITY	★★★★★
DIGESTION	☆☆☆☆☆
SKIN	★★★★☆

182 grape & green

4 large kale leaves

2 handfuls spinach

2 sticks celery

1 grapefruit

The tangy grapefruit and salty celery cut right through the earthy taste of the greens in this rejuvenating juice.

NUTRIENTS
Beta-carotene, folic acid, vitamin C; calcium, magnesium, manganese, phosphorus, potassium, sodium, sulphur

ENERGY ★★☆☆☆
DETOX ★★★★☆
IMMUNITY ★★★★☆
DIGESTION ★★☆☆☆
SKIN ★★★★☆

183 creamy green

1 bunch fresh parsley

1 handful watercress

4 carrots

1 lime

The sweet, creamy carrot juice carries the greens very well, and the lime gives it a good, sharp kick.

NUTRIENTS
Beta-carotene, folic acid, vitamins B3, C and E; calcium, iron, magnesium, phosphorus, potassium, sodium, sulphur

ENERGY	★★★☆☆
DETOX	★★★★★
IMMUNITY	★★★★★
DIGESTION	★★★☆☆
SKIN	★★★★☆

184 red & green

1 bunch fresh parsley

1 lemon

5 tomatoes

This is a fantastically cleansing juice, and another one with Middle Eastern salad undertones.

NUTRIENTS
Beta-carotene, biotin, folic acid,
vitamin B3, vitamin C; calcium, iron,
magnesium, phosphorus, potassium,
sodium, sulphur

ENERGY ★★★☆☆
DETOX ★★★★☆
IMMUNITY ★★★★☆
DIGESTION ★☆☆☆☆
SKIN ★★★★☆

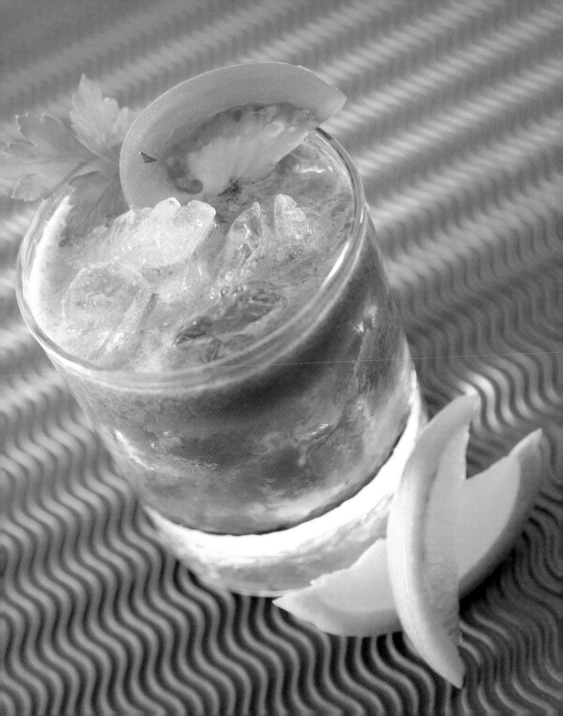

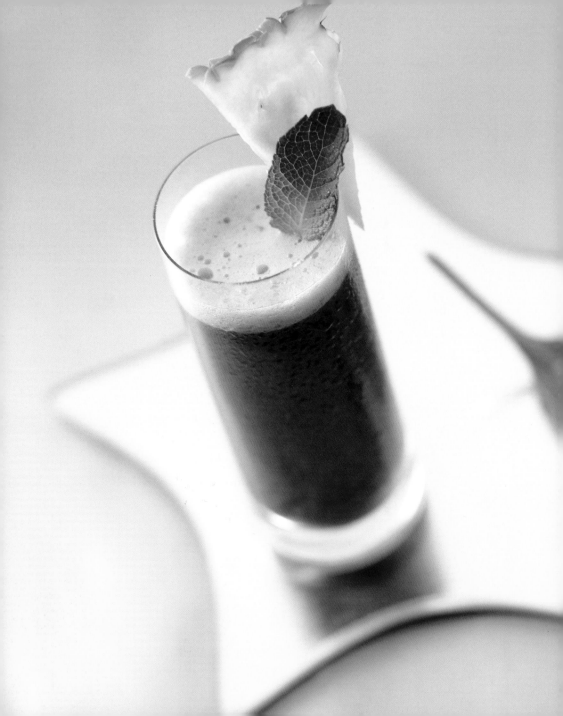

185 green piney hit

1 large handful spinach

1 large handful fresh parsley

1 large handful fresh mint leaves

½ pineapple

Although this is seriously green, the fresh parsley, mint and, of course, the pineapple make it less earthy than it could be.

NUTRIENTS
Beta-carotene, folic acid, vitamin B3, vitamin C; calcium, iron, magnesium, phosphorus, potassium, sodium

ENERGY	★★☆☆☆
DETOX	★★★★★
IMMUNITY	★★★☆☆
DIGESTION	★★★★☆
SKIN	★★★★☆

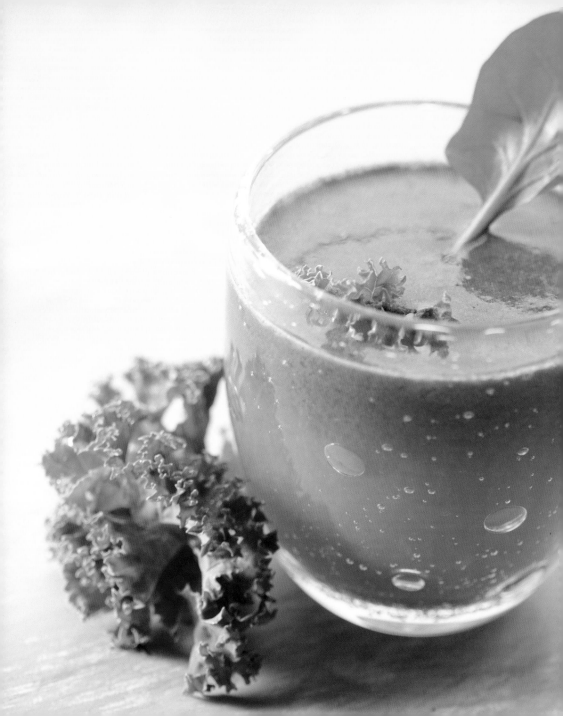

186   eye opener

1 handful kale

1 large handful spinach

1 carrot

1 grapefruit

This is a serious hit of carotene, essential for eye health and immunity.

NUTRIENTS
Beta-carotene, folic acid, vitamin B3, vitamin C; calcium, iron, magnesium, phosphorus, potassium, sodium, sulphur

ENERGY   ★★☆☆☆
DETOX   ★★★★☆
IMMUNITY   ★★★★★
DIGESTION   ★☆☆☆☆
SKIN   ★★★★☆

187 beet basic

2 beets (beetroot)

2 carrots

1 apple

1 orange

1 stick celery

½ inch (1 cm) ginger root

If I have beets in the refrigerator, this is one of my standard morning juices. It's a supreme energy-lifting, cleansing and immunity-boosting blend.

NUTRIENTS
Beta-carotene, folic acid, vitamin C; calcium, magnesium, phosphorus, potassium, sodium, sulphur

ENERGY	★★★★☆
DETOX	★★★★☆
IMMUNITY	★★★★☆
DIGESTION	★★★☆☆
SKIN	★★★★☆

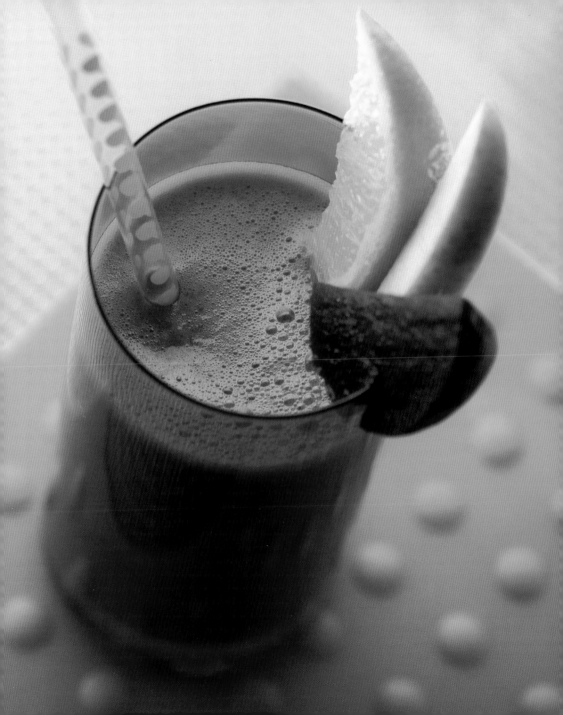

188 beetles

2 beets (beetroot)

2 apples

3 sticks celery

Another great combination of beet and fruit, enhanced by the celery.

NUTRIENTS
Beta-carotene, folic acid, vitamin C;
calcium, magnesium, phosphorus,
potassium, sodium, sulphur

ENERGY	★★★★☆
DETOX	★★★★★
IMMUNITY	★★★☆☆
DIGESTION	★★★☆☆
SKIN	★★★★☆

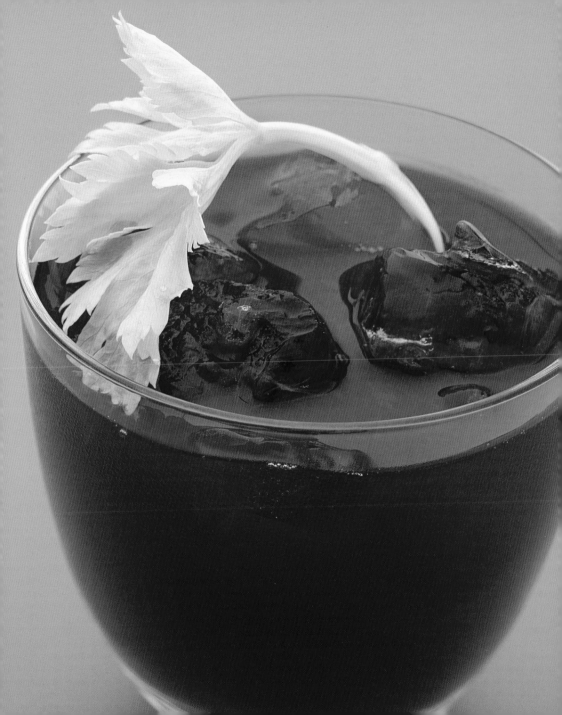

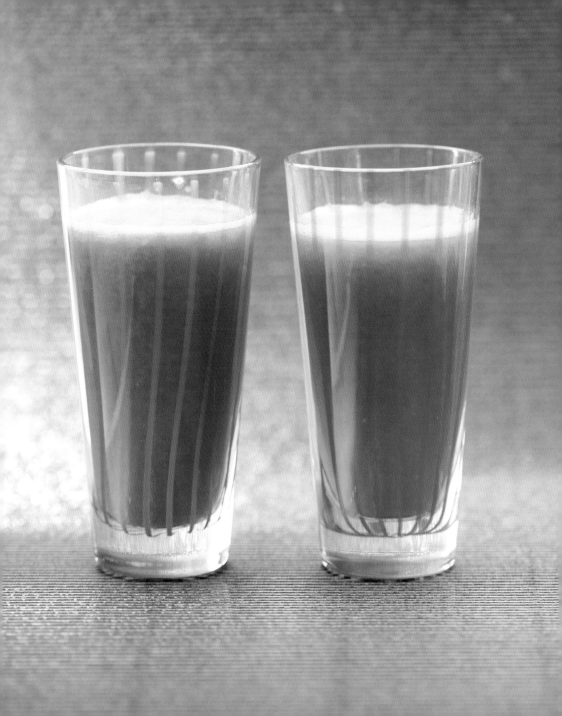

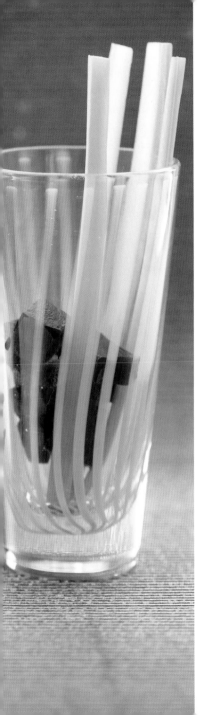

189 blood 'n' grape

2 beets (beetroot)

1 grapefruit

2 sticks celery

Grapefruit carries that earthy, sweet beet well and both are lifted by the salty celery – a convincing introduction to beet, if you need one.

NUTRIENTS
Beta-carotene, folic acid, vitamin C; calcium, magnesium, phosphorus, potassium, sodium, sulphur

ENERGY	★★★★☆
DETOX	★★★★☆
IMMUNITY	★★★★☆
DIGESTION	★★☆☆☆
SKIN	★★★★☆

190 blood & carrots

2 beets (beetroot)

2 oranges (ideally blood oranges)

4 carrots

Blood oranges or not, this sumptuous juice is going to be a rich, purple colour, swirling with the creamy orange from the carrots.

NUTRIENTS
Beta-carotene, folic acid, vitamin C; calcium, magnesium, phosphorus, potassium, sodium, sulphur

ENERGY ★★★★☆
DETOX ★★★☆☆
IMMUNITY ★★★★★
DIGESTION ★★☆☆☆
SKIN ★★★★☆

191 rooty pear

3 parsnips

3 pears

1 lime

A blend of very delicate, sweet flavours, sharpened by the lime.

NUTRIENTS
Beta-carotene, folic acid, vitamin C;
calcium, magnesium, phosphorus,
potassium, sodium, sulphur

ENERGY	★★★★☆
DETOX	★★☆☆☆
IMMUNITY	★★★☆☆
DIGESTION	★☆☆☆☆
SKIN	★★☆☆☆

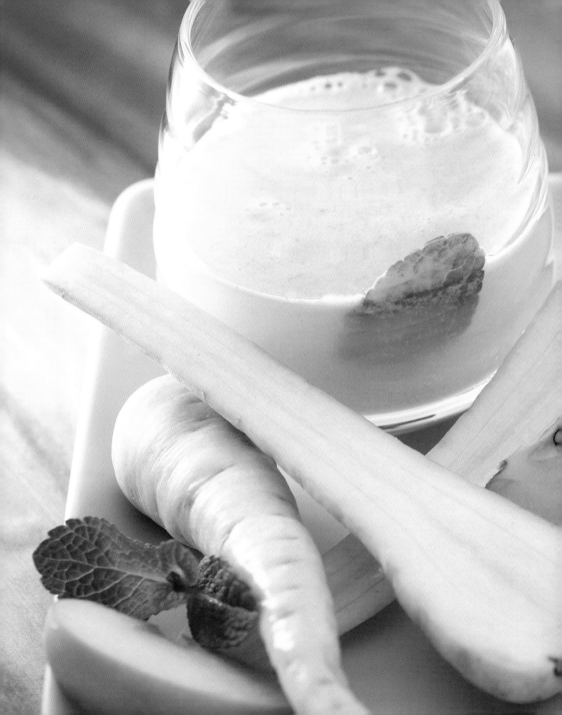

192 apples & neeps

3 parsnips

3 apples

½ lime

3 sprigs fresh mint

If you're at all hesitant to try root vegetable juice, this is a good one to start with. Add more lime if you want to give it more tang.

NUTRIENTS
Beta-carotene, folic acid, vitamin C; calcium, magnesium, phosphorus, potassium, sodium, sulphur

ENERGY	★★★★☆
DETOX	★★★☆☆
IMMUNITY	★★★☆☆
DIGESTION	★★☆☆☆
SKIN	★★☆☆☆

193 carotene kick

1 sweet potato

½ melon

3 carrots

Sweet potatoes are a delicious, rich source of carotene, as are the other ingredients in this vibrant orange drink.

NUTRIENTS
Beta-carotene, folic acid, vitamin C, vitamin E; calcium, magnesium, phosphorus, potassium, sodium, sulphur

ENERGY	★★★★★
DETOX	★★★☆☆
IMMUNITY	★★★★★
DIGESTION	★★★☆☆
SKIN	★★★★★

194 pineroot

1 sweet potato

1 carrot

½ pineapple

The root vegetables tone down the tangy pineapple for a sweet drink.

NUTRIENTS		
Beta-carotene, folic acid, vitamin C,	ENERGY	★★★★★
vitamin E; calcium, magnesium,	DETOX	★★★☆☆
manganese, phosphorus, potassium,	IMMUNITY	★★★★★
sodium, sulphur	DIGESTION	★★★★★
	SKIN	★★★★☆

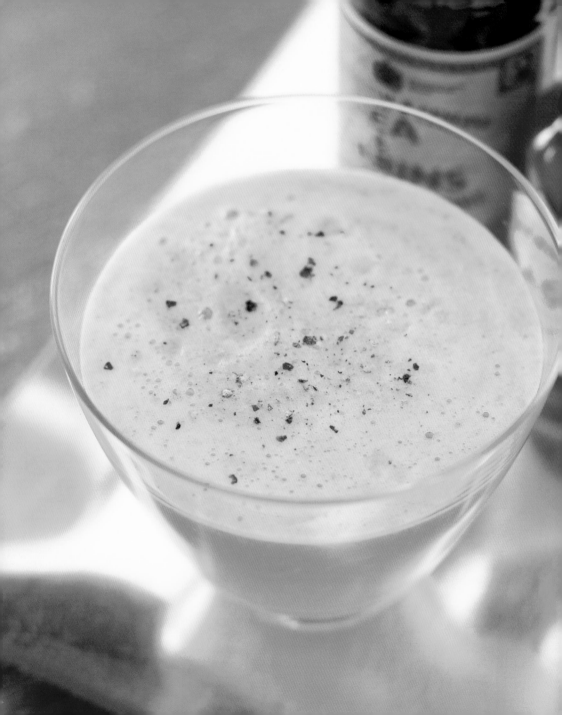

195 pure tomato

8 tomatoes

salt, pepper, Tabasco and
Worcestershire sauce to taste

One of the few vegetable juices that is
wonderful unadulterated. You can always
add a squeeze of lemon juice if you're not
into the pure stuff.

NUTRIENTS
Beta-carotene, biotin, folic acid,
vitamin C; calcium, magnesium,
phosphorus, potassium, sodium,
sulphur

ENERGY	★★★★☆
DETOX	★★☆☆☆
IMMUNITY	★★★★☆
DIGESTION	☆☆☆☆☆
SKIN	★★★★☆

196 ginger tom

6 tomatoes

2 sticks celery

1 inch (2.5 cm) ginger root

Celery is probably my favourite juice to combine with tomatoes – the light saltiness taking the edge off the richer tomato and the ginger in this one gives it all a sharp lift. You can be even more daring with the amount of ginger you use if you like.

NUTRIENTS
Beta-carotene, biotin, folic acid,
vitamin C; calcium, magnesium,
manganese, phosphorus, potassium,
sodium, sulphur

ENERGY	★★★★☆
DETOX	★★☆☆☆
IMMUNITY	★★★★☆
DIGESTION	★☆☆☆☆
SKIN	★★★★☆

197   tabouleh

6 tomatoes

1 large bunch fresh parsley

1 lemon

salt and pepper to taste

If you are a fan of tomato and parsley salad or tabouleh, you'll love this one.

NUTRIENTS
Beta-carotene, biotin, folic acid, vitamin B3, vitamin C; calcium, iron, magnesium, phosphorus, potassium, sodium, sulphur

ENERGY	★★★☆☆
DETOX	★★★☆☆
IMMUNITY	★★★★☆
DIGESTION	★☆☆☆☆
SKIN	★★★★☆

198 tomato bell

6 tomatoes

2 bell peppers

1 stick celery

½ lemon

salt, pepper, Tabasco and Worcestershire sauce to taste

I'd use only red or yellow peppers for this as the green ones tend to take over the other flavours. Season it well once you've made the juice, sit back and sip it slowly, nibbling from a bowl of potato chips, nuts and olives.

NUTRIENTS
Beta-carotene, biotin, folic acid, vitamin B3, vitamin C; calcium, iron, magnesium, phosphorus, potassium, sodium, sulphur

ENERGY	★★★★☆
DETOX	★★☆☆☆
IMMUNITY	★★★★☆
DIGESTION	☆☆☆☆☆
SKIN	★★★☆☆

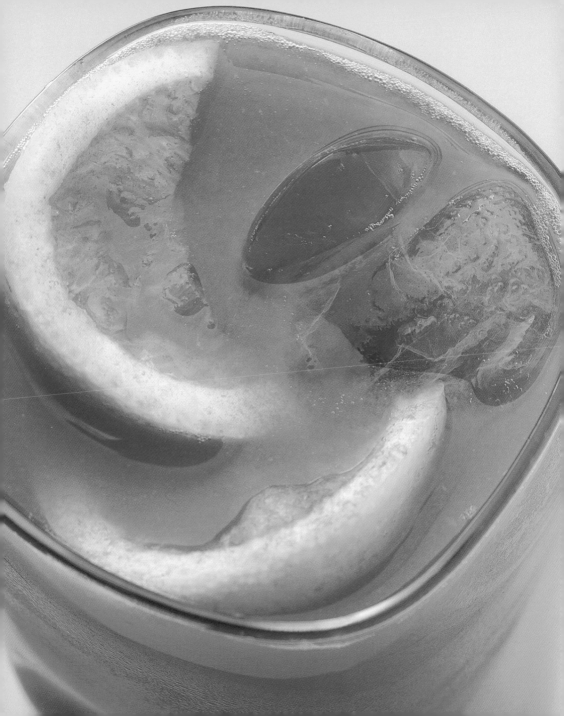

199 peppery tom

6 tomatoes

1 large bunch watercress

1 stick celery

The watercress in this acts as a seasoning all by itself,
and the celery lightens the rich taste of the tomatoes.

NUTRIENTS
Beta-carotene, biotin, folic acid,
vitamin C, vitamin E; calcium, iron,
magnesium, phosphorus, potassium,
sodium, sulphur

ENERGY	★★★★☆
DETOX	★★★★☆
IMMUNITY	★★★★☆
DIGESTION	★☆☆☆☆
SKIN	★★★★☆

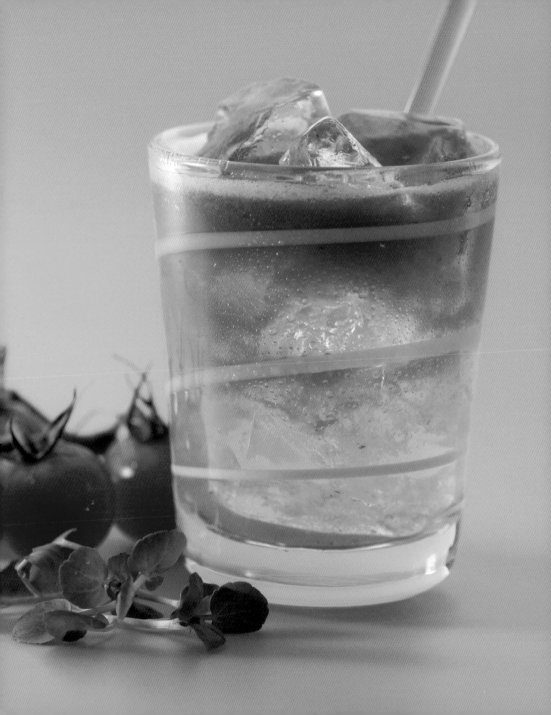

200 sweet 'n' fresh

6 tomatoes

1 red bell pepper

1 stick celery

1 large bunch fresh parsley

The wonderful sweetness of the tomatoes and peppers is heightened by the salty celery and freshened further by the parsley.

NUTRIENTS
Beta-carotene, biotin, folic acid,
vitamin B3, vitamin C; calcium, iron,
magnesium, manganese, phosphorus,
potassium, sodium, sulphur

ENERGY	★★★★☆
DETOX	★★★☆☆
IMMUNITY	★★★★☆
DIGESTION	★☆☆☆☆
SKIN	★★★★☆

201 classic combo

6 tomatoes

3 carrots

1 lime

1 small bunch fresh mint

The two most popular and palatable of the vegetable juices combined
with a lift from the mint and lime.

NUTRIENTS
Beta-carotene, biotin, folic acid,
vitamin C; calcium, magnesium,
phosphorus, potassium, sodium,
sulphur

ENERGY	★★★★☆
DETOX	★★★☆☆
IMMUNITY	★★★★☆
DIGESTION	★☆☆☆☆
SKIN	★★★★☆

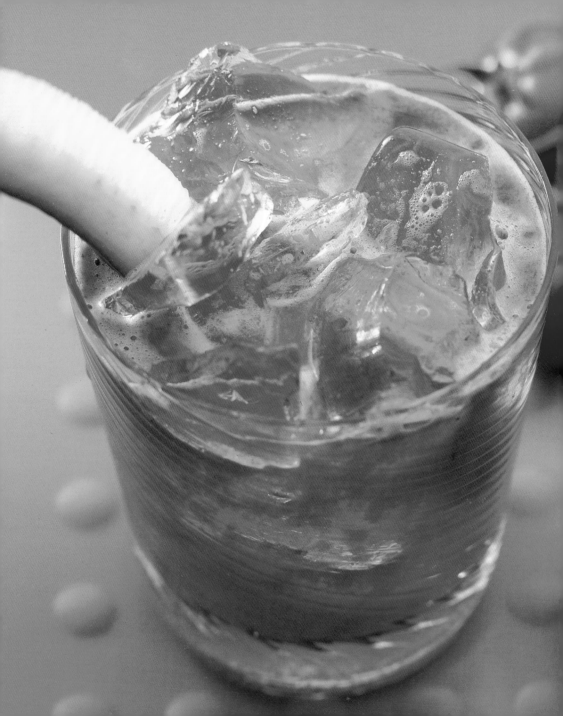

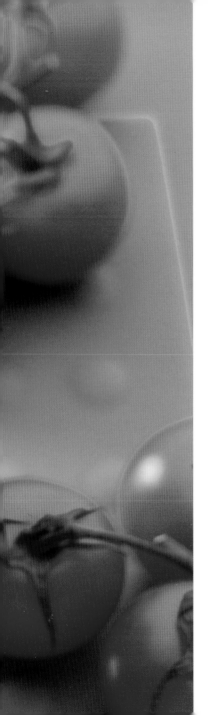

202 green tomatoes

4 tomatoes

½ long cucumber

1 large handful spinach leaves

4 broccoli spears

Not fried like at the Whistlestop Café, but blended with greens for a deep-cleansing juice. The earthy, green taste of the spinach and broccoli is nicely hidden by the other ingredients.

NUTRIENTS

Beta-carotene, biotin, folic acid, vitamin B3, vitamin C; calcium, iron, magnesium, phosphorus, potassium, sodium, sulphur

ENERGY	★★★☆☆
DETOX	★★★★☆
IMMUNITY	★★★☆☆
DIGESTION	☆☆☆☆☆
SKIN	★★☆☆☆

203 root tomato

4 tomatoes

4 carrots

1 handful radishes

salt, pepper and a squeeze of lemon to taste

No, not a tomato modified to grow underground, but a blend with wonderfully contrasting vegetables that do.

NUTRIENTS
Beta-carotene, biotin, folic acid,
vitamin C; calcium, magnesium,
phosphorus, potassium, sodium,
sulphur

ENERGY	★★★★☆
DETOX	★★☆☆☆
IMMUNITY	★★★★☆
DIGESTION	★☆☆☆☆
SKIN	★★★★☆

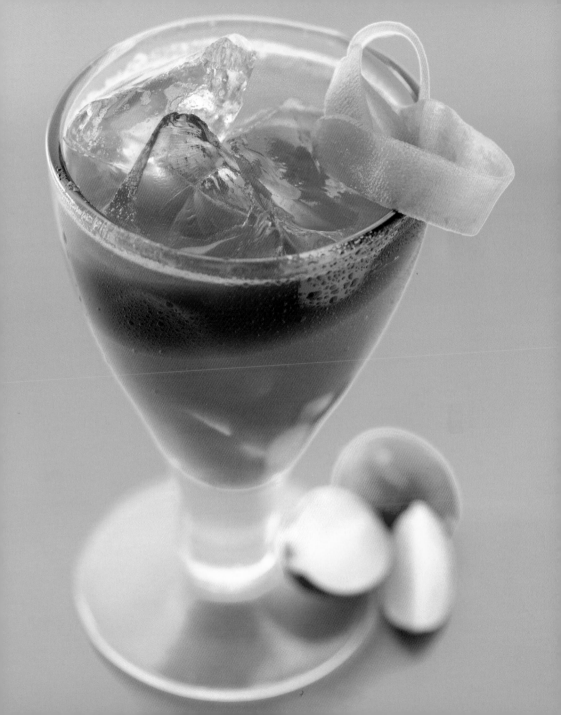

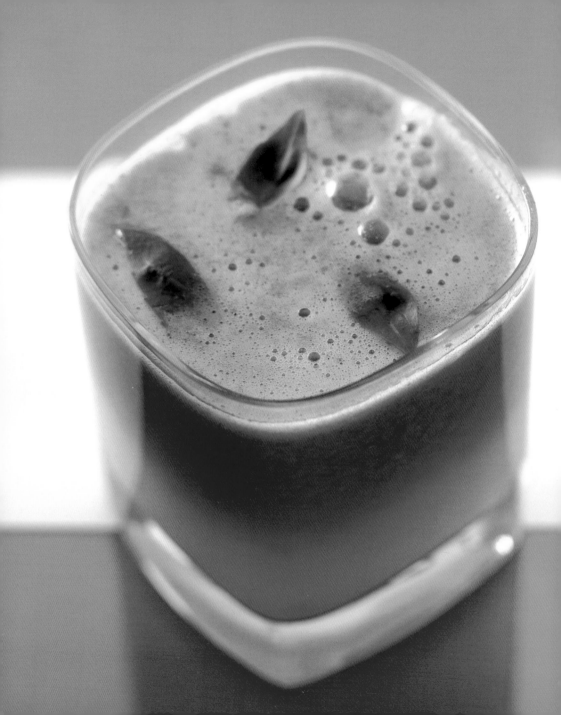

204 tricolore

6 tomatoes

2 parsnips

2 sticks celery

1 small handful fresh basil leaves

No mozzarella in here, but a red, white and green combination anyway, and the unusual touch from the basil will transport you straight to Italy.

NUTRIENTS
Beta-carotene, biotin, folic acid,
vitamin C; calcium, magnesium,
manganese, phosphorus, potassium,
sodium, sulphur

ENERGY	★★★★☆
DETOX	★★★☆☆
IMMUNITY	★★★☆☆
DIGESTION	★☆☆☆☆
SKIN	★★★☆☆

205 red tomato

6 tomatoes

1 beet (beetroot)

1 lemon

You may have found by now that, unlike tomato juice from a carton, the stuff you make at home is not red but pink, so the title may not be stating the obvious. Here it's the inimitable velvet red-purple of the beet that colours the juice.

NUTRIENTS
Beta-carotene, biotin, folic acid, vitamin C; calcium, magnesium, phosphorus, potassium, sodium, sulphur

ENERGY	★★★★☆
DETOX	★★★★☆
IMMUNITY	★★★★★
DIGESTION	☆☆☆☆☆
SKIN	★★★☆☆

206 black mud

5 tomatoes

1 beet (beetroot)

4 large kale leaves

1 lime

Not the most appetizing colour but it sure makes up for that in taste and some unbeatable health benefits.

NUTRIENTS
Beta-carotene, biotin, folic acid,
vitamin B3, vitamin C; calcium, iron,
magnesium, manganese, phosphorus,
potassium, sodium, sulphur

ENERGY	★★★★☆
DETOX	★★★★★
IMMUNITY	★★★★★
DIGESTION	★☆☆☆☆
SKIN	★★★☆☆

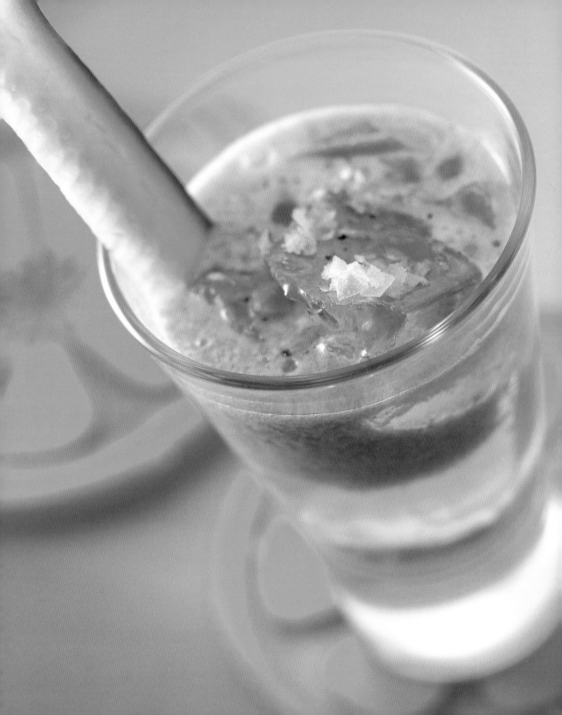

207 cool as a tomato

5 tomatoes

½ long cucumber

salt, pepper, Tabasco and
Worcestershire sauce to taste

As always with juices containing
cucumber, this is a light, refreshing
blend and another one which goes
down well with some seasoning.

NUTRIENTS
Beta-carotene, biotin, folic acid,
vitamin C; calcium, magnesium,
phosphorus, potassium, sodium,
sulphur

ENERGY	★★★☆☆
DETOX	★★☆☆☆
IMMUNITY	★★★☆☆
DIGESTION	☆☆☆☆☆
SKIN	★★☆☆☆

208 classic & green

6 tomatoes

3 carrots

1 large handful spinach

Classic with an earthy, green undertone, this juice is particularly good for the immune system as it's packed with carotene.

NUTRIENTS
Beta-carotene, biotin, folic acid, vitamin B3, vitamin C; calcium, iron, magnesium, phosphorus, potassium, sodium, sulphur

ENERGY ★★★★☆
DETOX ★★★☆☆
IMMUNITY ★★★★★
DIGESTION ☆☆☆☆☆
SKIN ★★★★☆

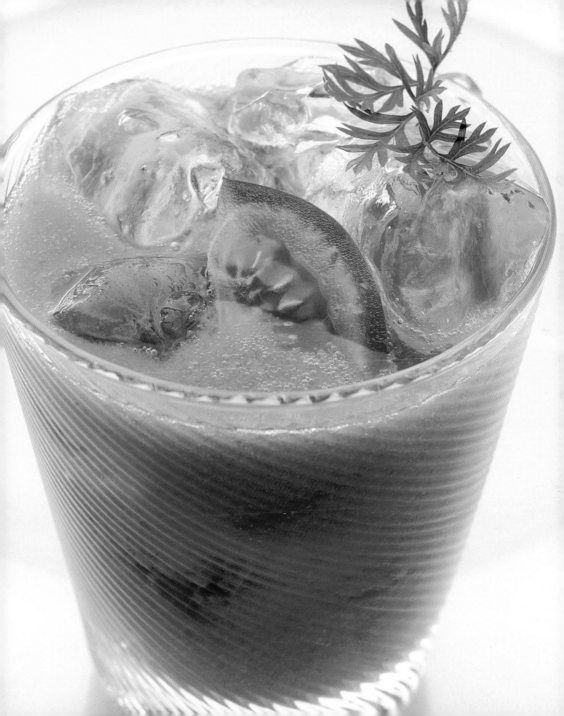

209 tomato cocktail

6 tomatoes

¼ long cucumber

½ inch (1 cm) ginger root

1 small bunch fresh mint leaves

1 lime

The cucumber is added to refresh, and then the mint, lime and ginger to take it all on to an even higher plane.

NUTRIENTS
Beta-carotene, biotin, folic acid, vitamin C; calcium, magnesium, phosphorus, potassium, sodium, sulphur

ENERGY	★★★☆☆
DETOX	★★☆☆☆
IMMUNITY	★★★☆☆
DIGESTION	★☆☆☆☆
SKIN	★★☆☆☆

210 old favourites

4 tomatoes

1 orange

2 carrots

Three of the most popular individual juices rolled into one to create an interesting-tasting juice that is great for your immune system.

NUTRIENTS
Beta-carotene, biotin, folic acid,
vitamin C; calcium, magnesium,
phosphorus, potassium, sodium,
sulphur

ENERGY ★★★★☆
DETOX ★★☆☆☆
IMMUNITY ★★★★★
DIGESTION ☆☆☆☆☆
SKIN ★★★★☆

211 tomorange

4 tomatoes

2 oranges

Probably the only combination of tomato juice with fruit that I think really works – very refreshing and very good for you.

NUTRIENTS
Beta-carotene, biotin, folic acid,
vitamin C; calcium, magnesium,
phosphorus, potassium, sodium,
sulphur

ENERGY	★★★★☆
DETOX	★★☆☆☆
IMMUNITY	★★★★★
DIGESTION	☆☆☆☆☆
SKIN	★★★☆☆

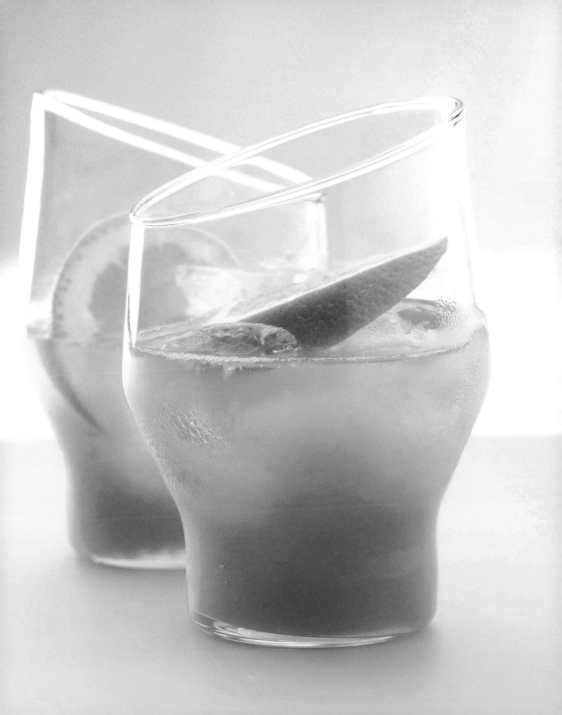

212 tomorange fresh

4 tomatoes

2 oranges

1 small handful fresh mint leaves

Basically a Tomorange (see blend 211), but with a hint of mint that takes it up a notch in the refreshing stakes. A great immunity-booster as well.

NUTRIENTS
Beta-carotene, biotin, folic acid, vitamin C; calcium, magnesium, phosphorus, potassium, sodium, sulphur

ENERGY	★★★★☆
DETOX	★★☆☆☆
IMMUNITY	★★★★★
DIGESTION	★☆☆☆☆
SKIN	★★★☆☆

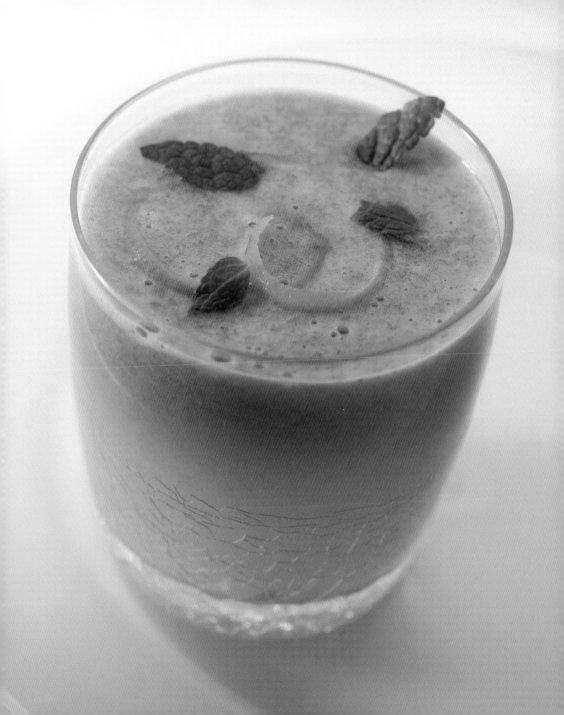

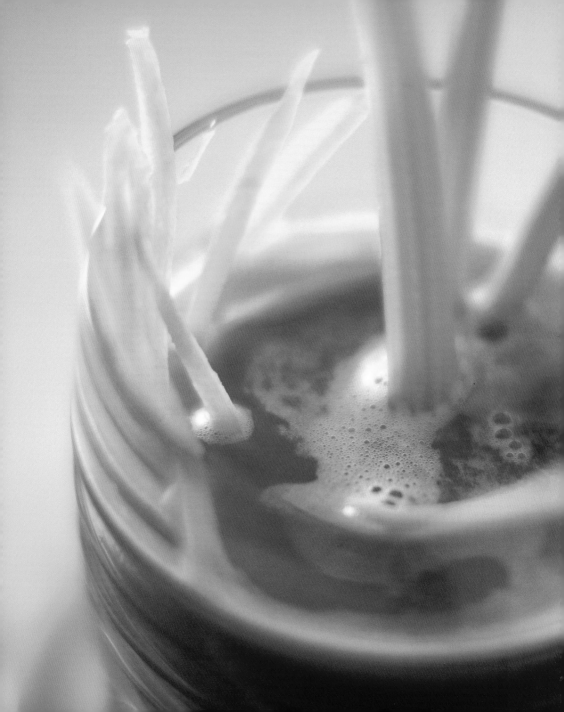

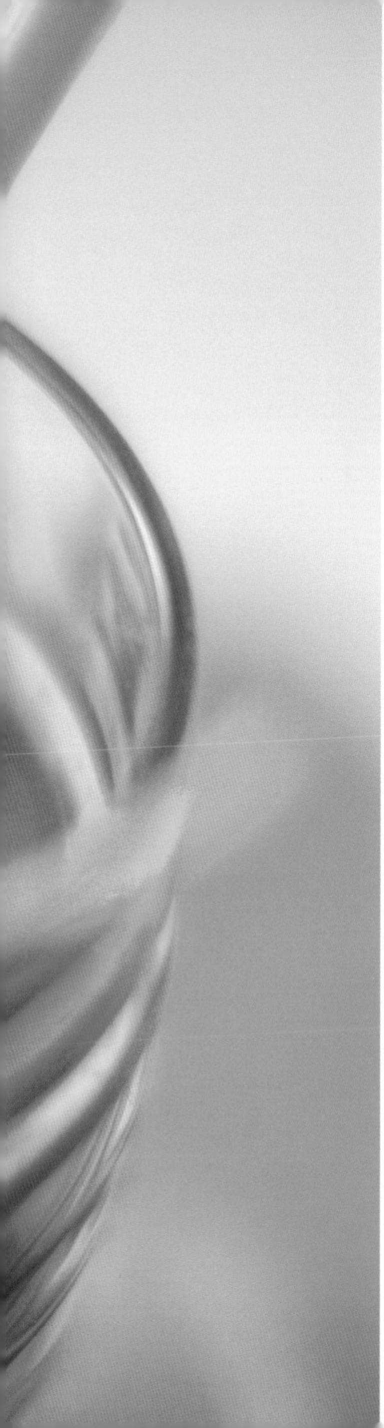

213 creamy crunch

4 sticks celery

3 carrots

Each of these juices brings out
the best in the other.

NUTRIENTS

Beta-carotene, folic acid, vitamin C;
calcium, magnesium, manganese,
phosphorus, potassium, sodium,
sulphur

ENERGY	★★★☆☆
DETOX	★★★★☆
IMMUNITY	★★★☆☆
DIGESTION	★★★☆☆
SKIN	★★★☆☆

214 cool 'n' pale II

4 sticks celery

2 apples

A dreamy shade of green, with a taste to match. Discovery apples make an ideal partner for the celery in this one.

NUTRIENTS
Beta-carotene, folic acid, vitamin C; calcium, magnesium, manganese, phosphorus, potassium, sodium, sulphur

ENERGY	★★☆☆☆
DETOX	★★★☆☆
IMMUNITY	★★☆☆☆
DIGESTION	★★★☆☆
SKIN	★★☆☆☆

215 savoury fruit

3 sticks celery

1 apple

1 orange

The celery here lifts the flavours of the fruit juices.

NUTRIENTS
Beta-carotene, folic acid, vitamin C;
calcium, magnesium, manganese,
phosphorus, potassium, sodium,
sulphur

ENERGY	★★★☆☆
DETOX	★★★☆☆
IMMUNITY	★★★☆☆
DIGESTION	★☆☆☆☆
SKIN	★★☆☆☆

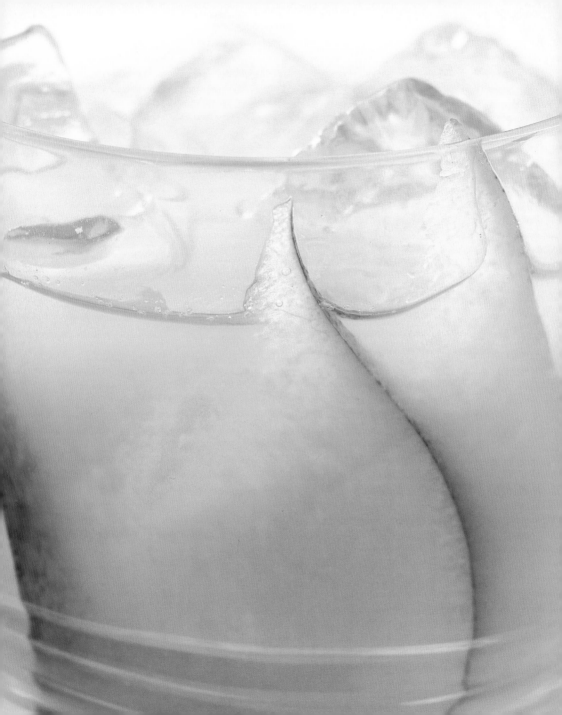

216 delicate pale

4 sticks celery

2 pears

Because pears tend to have a more delicate flavour than apples,
this one is even more subtle than Cool 'n' Pale II (see blend 214),
but is just as refreshing.

NUTRIENTS
Beta-carotene, folic acid, vitamin C;
calcium, magnesium, phosphorus,
potassium, sodium, sulphur

ENERGY ★★★☆☆
DETOX ★★★★☆
IMMUNITY ★★☆☆☆
DIGESTION ★★★☆☆
SKIN ★★☆☆☆

217   crunch morning favourite

3 sticks celery

1 grapefruit

½ inch (1 cm) ginger root

One of a few standard morning favourites to come out of my fruit bowl and refrigerator. Grapefruit always seems to go well with vegetable juices.

NUTRIENTS
Beta-carotene, folic acid, vitamin C; calcium, magnesium, manganese, phosphorus, potassium, sodium, sulphur

ENERGY	★★☆☆☆
DETOX	★★★☆☆
IMMUNITY	★★★☆☆
DIGESTION	★☆☆☆☆
SKIN	★★☆☆☆

218 celery jointaid

3 sticks celery

½ pineapple

1 inch (2.5 cm) ginger root

1 tablespoon (15 ml) flaxseed (linseed) oil

A combination of minerals, antioxidants and essential fats to help promote healthy joints, this fresh juice also offers the anti-inflammatory properties of pineapple and ginger.

NUTRIENTS
Beta-carotene, folic acid, vitamin C; calcium, magnesium, manganese, phosphorus, potassium, sodium, sulphur; essential fatty acids

ENERGY	★★★★☆
DETOX	★★★★☆
IMMUNITY	★★★★★
DIGESTION	★★★★★
SKIN	★★★☆☆

219 pink punch

3 sticks celery

2 apples

1 handful cranberries (or raspberries)

3 sprigs fresh mint

½ inch (1 cm) ginger root

Who needs alcohol on a hot summer's day?

NUTRIENTS
Beta-carotene, folic acid, vitamin C;
calcium, iron, magnesium, manganese,
phosphorus, potassium, sodium,
sulphur

ENERGY	★★★★☆
DETOX	★★★☆☆
IMMUNITY	★★★★☆
DIGESTION	★★☆☆☆
SKIN	★★☆☆☆

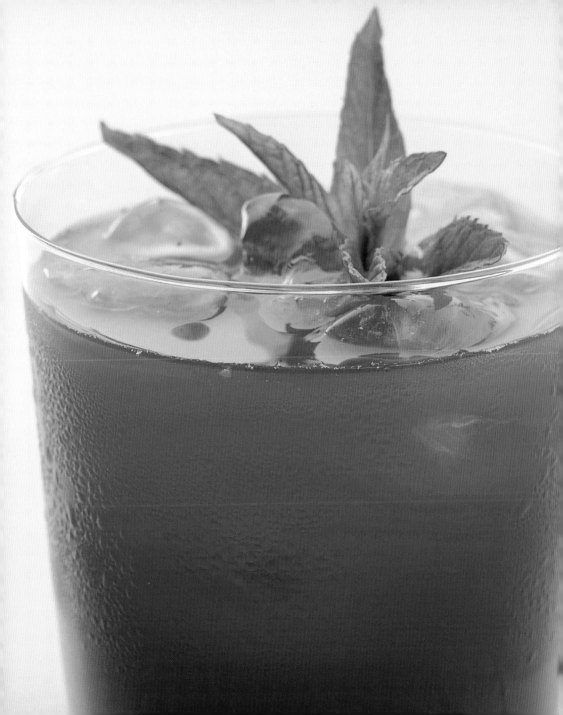

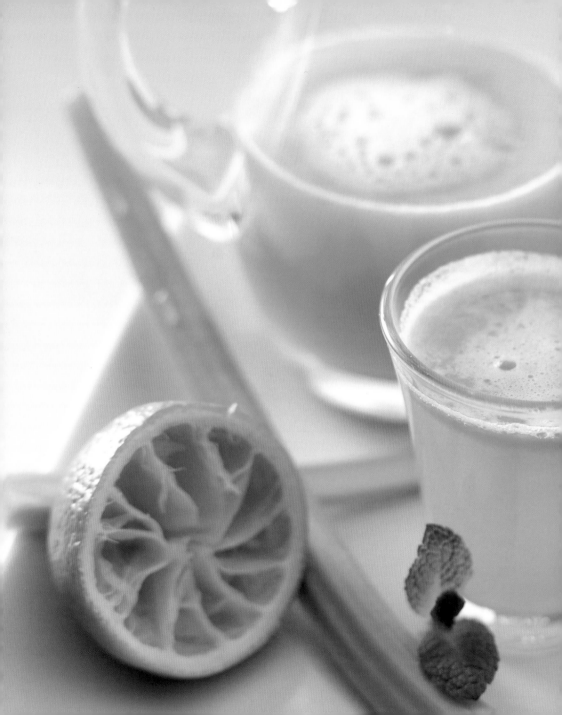

220 fresh crunch

4 sticks celery

1 apple

5 sprigs fresh mint

1 lime

A startling, fresh combination – use more lime
if you fancy giving it a sharper bite.

NUTRIENTS
Beta-carotene, folic acid, vitamin C;
calcium, magnesium, manganese,
phosphorus, potassium, sodium,
sulphur

ENERGY	★★☆☆☆
DETOX	★★★★☆
IMMUNITY	★★★☆☆
DIGESTION	★★☆☆☆
SKIN	★★★☆☆

221   salty sharp melon

3 sticks celery

½ melon

1 lime

Melon juice is so sweet and creamy – here the celery and lime lift
it to a sharper plane.

NUTRIENTS
Beta-carotene, folic acid, vitamin C;
calcium, magnesium, manganese,
phosphorus, potassium, sodium,
sulphur

ENERGY	★★★☆☆
DETOX	★★★☆☆
IMMUNITY	★★★★☆
DIGESTION	☆☆☆☆☆
SKIN	★★★☆☆

222 soft and sharp

3 sticks celery

2 pears

1 large bunch watercress

The sharp contrast between the pear and the watercress goes well with the fresh, salty celery in this pretty, green drink.

NUTRIENTS
Beta-carotene, folic acid, vitamin C, vitamin E; calcium, iron, magnesium, phosphorus, potassium, sodium, sulphur

ENERGY	★★☆☆☆
DETOX	★★★★★
IMMUNITY	★★★★☆
DIGESTION	★★★☆☆
SKIN	★★★☆☆

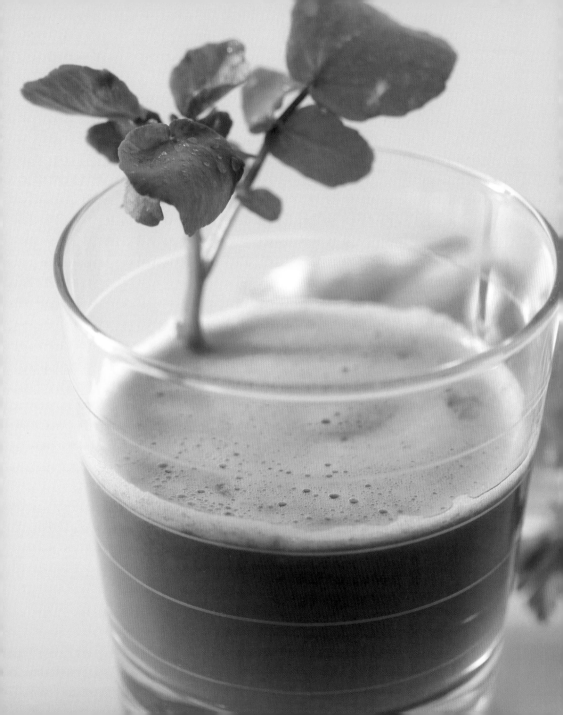

223 tricolore cruncher

3 sticks celery

3 tomatoes

1 small bunch fresh parsley

1 handful watercress

½ lemon

Fresh and cleansing, with a kick from the watercress and lemon, this is a delicious, salad-like combination.

NUTRIENTS
Beta-carotene, biotin, folic acid, vitamins B3, C and E; calcium, iron, magnesium, manganese, phosphorus, potassium, sodium, sulphur

ENERGY	★★☆☆☆
DETOX	★★★★☆
IMMUNITY	★★★☆☆
DIGESTION	☆☆☆☆☆
SKIN	★★★★★

224 grape crunch

4 sticks celery

1 large bunch seedless grapes (about 50)

There's something about the sweetness of grapes that goes fantastically well with celery. Use either green or red grapes, although red are richer in antioxidants.

NUTRIENTS
Folic acid, vitamin C, vitamin E; calcium, manganese, phosphorus, potassium, sodium, sulphur

ENERGY	★★★★☆
DETOX	★★★★☆
IMMUNITY	★★★☆☆
DIGESTION	★★☆☆☆
SKIN	★★★☆☆

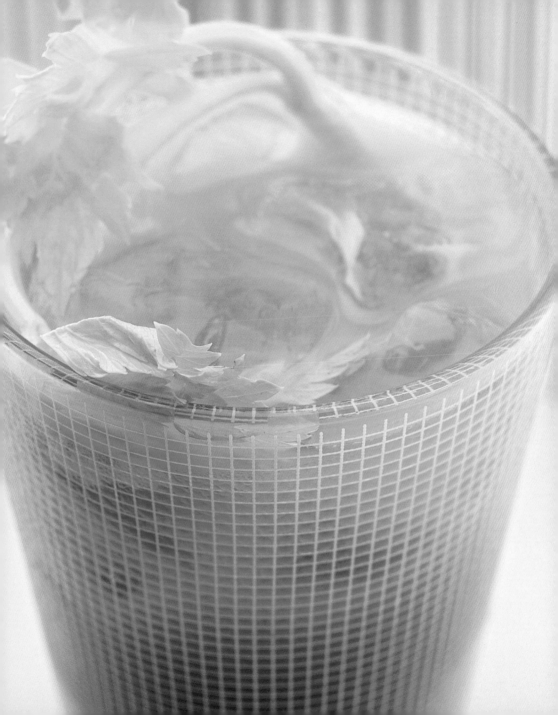

225 chlorophyll crunch

3 sticks celery

3 carrots

1 bunch fresh parsley

Creamy carrots, salty celery and perky parsley combine in
this substantial drink that is a good detoxifier and all-round
immunity-boosting tonic. You really can taste the goodness.

NUTRIENTS
Beta-carotene, folic acid, vitamin B3,
vitamin C; calcium, iron, magnesium,
manganese, phosphorus, potassium,
sodium, sulphur

ENERGY	★★☆☆☆
DETOX	★★★★★
IMMUNITY	★★★★★
DIGESTION	★★★☆☆
SKIN	★★★★☆

226 celery blood cleanser

3 sticks celery

1 apple

1 beet (beetroot)

1 teaspoon spirulina

This has such a fantastic taste that you'll hardly believe it's so good for you. Put in a little less beet if you're not a hardened fan. Shake the spirulina with some of the juice in a jar before mixing in with the rest.

NUTRIENTS
Beta-carotene, folic acid, vitamins B1, B3, B5, B6 and C; calcium, iron, magnesium, manganese, phosphorus, potassium, sodium, sulphur; protein; essential fatty acids

ENERGY ★★★☆☆
DETOX ★★★★★
IMMUNITY ★★★☆☆
DIGESTION ★★★★☆
SKIN ★★★★☆

227 take heart

4 sticks celery

1 apple

1 handful blackcurrants

½ inch (1 cm) ginger root

1 tablespoon (15 ml) flaxseed (linseed) oil

Each of the ingredients in this bright juice has properties that can help support healthy blood pressure and blood vessels – and it tastes great.

NUTRIENTS
Beta-carotene, biotin, folic acid, vitamin C, vitamin E; calcium, magnesium, manganese, phosphorus, potassium, sodium, sulphur; essential fatty acids

ENERGY	★★★☆☆
DETOX	★★★★☆
IMMUNITY	★★★★☆
DIGESTION	★★☆☆☆
SKIN	★★★★☆

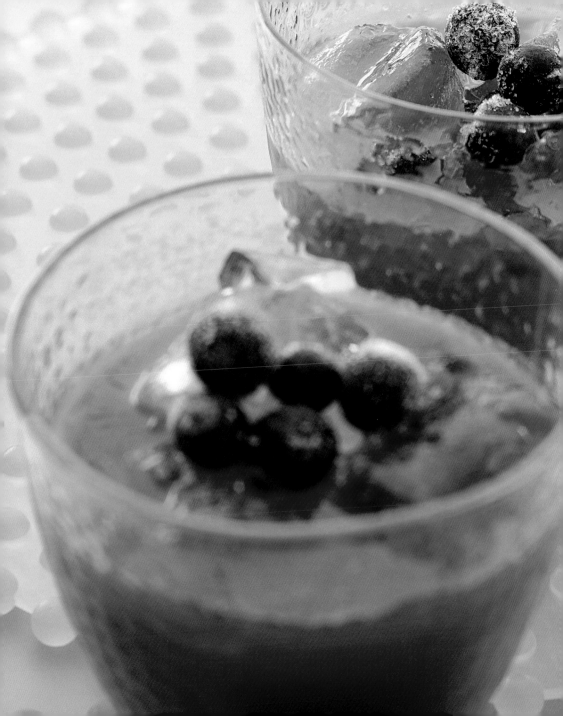

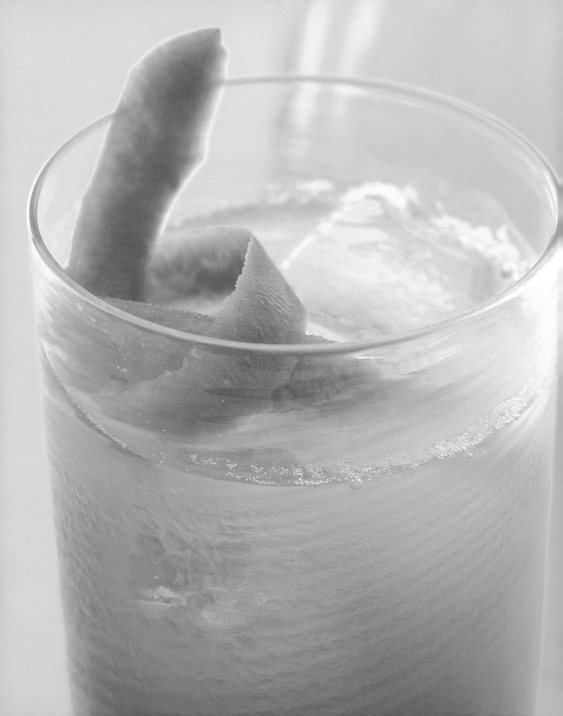

228 veggie cocktail

3 sticks celery

3 tomatoes

2 carrots

½ lemon

A sweet, pale orange vegetable juice – you could add some parsley too if you want that green, cleansing taste.

NUTRIENTS
Beta-carotene, biotin, folic acid,
vitamin C; calcium, magnesium,
manganese, phosphorus, potassium,
sodium, sulphur

ENERGY	★★★★☆
DETOX	★★★☆☆
IMMUNITY	★★★★★
DIGESTION	★☆☆☆☆
SKIN	★★★★☆

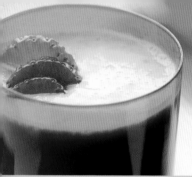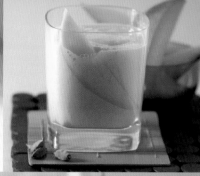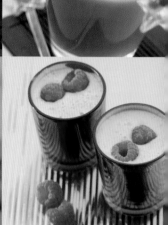
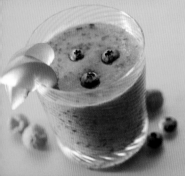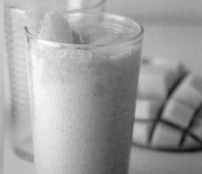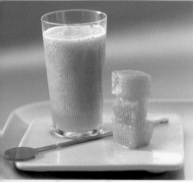
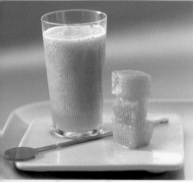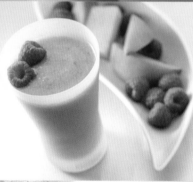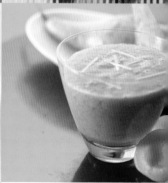
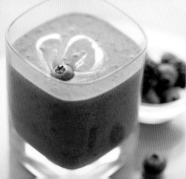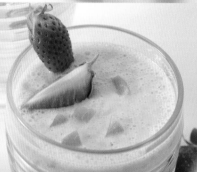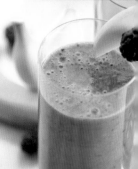

making
smoothies

Making a smoothie couldn't be easier – just prepare your ingredients (see pages 16–30), throw them into a blender and press "on".

In this chapter, fruity smoothies are thick drinks made from fresh fruits blended together with a little added fruit juice; and creamy smoothies are richer, creamier drinks because they contain yogurt. All of the creamy smoothie recipes list yogurt, but you can use milk or soy (soya) milk instead if you prefer a runnier drink. Either way, a creamy smoothie provides a rich source of protein.

Each recipe suggests which juice to add to help make your smoothie a drink, rather than a pudding, but feel free to experiment with different juices and different amounts according to your tastes and preferences. The recipes each make two generous portions, and provide a delicious, substantial drink, snack or even a light meal for any time of the day.

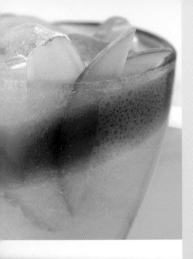

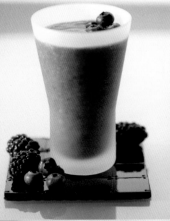

top tips

Below are a few reminders and helpful hints, tips and suggestions to enable you to get the most from your smoothie making.

1 Choose fruit for a smoothie at its peak of ripeness for the best taste and most goodness in a glass.

2 When adding juice to your smoothie, use fresh, home-made juice in preference to commercially produced juices (which often contain artificial sweeteners and other additives).

3 When adding juice to your smoothie, you don't have to stick rigidly to the one listed in the ingredients – try using whichever juice you have available rather than go without.

4 Add more or less juice to your smoothie, according to your own tastes and preferences, to make a thinner or thicker drink.

5 For creamy smoothies, the recipes suggest using yogurt. For thinner, runnier drinks, use milk or a milk alternative made from soy (soya), rice or nuts.

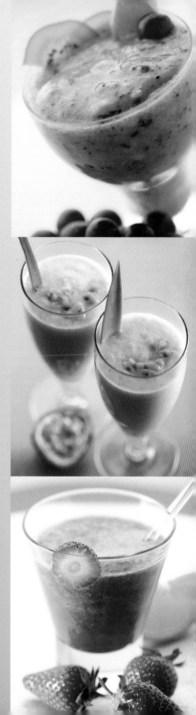

6 Use soy (soya) yogurt or soy (soya) milk as a non-dairy alternative when making creamy smoothies.

7 For a more refreshing smoothie, blend a few crushed cubes of ice in with the other ingredients.

8 Any smoothie can be frozen to be eaten as a delicious popsicle (ice-lolly). Either use special popsicle moulds or ice-cube trays.

9 Try adding some of the extra ingredients listed on pages 31–3 to give your smoothie an even greater healthy boost.

10 Even if you don't have all the fruits needed for a particular recipe, or the exact amounts, give it a try anyway and have some fun creating your own blends.

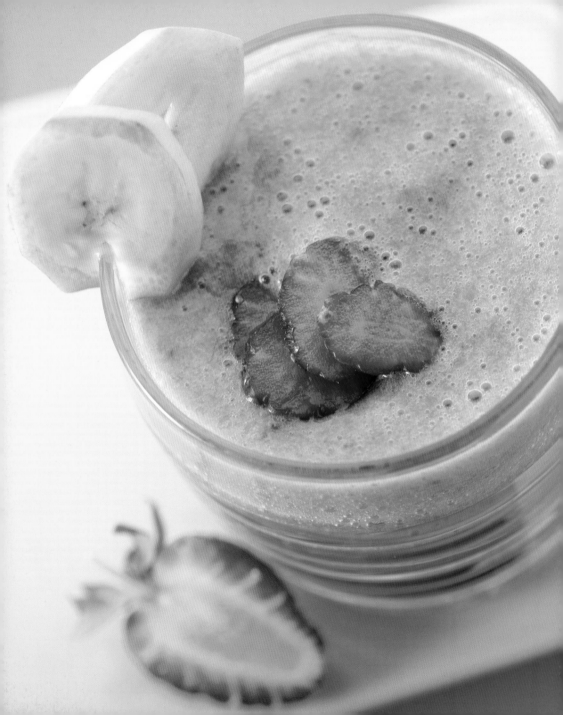

229 pink banana

2 bananas

8 medium strawberries

10 tablespoons (150 ml) apple juice

This one is a summer favourite – best to use fresh organic strawberries.

NUTRIENTS
Beta-carotene, biotin, folic acid, vitamins B1, B3, B6 and C; calcium, magnesium, phosphorus, potassium, sulphur

ENERGY ★★★★★
DETOX ★☆☆☆☆
IMMUNITY ★★★☆☆
DIGESTION ★☆☆☆☆
SKIN ★★★☆☆

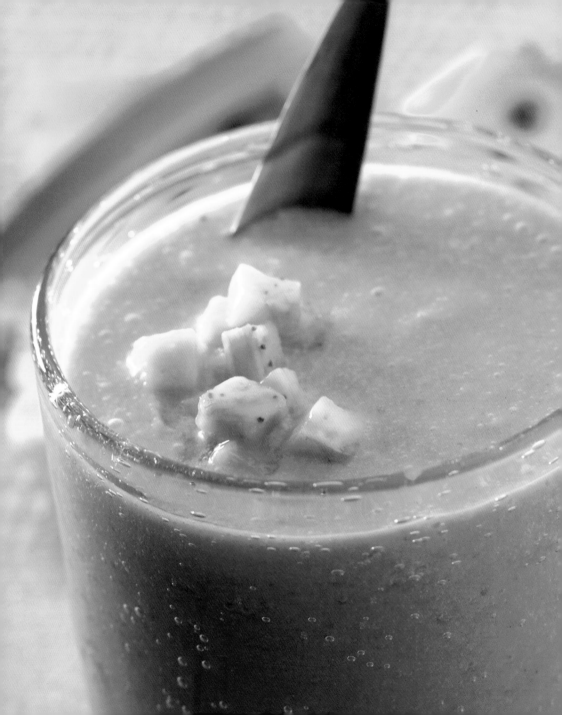

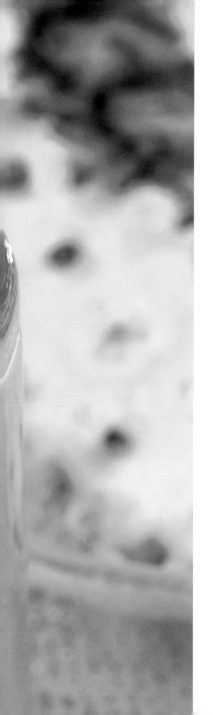

230 green banana smoothie

1 banana

½ pineapple

8 tablespoons (120 ml) pineapple juice

2 tablespoons (30 ml) coconut milk

1 heaped teaspoon spirulina

The spirulina turns this delicious, pastel-yellow drink into a green delight.

NUTRIENTS
Beta-carotene, folic acid, vitamins
B1, B3, B6 and C; calcium, iron,
magnesium, manganese, phosphorus,
potassium, sodium, sulphur; protein;
essential fatty acids

ENERGY	★★★★★
DETOX	★★★☆☆
IMMUNITY	★★★☆☆
DIGESTION	★★★★☆
SKIN	★★★☆☆

231 green banana too

2 bananas

2 kiwi fruits

1 handful seedless red grapes

10 tablespoons (150 ml) apple juice

This juice is a pretty, green colour because of the delicious, tangy, vitamin C-rich kiwi fruit.

NUTRIENTS
Beta-carotene, folic acid, vitamins B1, B3, B6, C and E; calcium, magnesium, manganese, phosphorus, potassium, sodium, sulphur

ENERGY ★★★★★
DETOX ★★★★☆
IMMUNITY ★★★★☆
DIGESTION ★★★☆☆
SKIN ★★★★☆

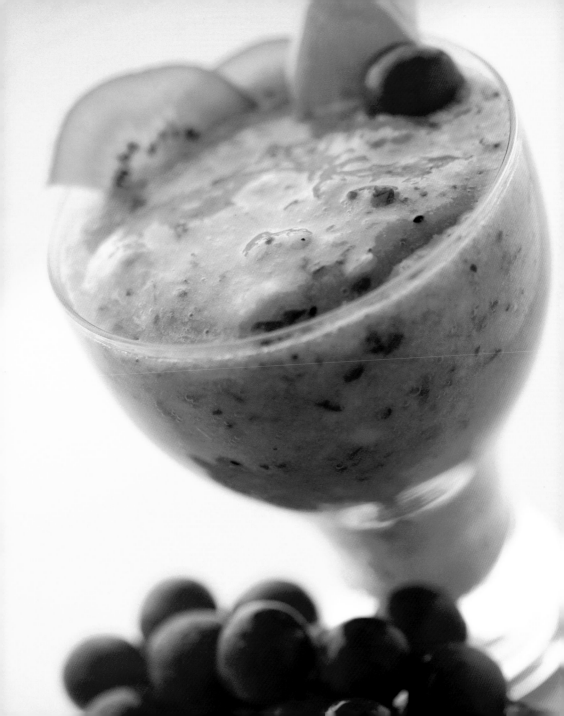

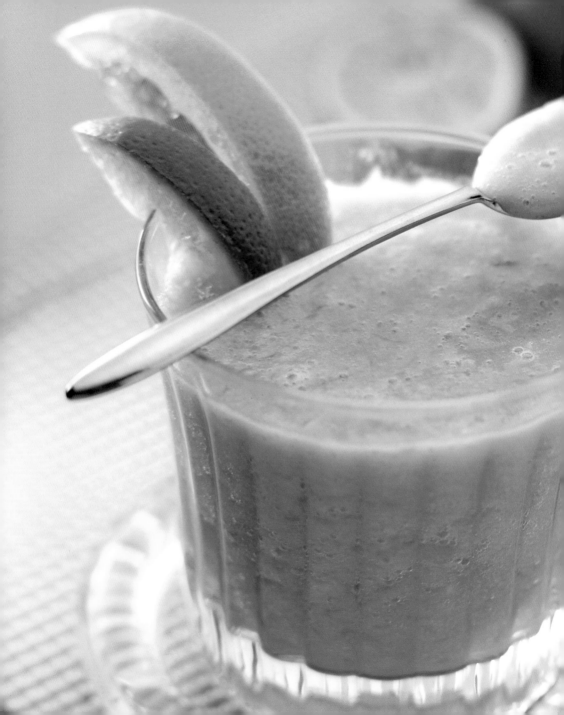

419

FRUITY SMOOTHIES – BANANA

232 banana sharp

2 bananas

1 pink grapefruit

8 tablespoons (120 ml) orange juice

juice of a lime

A great contrast between the tangy citrus and sweet banana.

NUTRIENTS
Beta-carotene, folic acid, vitamins B1, B3, B6 and C; calcium, magnesium, phosphorus, potassium, sodium, sulphur

ENERGY	★★★★★
DETOX	★☆☆☆☆
IMMUNITY	★★★☆☆
DIGESTION	★☆☆☆☆
SKIN	★★★☆☆

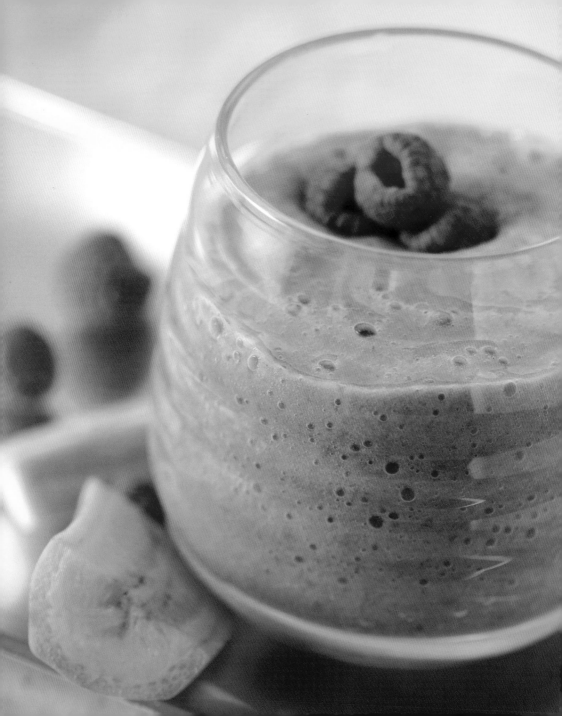

233 pink lady

2 bananas

2 handfuls raspberries

10 tablespoons (150 ml) cranberry juice

This one is certainly heaven-sent and gives a great energy boost too.

NUTRIENTS
Beta-carotene, biotin, folic acid, vitamins B1, B3, B6 and C; calcium, iron, magnesium, manganese, phosphorus, potassium, sodium, sulphur

ENERGY	★★★★★
DETOX	★☆☆☆☆
IMMUNITY	★★★☆☆
DIGESTION	★★☆☆☆
SKIN	★★★☆☆

234 pure passion

3 bananas

4 passion fruits

10 tablespoons (150 ml) guava juice

Surely one of the most exquisite combinations of fruit ever.

NUTRIENTS
Beta-carotene, folic acid, vitamins B1,
B3, B6 and C; calcium, iron, magnesium,
phosphorus, potassium, sodium,
sulphur

ENERGY ★★★★★
DETOX ★☆☆☆☆
IMMUNITY ★★★☆☆
DIGESTION ★☆☆☆☆
SKIN ★★★☆☆

235 banana nectar

2 bananas

4 apricots

10 tablespoons (150 ml) apricot or apple juice

Nothing to do with nectarines – I always think the pulp or juice of apricots conjures up the word "nectar" more than that of most fruits.

NUTRIENTS
Beta-carotene, folic acid, vitamins B1,
B3, B6 and C; calcium, magnesium,
phosphorus, potassium, sulphur

ENERGY	★★★★★
DETOX	★☆☆☆☆
IMMUNITY	★★★☆☆
DIGESTION	★★☆☆☆
SKIN	★★★☆☆

236 black banana

2 bananas

2 heaped tablespoons blackcurrants

10 tablespoons (150 ml) apple juice (or the juice from
the blackcurrants, if they come from a can)

A wonderful contrast between the sweet bananas and the tangy
blackcurrants. Use blackcurrants canned in natural juice if you don't
have fresh ones – a good standby to keep in the cupboard in winter.

NUTRIENTS
Beta-carotene, biotin, vitamins B1, B3,
B6, C and E; calcium, iron, magnesium,
phosphorus, potassium, sodium,
sulphur

ENERGY	★★★★★
DETOX	★☆☆☆☆
IMMUNITY	★★★☆☆
DIGESTION	★☆☆☆☆
SKIN	★★★☆☆

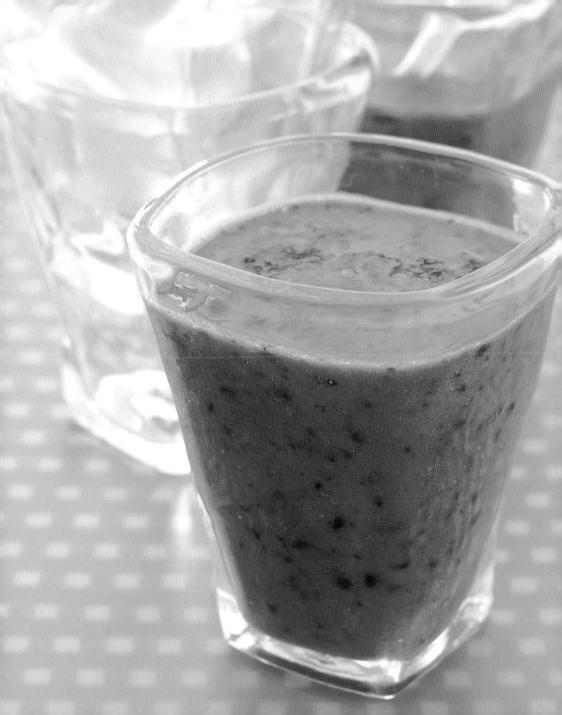

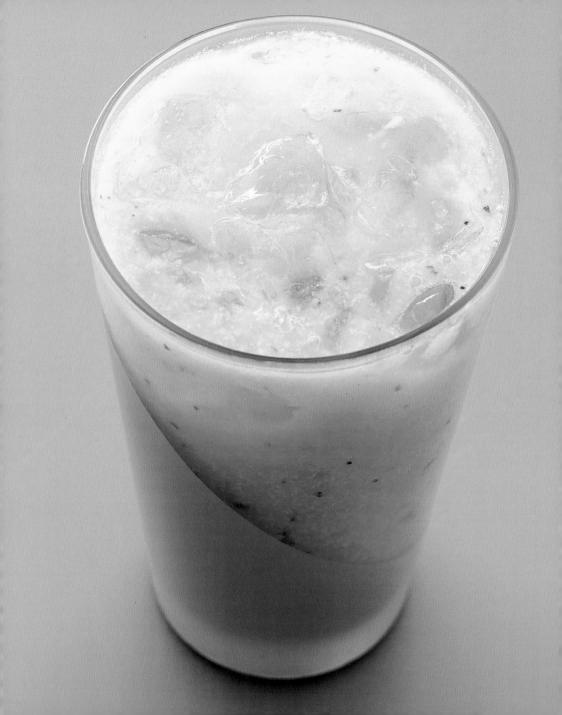

237   easy morning mash

2 bananas

1 pear

1 orange

8 tablespoons (120 ml) apple juice

Just reach into the fruit bowl and whiz it all up. Easy.

NUTRIENTS
Beta-carotene, folic acid, vitamins B1,
B3, B6 and C; calcium, magnesium,
phosphorus, potassium, sulphur

ENERGY	★★★★★
DETOX	★☆☆☆☆
IMMUNITY	★★★☆☆
DIGESTION	★★☆☆☆
SKIN	★★☆☆☆

238 banana pie

2 bananas

1 apple

1 handful blackberries (or blackcurrants)

10 tablespoons (150 ml) apple juice

Well, not literally, but I always think of the apple-
and-blackberry pie combination when the two are
blended, and they cut deliciously through the dense
flavour of the banana.

NUTRIENTS
Beta-carotene, folic acid, vitamins B1,
B3, B5, B6, C and E; calcium, iron,
magnesium, phosphorus, potassium,
sodium, sulphur

ENERGY	★★★★★
DETOX	★☆☆☆☆
IMMUNITY	★★★☆☆
DIGESTION	★★☆☆☆
SKIN	★★☆☆☆

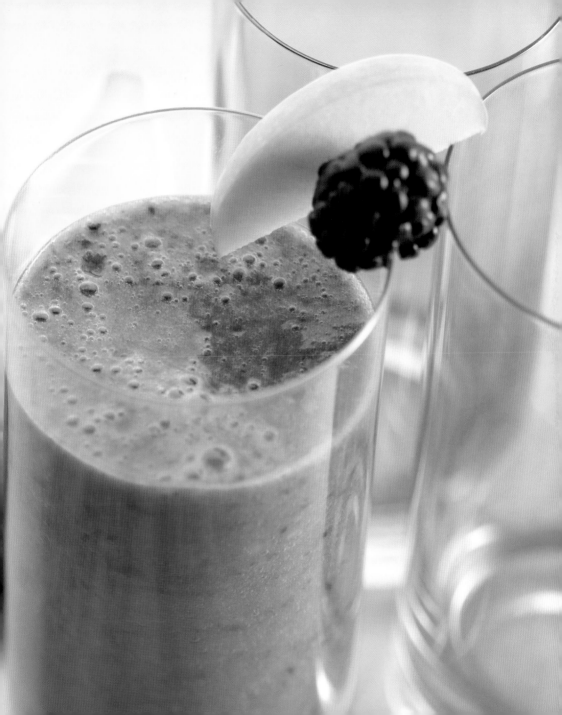

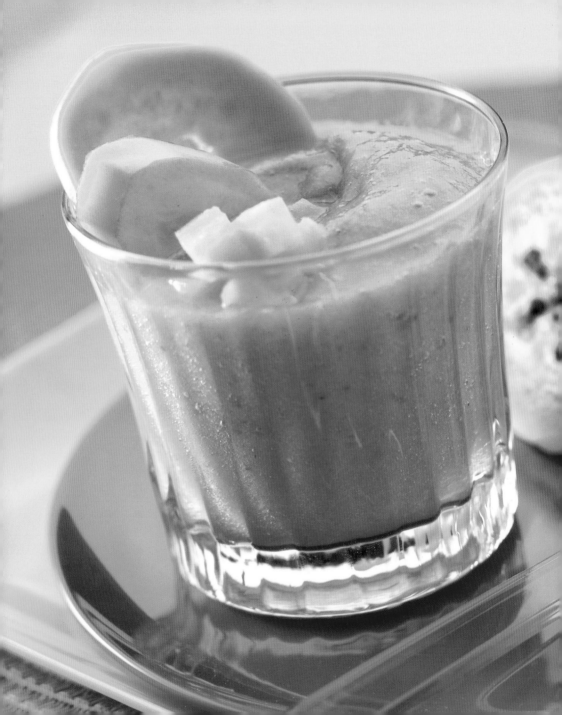

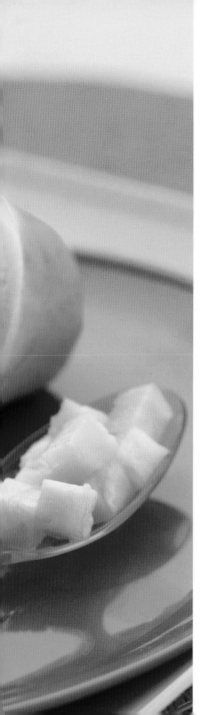

239 tropical treat

1 banana

½ pineapple

½ papaya

8 tablespoons (120 ml) guava juice

Fancy being transported to a fresh fruit salad on a beach in Thailand?

NUTRIENTS

Beta-carotene, folic acid, vitamin B3, vitamin C; calcium, magnesium, manganese, phosphorus, potassium, sodium, sulphur

ENERGY	★★★★★
DETOX	★☆☆☆☆
IMMUNITY	★★★☆☆
DIGESTION	★★★★☆
SKIN	★★★☆☆

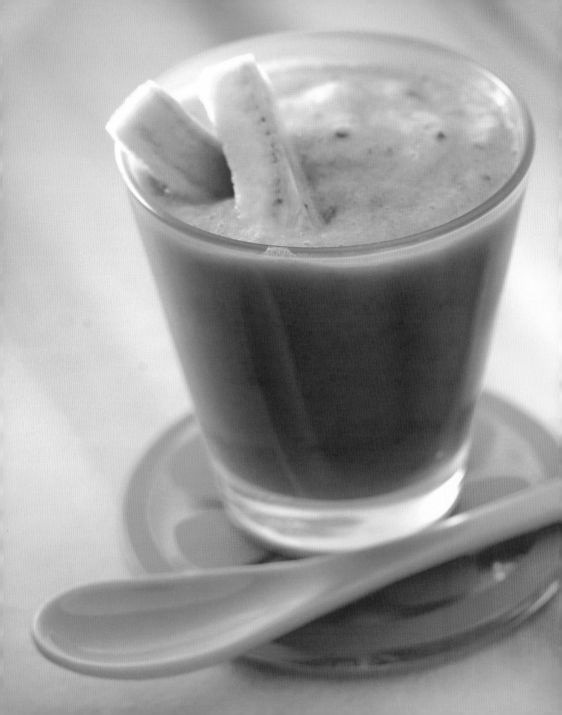

240 peaches 'n' dream

2 bananas

2 peaches

2 tangerines

8 tablespoons (120 ml) orange juice

Juicy, ripe peaches (or nectarines) make this one a dream combination.

NUTRIENTS
Beta-carotene, folic acid, vitamins B1, B3, B6 and C; calcium, magnesium, phosphorus, potassium, sodium, sulphur

ENERGY	★★★★★
DETOX	★☆☆☆☆
IMMUNITY	★★★☆☆
DIGESTION	★★☆☆☆
SKIN	★★☆☆☆

241 mellow bite

2 bananas

½ melon

8 tablespoons (120 ml) apple juice

juice of a lime

The contrasting mild melon and sharp lime make quite an impact on your tastebuds but are mellowed by the banana.

NUTRIENTS
Beta-carotene, folic acid, vitamins B1,
B3, B6 and C; calcium, iron, magnesium,
phosphorus, potassium, sodium,
sulphur

ENERGY	★★★★★
DETOX	★☆☆☆☆
IMMUNITY	★★★☆☆
DIGESTION	★☆☆☆☆
SKIN	★★☆☆☆

242 regular banana

2 bananas

10 prunes (soaked and pitted)

½ teaspoon vanilla essence

10 tablespoons (150 ml) apple juice

You'd barely believe this was so good for keeping your guts going, it tastes so delicious. Use particularly ripe bananas.

NUTRIENTS
Beta-carotene, folic acid, vitamins B1, B3, B6 and C; calcium, magnesium, phosphorus, potassium, sulphur

ENERGY	★★★★☆
DETOX	★☆☆☆☆
IMMUNITY	★★★☆☆
DIGESTION	★★★☆☆
SKIN	★★☆☆☆

243 coconutty 'nana

2 bananas

½ pineapple

2 tablespoons (30 ml) coconut milk

8 tablespoons (120 ml) pineapple juice

If you're a fan of coconut, you'll love this one and the way it conjures up the feeling of being on a warm, palm-fringed beach.

NUTRIENTS
Beta-carotene, folic acid, vitamins B1, B3, B6, C and E; calcium, magnesium, manganese, phosphorus, potassium, sodium, sulphur

ENERGY	★★★★★
DETOX	★☆☆☆☆
IMMUNITY	★★★☆☆
DIGESTION	★★★★☆
SKIN	★★☆☆☆

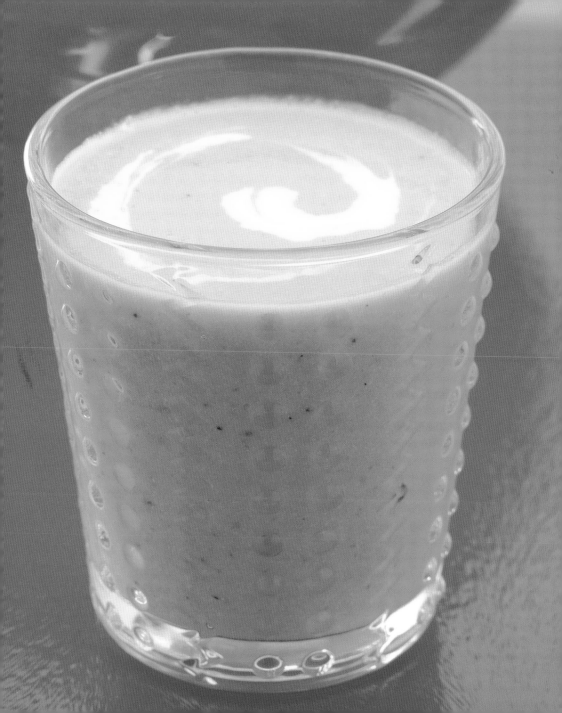

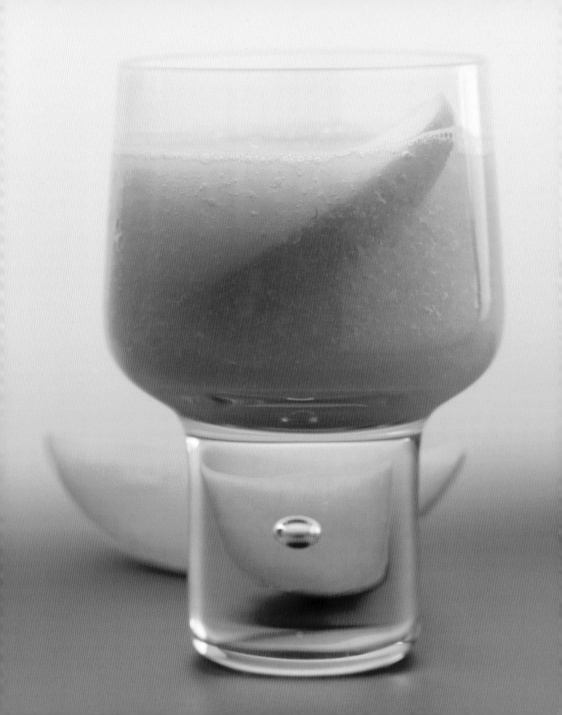

244   eve's delight

2 mangoes

2 apples

8 tablespoons (120 ml) apple juice

If Eve had had anything to blend the apple with in Eden, it would have been a juicy, ripe mango. This is one of my all-time favourite smoothies.

NUTRIENTS
Beta-carotene, folic acid, vitamin C,
vitamin E; calcium, iron, magnesium,
phosphorus, potassium, sodium,
sulphur

ENERGY	★★★★★
DETOX	★☆☆☆☆
IMMUNITY	★★★★☆
DIGESTION	★★★★☆
SKIN	★★☆☆☆

245 mango crush

2 mangoes

2 oranges

juice of a lime

8 tablespoons (120 ml) apple juice

One pure orange colour, two different tastes, one result – a fabulous smoothie where the creamy, sweet mango contrasts well with the tangy orange.

NUTRIENTS
Beta-carotene, folic acid, vitamin C, vitamin E; calcium, iron, magnesium, phosphorus, potassium, sodium, sulphur

ENERGY ★★★★★
DETOX ★☆☆☆☆
IMMUNITY ★★★★★
DIGESTION ★☆☆☆☆
SKIN ★★★☆☆

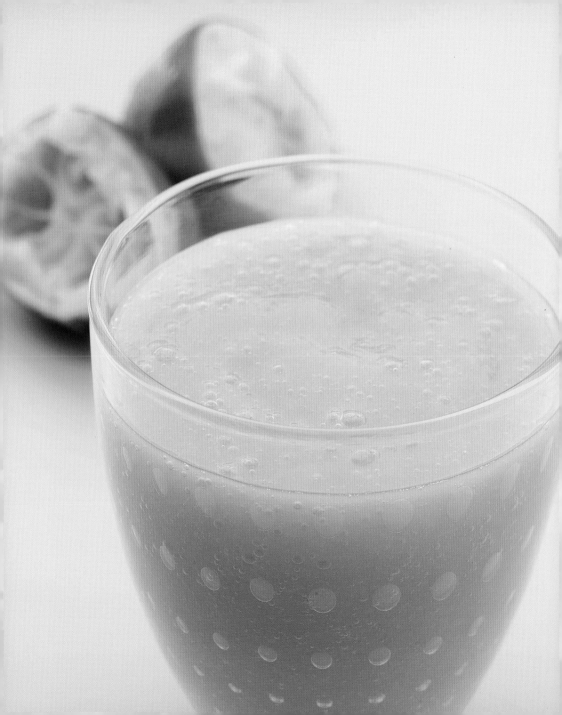

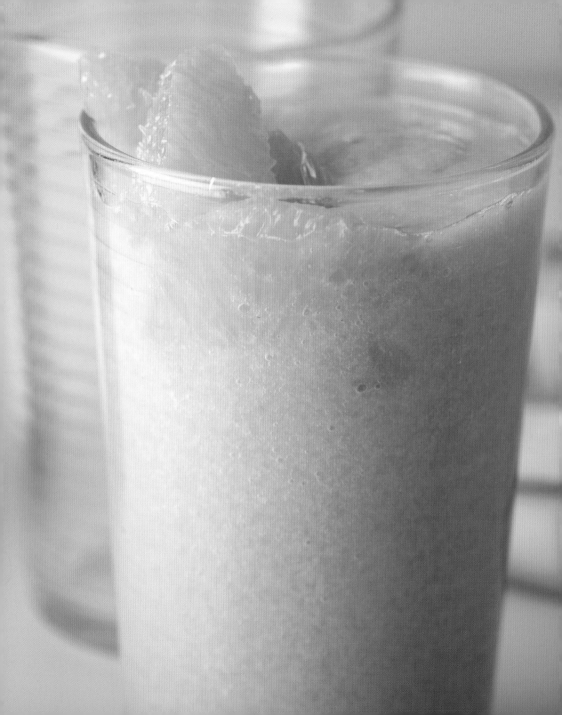

246 simple tropical

2 mangoes

1 banana

10 tablespoons (150 ml) orange juice

Dense and rich, this is a high-energy blend. You can use pineapple juice as an alternative to the orange for an extra tropical touch.

NUTRIENTS
Beta-carotene, folic acid, vitamins B1, B3, B6, C and E; calcium, iron, magnesium, phosphorus, potassium, sodium, sulphur

ENERGY	★★★★★
DETOX	★☆☆☆☆
IMMUNITY	★★★☆☆
DIGESTION	★★☆☆☆
SKIN	★★★☆☆

247 mango passion

2 mangoes

½ pineapple

2 passion fruits

8 tablespoons (120 ml) pineapple juice

I love any blend with passion fruit, but with pineapple and mango – mmm!

NUTRIENTS
Beta-carotene, folic acid, vitamins B3,
C and E; calcium, iron, magnesium,
manganese, phosphorus, potassium,
sodium, sulphur

ENERGY	★★★★★
DETOX	★☆☆☆☆
IMMUNITY	★★★★☆
DIGESTION	★★★★☆
SKIN	★★★☆☆

248   manilla

2 mangoes

4 tangerines

½ teaspoon vanilla essence

8 tablespoons (120 ml) orange juice

Somehow the vanilla makes this taste even sweeter.

NUTRIENTS
Beta-carotene, folic acid, vitamin C,
vitamin E; calcium, iron, magnesium,
phosphorus, potassium, sodium,
sulphur

ENERGY	★★★★★
DETOX	★☆☆☆☆
IMMUNITY	★★★★★
DIGESTION	★☆☆☆☆
SKIN	★★★☆☆

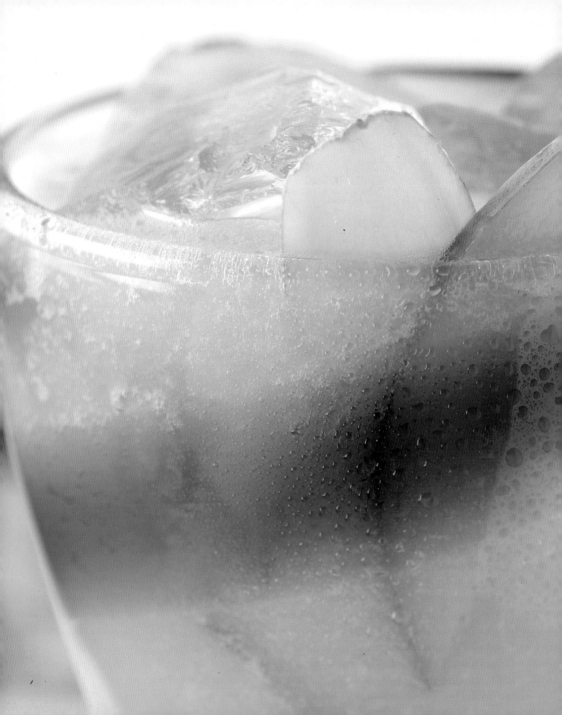

249 mango zingo

2 mangoes

1 grapefruit

¼ inch (0.5 cm) ginger root, grated

8 tablespoons (120 ml) apple juice

The slightly bitter grapefruit and spicy ginger blend beautifully with sweet, creamy mango to create this energy- and immunity-boosting drink.

NUTRIENTS
Beta-carotene, folic acid, vitamin C, vitamin E; calcium, iron, magnesium, phosphorus, potassium, sodium, sulphur

ENERGY	★★★★★
DETOX	★☆☆☆☆
IMMUNITY	★★★★★
DIGESTION	★★☆☆☆
SKIN	★★★☆☆

250 summer mango special

2 mangoes

2 handfuls raspberries

juice of half a lemon

8 tablespoons (120 ml) apple juice

Just as those fantastic Indian mangoes are at the tail end of their season, the raspberries come in – catch this divine combination if you can, otherwise use any good mango.

NUTRIENTS		
Beta-carotene, biotin, folic acid,	ENERGY	★★★★★
vitamin C, vitamin E; calcium, iron,	DETOX	★★☆☆☆
magnesium, manganese, phosphorus,	IMMUNITY	★★★☆☆
potassium, sodium, sulphur	DIGESTION	★★☆☆☆
	SKIN	★★☆☆☆

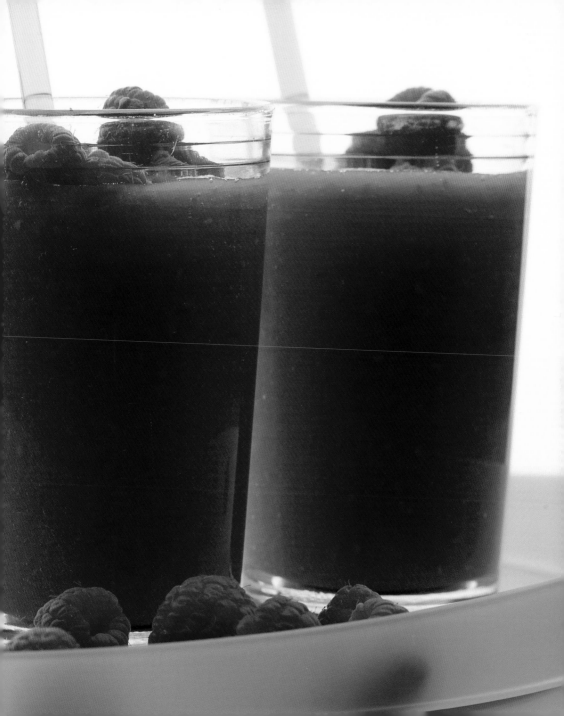

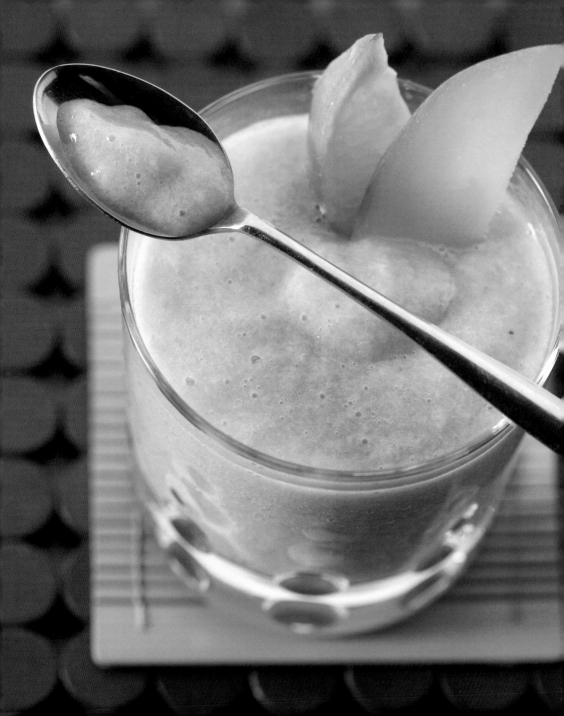

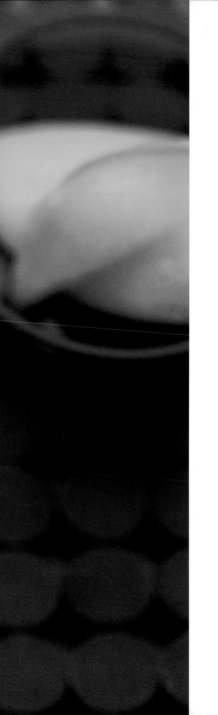

251 tropical deluxe

2 mangoes

2 bananas

juice of a lime

8 tablespoons (120 ml) guava juice

There have to be very few, if any, smoothies that go down this well.

NUTRIENTS
Beta-carotene, folic acid, vitamins B1, B3, B6, C and E; calcium, iron, magnesium, phosphorus, potassium, sodium, sulphur

ENERGY   ★★★★★
DETOX   ★☆☆☆☆
IMMUNITY ★★★★☆
DIGESTION ★★☆☆☆
SKIN   ★★★☆☆

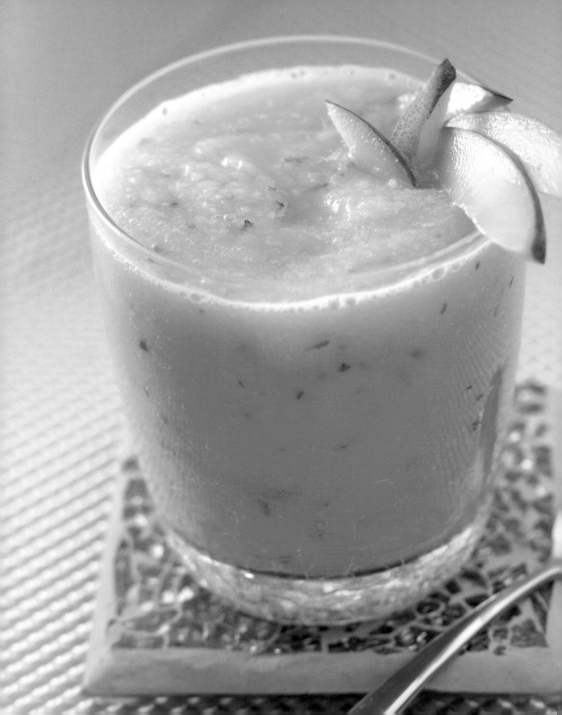

252   nectargo

2 mangoes

2 nectarines

1 orange

8 tablespoons (120 ml) orange juice

A triple-orange whammy with a taste to match. This is also an excellent booster blend for the body's defences.

NUTRIENTS
Beta-carotene, folic acid, vitamin C, vitamin E; calcium, iron, magnesium, phosphorus, potassium, sodium, sulphur

ENERGY ★★★★★

DETOX ★☆☆☆☆

IMMUNITY ★★★★★

DIGESTION ★☆☆☆☆

SKIN ★★★★☆

253 mango blues

2 mangoes

2 handfuls blueberries

juice of a lime

8 tablespoons (120 ml) apple juice

Tropic and temperate fruits kicking up a storm in frothy red.

NUTRIENTS
Beta-carotene, biotin, folic acid,
vitamins B1, B2, B6, C and E; calcium,
chromium, iron, magnesium, phosphorus,
potassium, sodium, sulphur

ENERGY	★★★★★
DETOX	★★☆☆☆
IMMUNITY	★★★★★
DIGESTION	★★☆☆☆
SKIN	★★★★☆

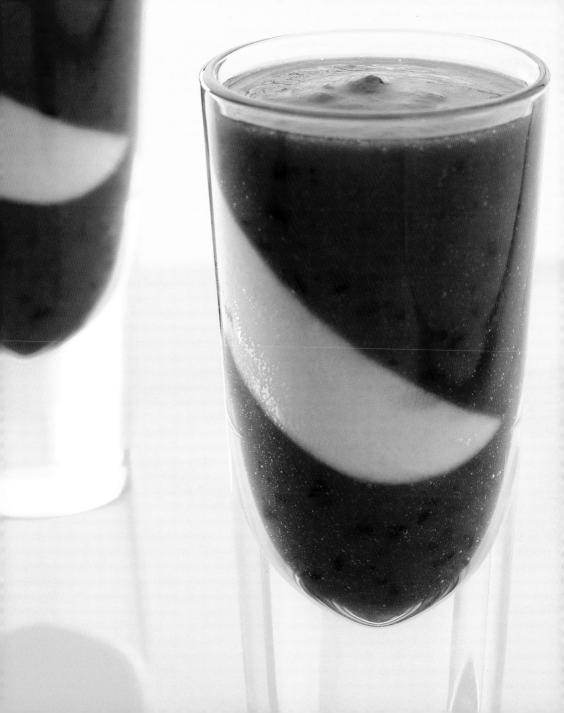

254 pineapple classic

½ pineapple

2 bananas

2 passion fruits

8 tablespoons (120 ml) pineapple juice

An idyllic tropical combo.

NUTRIENTS
Beta-carotene, folic acid, vitamin B3,
vitamin C; calcium, iron, magnesium,
manganese, phosphorus, potassium,
sodium, sulphur

ENERGY	★★★★★
DETOX	★☆☆☆☆
IMMUNITY	★★★☆☆
DIGESTION	★★★☆☆
SKIN	★★★☆☆

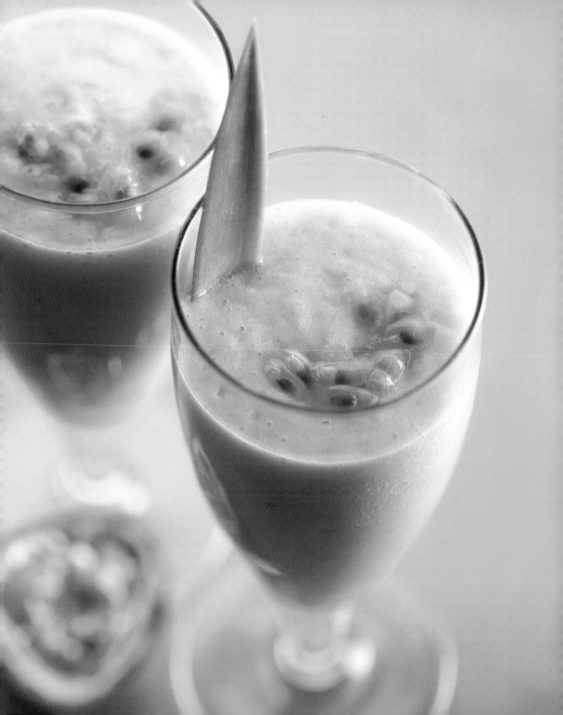

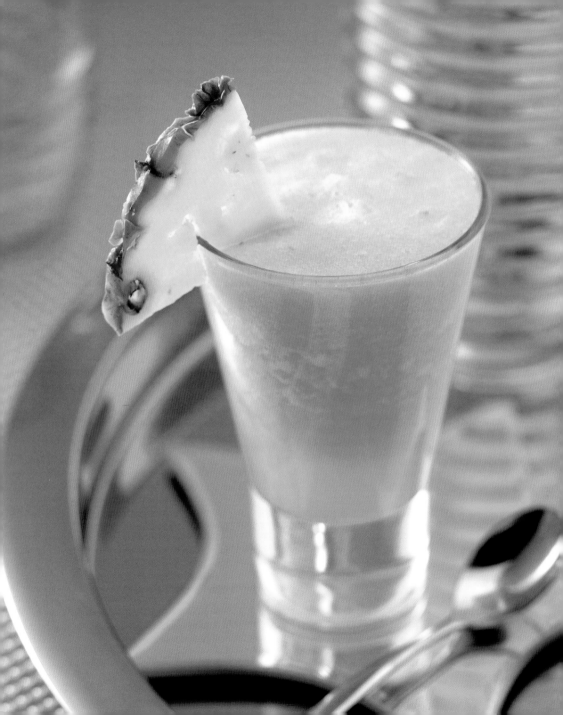

255 citrus pineapple

½ pineapple

2 oranges

juice of a lime

6 tablespoons (90 ml) orange juice

A blend of three tangy flavours
to get your tastebuds singing.

NUTRIENTS
Beta-carotene, folic acid, vitamin C;
calcium, magnesium, manganese,
phosphorus, potassium, sodium

ENERGY	★★★★★
DETOX	★☆☆☆☆
IMMUNITY	★★★★☆
DIGESTION	★★☆☆☆
SKIN	★★☆☆☆

256 pineapple zing

½ pineapple

1 grapefruit

¼ inch (0.5 cm) ginger root, grated

8 tablespoons (120 ml) pineapple juice

If you don't use a sweet, pink grapefruit for this one, you'll be in for a sharp surprise. You decide.

NUTRIENTS
Beta-carotene, folic acid, vitamin C;
calcium, magnesium, manganese,
phosphorus, potassium, sodium,
sulphur

ENERGY	★★★★★
DETOX	★☆☆☆☆
IMMUNITY	★★★★☆
DIGESTION	★★★☆☆
SKIN	★★★☆☆

257 summer refresher

¾ pineapple

1 handful raspberries

5–6 fresh mint leaves

8 tablespoons (120 ml) pineapple juice

A tropical-temperate blend of fruits lifted even higher by the refreshing mint.

NUTRIENTS
Beta-carotene, biotin, folic acid,
vitamin C; calcium, magnesium,
manganese, phosphorus, potassium,
sodium, sulphur

ENERGY	★★★★★
DETOX	★☆☆☆☆
IMMUNITY	★★★☆☆
DIGESTION	★★★☆☆
SKIN	★★★☆☆

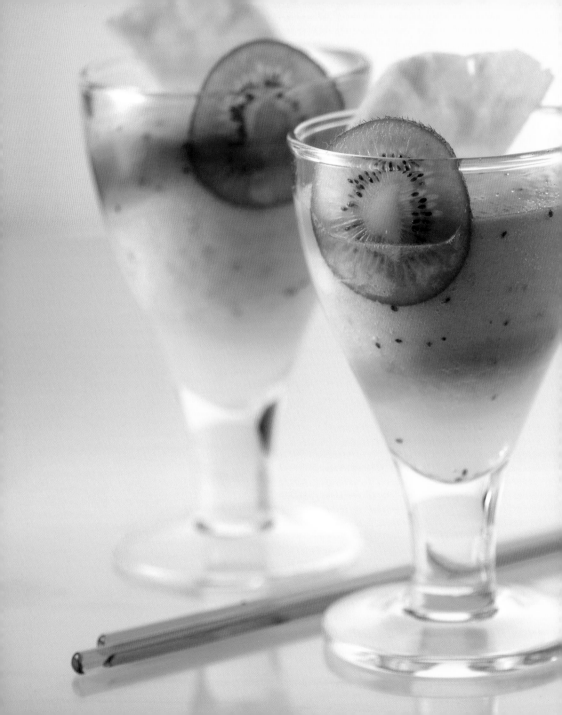

258 pastel perfect

½ pineapple

3 kiwi fruits

8 tablespoons (120 ml) pineapple juice

A delicious mix that can be sharp on the tongue if the fruits aren't nice and ripe, so pick your moment well.

NUTRIENTS
Beta-carotene, folic acid, vitamin C; calcium, magnesium, manganese, phosphorus, potassium, sodium

ENERGY	★★★★★
DETOX	★★☆☆☆
IMMUNITY	★★★★☆
DIGESTION	★★★☆☆
SKIN	★★★☆☆

259 malibu mix

1 pineapple

2 tablespoons (30 ml) coconut milk

½ teaspoon vanilla essence

juice of half a lemon

5 tablespoons (75 ml) pineapple juice

Sit back and enjoy the sunshine. Well, perhaps the central heating... either way, this smoothie is very good and will transport you to tropical climes.

NUTRIENTS
Beta-carotene, folic acid, vitamin C, vitamin E; calcium, magnesium, manganese, phosphorus, potassium, sodium, sulphur

ENERGY	★★★★★
DETOX	★★☆☆☆
IMMUNITY	★★☆☆☆
DIGESTION	★★★☆☆
SKIN	★★☆☆☆

260 apple squared

½ pineapple

2 apples

8 tablespoons (120 ml) apple juice

I was surprised at how well this combination worked out!
Use a relatively sweet apple variety, such as Pink Lady or
Empire, for the perfect contrast.

NUTRIENTS
Beta-carotene, folic acid, vitamin C;
calcium, magnesium, manganese,
phosphorus, potassium, sodium,
sulphur

ENERGY	★★★★★
DETOX	★☆☆☆☆
IMMUNITY	★★★☆☆
DIGESTION	★★★★☆
SKIN	★★★☆☆

.261 **pineberry**

½ pineapple

1 handful cranberries

1 handful strawberries

8 tablespoons (120 ml) pineapple juice

The sharp taste of the cranberries is well balanced by the sweetness of all the other ingredients.

NUTRIENTS
Beta-carotene, biotin, folic acid,
vitamin C; calcium, iron, magnesium,
manganese, phosphorus, potassium,
sodium, sulphur

ENERGY	★★★★★
DETOX	★★☆☆☆
IMMUNITY	★★★★☆
DIGESTION	★★☆☆☆
SKIN	★★★☆☆

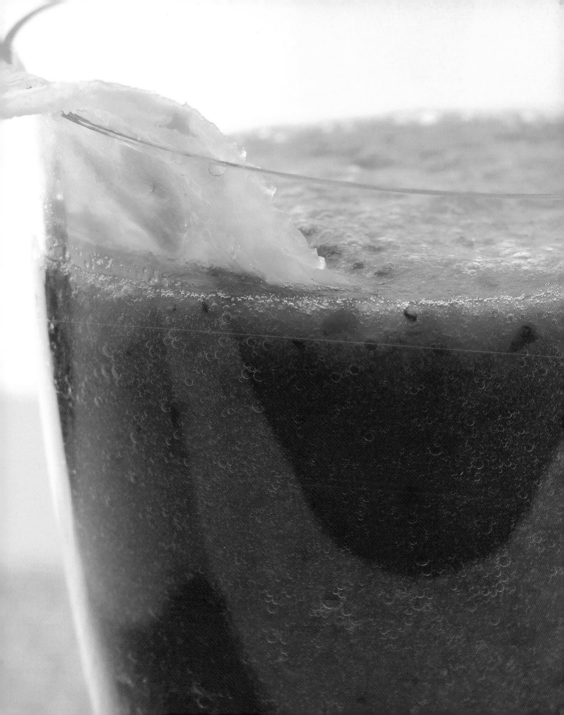

262 sunset crush

½ pineapple

2 thick slices watermelon

a dash orange juice

This is a very juicy combo.

NUTRIENTS
Beta-carotene, folic acid, vitamin
B5, vitamin C; calcium, magnesium,
phosphorus, potassium, sodium; fibre

ENERGY	★★★★★
DETOX	★☆☆☆☆
IMMUNITY	★★★☆☆
DIGESTION	★★★☆☆
SKIN	★★★☆☆

263 scrum

½ pineapple

1 banana

1 handful strawberries

10 tablespoons (150 ml) pineapple (or apple) juice

An absolutely delicious, uncomplicated blend.

NUTRIENTS
Beta-carotene, biotin, folic acid,
vitamin B3, vitamin C; calcium,
magnesium, phosphorus, potassium,
sodium, sulphur; fibre

ENERGY	★★★★★
DETOX	☆☆☆☆☆
IMMUNITY	★★☆☆☆
DIGESTION	★★★★☆
SKIN	★★☆☆☆

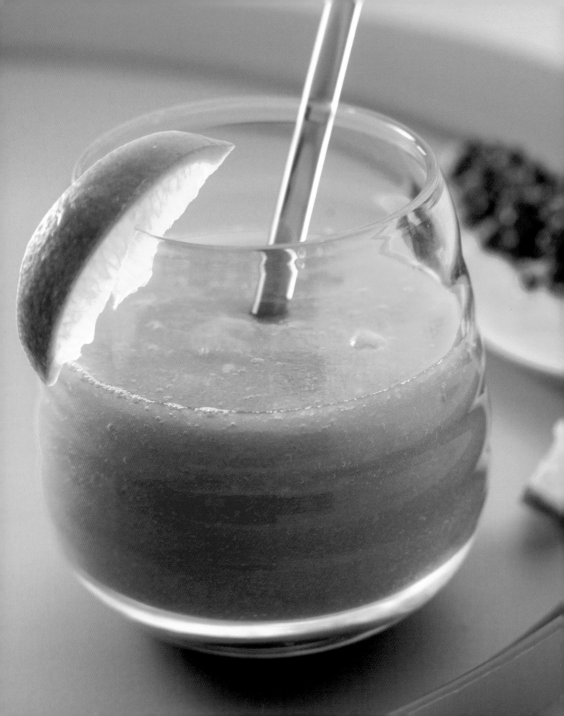

264 papaya pure

2 papayas

juice of a lime

8 tablespoons (120 ml) apple juice

This, the first of three Thai-inspired recipes, is pure Thailand in a glass – whenever you buy a slice of fresh papaya from a street stall in this tropical country, it is always served with a wedge of lime.

NUTRIENTS
Beta-carotene, folic acid, vitamin C; calcium, magnesium, phosphorus, potassium, sodium, sulphur

ENERGY	★★★★★
DETOX	★★★★☆
IMMUNITY	★★★★☆
DIGESTION	★★★★☆
SKIN	★★★★☆

265 papaya salad

1 papaya

¼ pineapple

1 slice watermelon

1 banana

8 tablespoons (120 ml) pineapple juice

This classic combo served to tropical-fruit-hungry foreigners for breakfast in Thailand is a delicious smoothie in any corner of the globe.

NUTRIENTS
Beta-carotene, folic acid, vitamins B1, B3, B5, B6 and C; calcium, magnesium, manganese, phosphorus, potassium, sodium, sulphur

ENERGY	★★★★★
DETOX	★★★☆☆
IMMUNITY	★★★★☆
DIGESTION	★★★★☆
SKIN	★★★★☆

266 identity crisis

1 papaya

3 tangerines

8 tablespoons (120 ml) orange juice

In Thailand, "oranges" are usually green and taste like tangerines. Whatever… this is a wonderfully refreshing blend.

NUTRIENTS
Beta-carotene, folic acid, vitamin C; calcium, magnesium, phosphorus, potassium, sodium

ENERGY	★★★★★
DETOX	★☆☆☆☆
IMMUNITY	★★★★★
DIGESTION	★★☆☆☆
SKIN	★★★☆☆

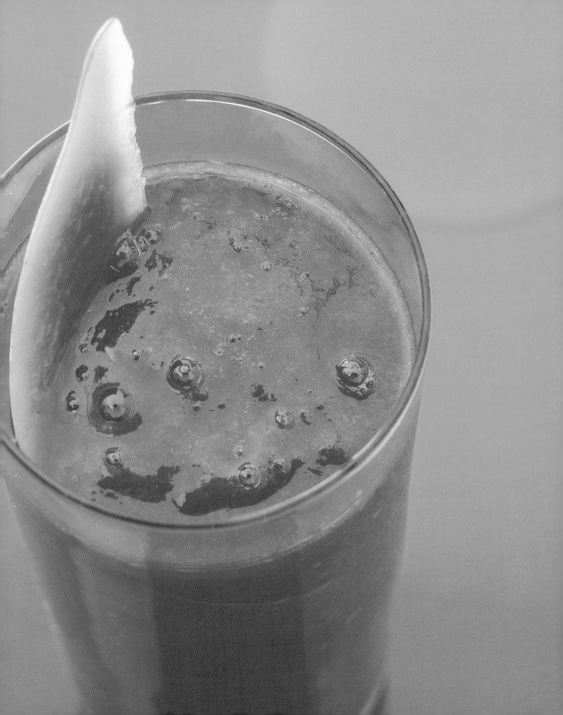

267 heaven scent

1 papaya

1 grapefruit

1 handful raspberries

juice of a lime

8 tablespoons (120 ml) grapefruit juice

A quite magnificent combination of tastes.

NUTRIENTS
Beta-carotene, biotin, folic acid,
vitamin C; calcium, magnesium,
manganese, phosphorus, potassium,
sodium, sulphur

ENERGY	★★★★★
DETOX	★☆☆☆☆
IMMUNITY	★★★★★
DIGESTION	★☆☆☆☆
SKIN	★★★★☆

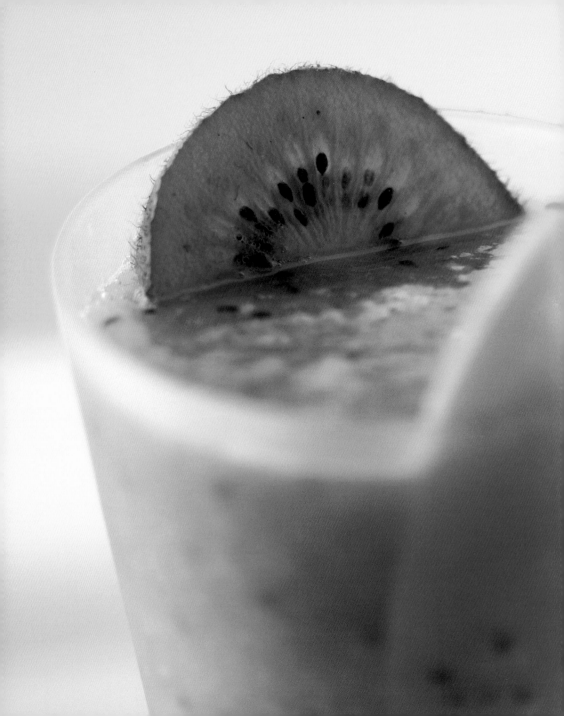

268 globe trotter

1 papaya

2 kiwi fruits

1 pear

8 tablespoons (120 ml) apple juice

This one is certainly a sign of the times – fruit from around the world in one big taste.

NUTRIENTS
Beta-carotene, folic acid, vitamin C; calcium, magnesium, phosphorus, potassium, sodium, sulphur

ENERGY	★★★★★
DETOX	★☆☆☆☆
IMMUNITY	★★★★☆
DIGESTION	★★★☆☆
SKIN	★★★★☆

269 supreme strawberry

2 handfuls strawberries

2 oranges

8 tablespoons (120 ml) guava juice

The most popular berry just got even better.

NUTRIENTS
Beta-carotene, biotin, folic acid,
vitamin B3, vitamin C; calcium,
magnesium, phosphorus, potassium,
sodium, sulphur

ENERGY	★★★★★
DETOX	★☆☆☆☆
IMMUNITY	★★★★★
DIGESTION	☆☆☆☆☆
SKIN	★★★★☆

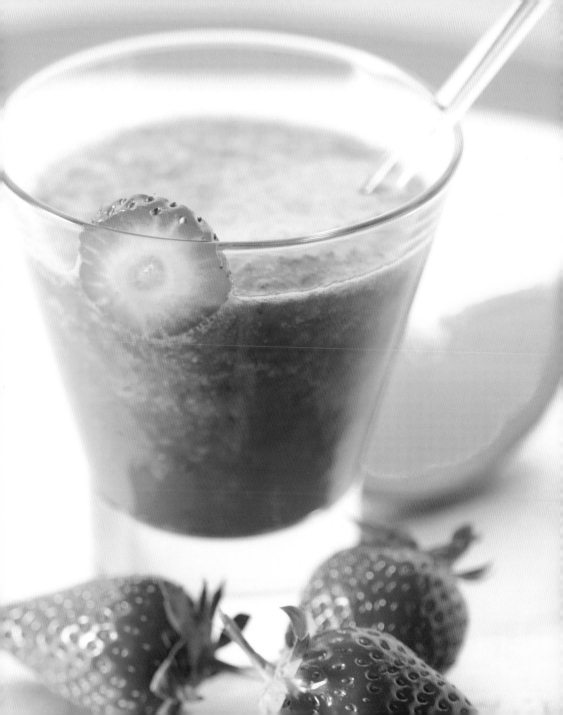

270 strawblend classic

2 handfuls strawberries

1 banana

¼ pineapple

8 tablespoons (120 ml) pineapple juice

Classic favourites, strawberries and banana, with a touch of tang from the tropics create this fabulous staple blend.

NUTRIENTS
Beta-carotene, biotin, folic acid,
vitamins B1, B3, B6 and C; calcium,
magnesium, manganese, phosphorus,
potassium, sodium, sulphur

ENERGY	★★★★★
DETOX	★☆☆☆☆
IMMUNITY	★★★★☆
DIGESTION	★★☆☆☆
SKIN	★★★★☆

271 peachy strawbs

2 handfuls strawberries

3 peaches (or nectarines)

juice of a lime

8 tablespoons (120 ml) orange juice

Summer delight in a glass, and laden with antioxidants for better immunity and healthy skin.

NUTRIENTS
Beta-carotene, biotin, folic acid,
vitamin B3, vitamin C; calcium,
magnesium, phosphorus, potassium,
sodium, sulphur

ENERGY	★★★★★
DETOX	★★☆☆☆
IMMUNITY	★★★★★
DIGESTION	☆☆☆☆☆
SKIN	★★★★★

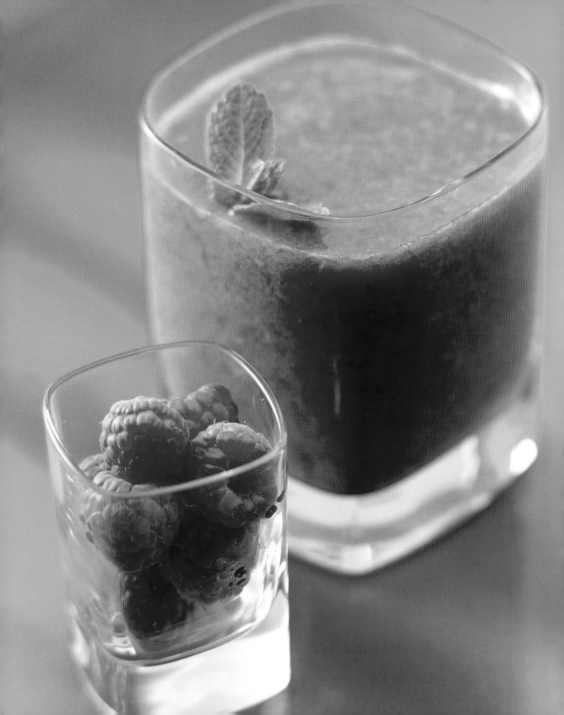

272 pink berry crush

2 handfuls raspberries

2 handfuls strawberries

1 orange

3–4 fresh mint leaves

8 tablespoons (120 ml) orange juice

An easy summer favourite with a hint of mint.

NUTRIENTS
Beta-carotene, biotin, folic acid,
vitamin C; calcium, magnesium,
manganese, phosphorus, potassium,
sodium, sulphur

ENERGY	★★★★★
DETOX	★★☆☆☆
IMMUNITY	★★★★★
DIGESTION	★☆☆☆☆
SKIN	★★★★★

273 citrus strawbs

2 handfuls strawberries

1 pink grapefruit

2 oranges

6 tablespoons (90 ml) orange juice

Another strawberry blend that'll have you coming back for more and more.

NUTRIENTS
Beta-carotene, biotin, folic acid,
vitamin C; calcium, magnesium,
phosphorus, potassium, sulphur

ENERGY	★★★★★
DETOX	★★☆☆☆
IMMUNITY	★★★★☆
DIGESTION	☆☆☆☆☆
SKIN	★★★☆☆

274 berry bonanza II

1 handful raspberries

1 handful strawberries

1 handful blueberries

1 handful blackberries

8 tablespoons (120 ml) apple juice

Just use every type of berry they've got at the shop to create this high-energy, immunity-boosting combo.

NUTRIENTS
Beta-carotene, biotin, folic acid, vitamins B1, B2, B6, C and E; calcium, chromium, iron, magnesium, manganese, phosphorus, potassium, sodium, sulphur

ENERGY	★★★★★
DETOX	★★☆☆☆
IMMUNITY	★★★★★
DIGESTION	★☆☆☆☆
SKIN	★★★★☆

275　blue healer

1 handful blueberries

1 handful blackberries

1 handful blackcurrants

1 banana

10 tablespoons (150 ml) apple juice

Named after a boisterous breed of dog in Australia, this is a rich mix.

NUTRIENTS
Beta-carotene, biotin, folic acid, vitamins
B1, B2, B3, B5, B6, C and E; calcium,
chromium, iron, magnesium, manganese,
phosphorus, potassium, sodium, sulphur

ENERGY ★★★★★
DETOX ★☆☆☆☆
IMMUNITY ★★★★★
DIGESTION ★★☆☆☆
SKIN ★★★★☆

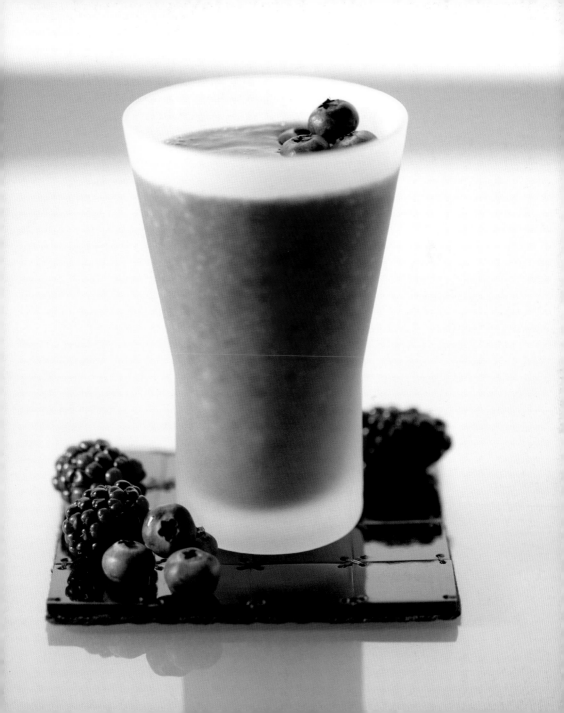

276 apple and black

2 handfuls blackberries

1 handful blackcurrants

2 apples

10 tablespoons (150 ml) apple juice

It's that favourite pie or crumble combination again, without the topping.

NUTRIENTS
Beta-carotene, biotin, folic acid,
vitamins B5, C and E; calcium, iron,
magnesium, phosphorus, potassium,
sodium, sulphur

ENERGY	★★★★★
DETOX	★☆☆☆☆
IMMUNITY	★★★★☆
DIGESTION	★★☆☆☆
SKIN	★★★★★

277 cranapple crush

2 handfuls raspberries

1 handful cranberries

2 apples

10 tablespoons (150 ml) apple juice

Contrasting berries and sweet apples make a delicious drink.

NUTRIENTS
Beta-carotene, biotin, folic acid,
vitamin C; calcium, iron, magnesium,
manganese, phosphorus, potassium,
sodium, sulphur

ENERGY	★★★★★
DETOX	★★☆☆☆
IMMUNITY	★★★★★
DIGESTION	☆☆☆☆☆
SKIN	★★★☆☆

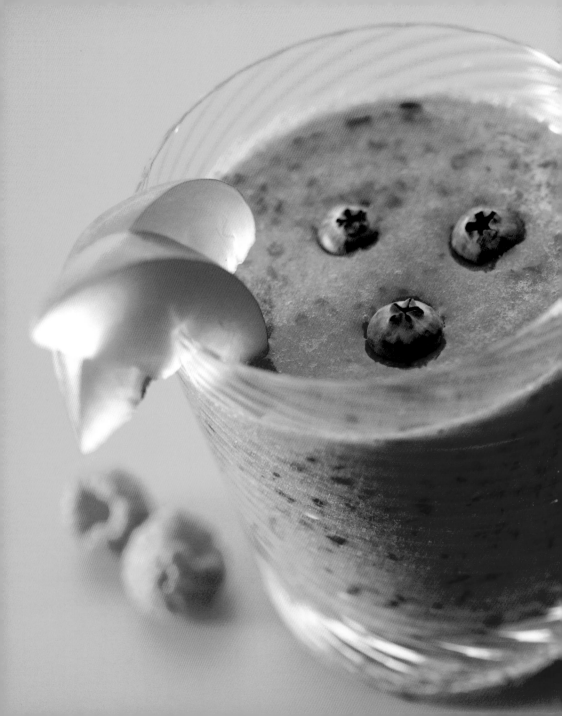

278 raspberry roller

2 handfuls raspberries

1 handful blueberries

1 nectarine (or peach)

10 tablespoons (150 ml) grapefruit juice

A lovely speckled summer blend.

NUTRIENTS
Beta-carotene, biotin, folic acid,
vitamins B1, B2, B6, C and E; calcium,
chromium, magnesium, phosphorus,
potassium, sulphur; fibre

ENERGY	★★★★★
DETOX	★★☆☆☆
IMMUNITY	★★★★☆
DIGESTION	★☆☆☆☆
SKIN	★★★★★

279 panana

3 peaches (or nectarines)

2 bananas

10 tablespoons (150 ml) apple juice

Creamy and sweet – a complete treat.

NUTRIENTS
Beta-carotene, folic acid, vitamins B1,
B3, B6 and C; calcium, magnesium,
phosphorus, potassium, sodium,
sulphur

ENERGY	★★★★★
DETOX	★☆☆☆☆
IMMUNITY	★★★★☆
DIGESTION	★★★☆☆
SKIN	★★★★☆

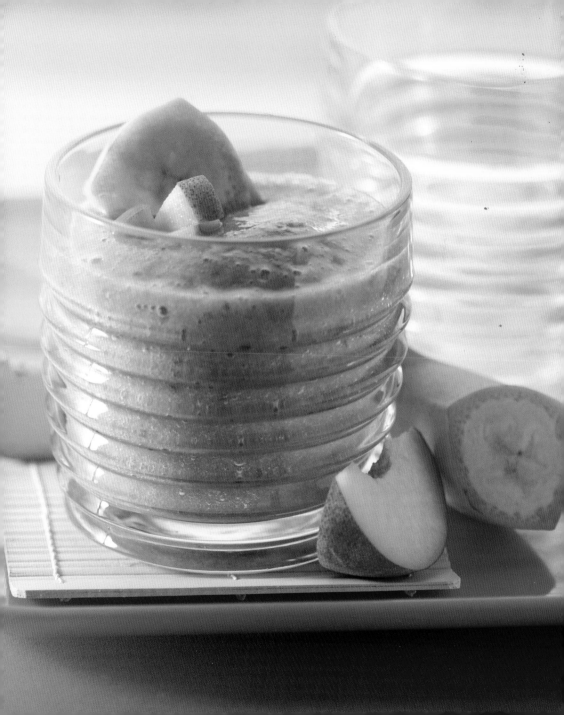

280 peach melba

3 peaches (or nectarines)

1 banana

1 handful raspberries

10 tablespoons (150 ml) apple juice

An exquisite combination bursting with energy and taste.

NUTRIENTS
Beta-carotene, biotin, folic acid,
vitamins B1, B3, B6 and C; calcium,
magnesium, manganese, phosphorus,
potassium, sodium, sulphur

ENERGY	★★★★★
DETOX	★☆☆☆☆
IMMUNITY	★★★★☆
DIGESTION	★★☆☆☆
SKIN	★★★☆☆

281 summer sunset

3 peaches (or nectarines)

2 handfuls strawberries

10 tablespoons (150 ml) guava juice

You won't be able to stop drinking this one – heaven on a summer's day.

NUTRIENTS
Beta-carotene, biotin, folic acid, vitamin B3, vitamin C; calcium, magnesium, phosphorus, potassium, sodium, sulphur

ENERGY ★★★★★
DETOX ★☆☆☆☆
IMMUNITY ★★★★★
DIGESTION ☆☆☆☆☆
SKIN ★★★★★

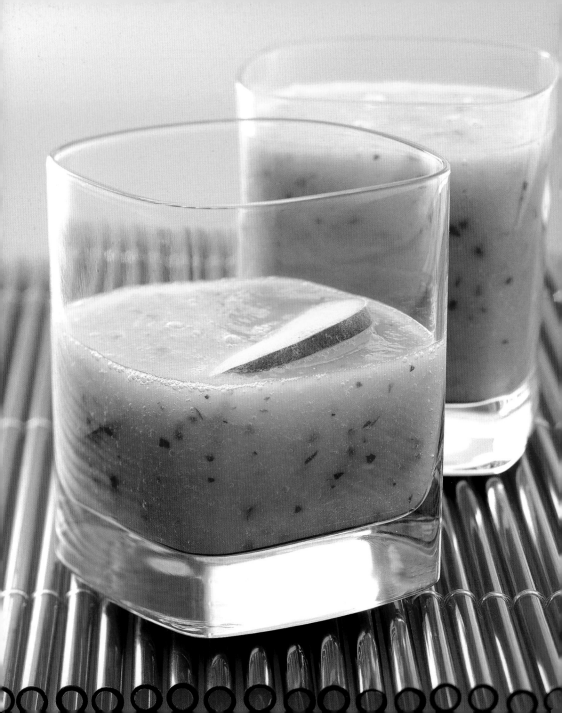

282   creamy orange dream

3 peaches (or nectarines)

1 mango

1 orange

8 tablespoons (120 ml) orange juice

Three different orange-coloured fruits, with wonderfully contrasting tastes and textures.

NUTRIENTS
Beta-carotene, folic acid, vitamin B3,
vitamin C; calcium, iron, magnesium,
phosphorus, potassium, sodium,
sulphur

ENERGY	★★★★★
DETOX	★☆☆☆☆
IMMUNITY	★★★★★
DIGESTION	★☆☆☆☆
SKIN	★★★★★

283   orange peaches

3 peaches (or nectarines)

½ papaya

juice of half a lime

8 tablespoons (120 ml) orange juice

A super hit of beta-carotene for your skin and immune system.

NUTRIENTS
Beta-carotene, folic acid, vitamin
B3, vitamin C; calcium, magnesium,
phosphorus, potassium, sodium,
sulphur; fibre

ENERGY	★★★★★
DETOX	☆☆☆☆☆
IMMUNITY	★★★★★
DIGESTION	★★★★☆
SKIN	★★★★☆

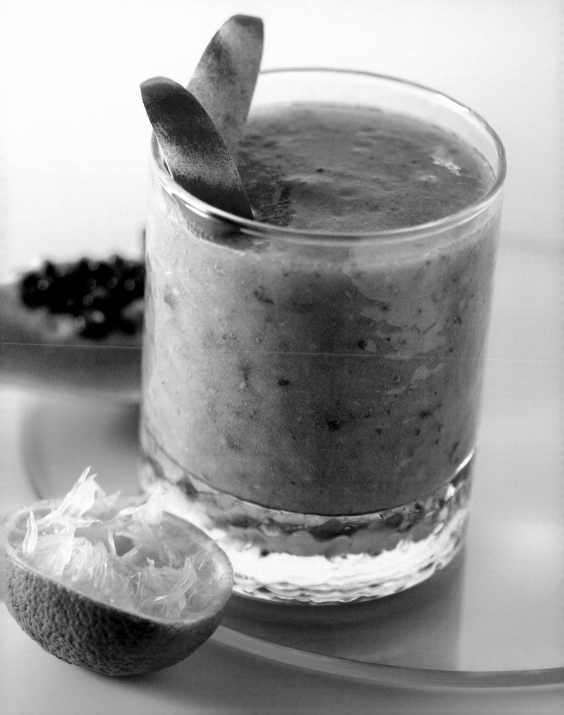

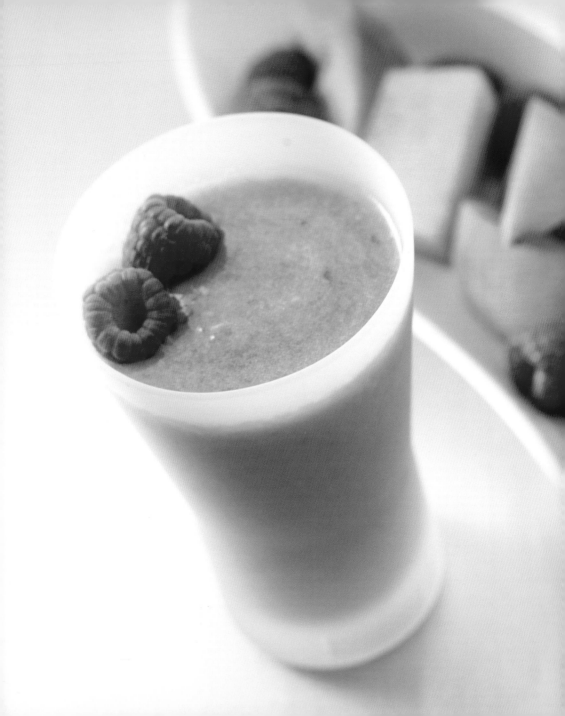

284 pinky peach

3 peaches (or nectarines)

1 thick slice melon

1 handful raspberries

10 tablespoons (150 ml) orange juice

Another wonderful summer combination.

NUTRIENTS
Beta-carotene, biotin, folic acid,
vitamin B3, vitamin C; calcium,
magnesium, phosphorus, potassium,
sodium, sulphur; fibre

ENERGY	★★★★★
DETOX	☆☆☆☆☆
IMMUNITY	★★★★☆
DIGESTION	☆☆☆☆☆
SKIN	★★★★☆

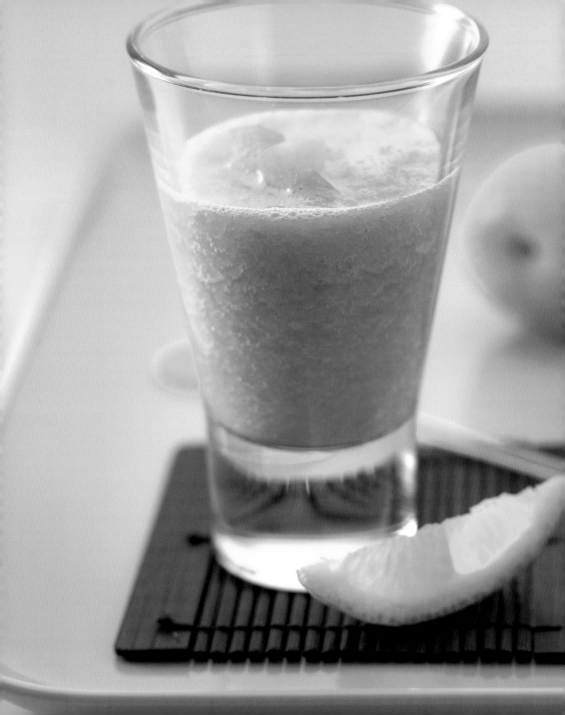

285 orangicot

5 apricots

2 oranges

8 tablespoons (120 ml) orange juice

Tangy and refreshing, with creamy apricots to take the edge off the sharper oranges. Brimming with antioxidants.

NUTRIENTS
Beta-carotene, folic acid, vitamins B1, B3, B5 and C; calcium, magnesium, phosphorus, potassium, sulphur

ENERGY	★★★★★
DETOX	★☆☆☆☆
IMMUNITY	★★★★★
DIGESTION	★☆☆☆☆
SKIN	★★★★★

286 apricot zinger

5 apricots

2 pears

¼ inch (0.5 cm) ginger root, grated

10 tablespoons (150 ml) apple juice

A surprising combination which blends beautifully, thanks to the hot ginger contrasting with the rich, sweeter apricots.

NUTRIENTS
Beta-carotene, folic acid, vitamins
B3, B5 and C; calcium, magnesium,
phosphorus, potassium, sulphur

ENERGY ★★★★★
DETOX ★☆☆☆☆
IMMUNITY ★★★★★
DIGESTION ★★★☆☆
SKIN ★★★★★

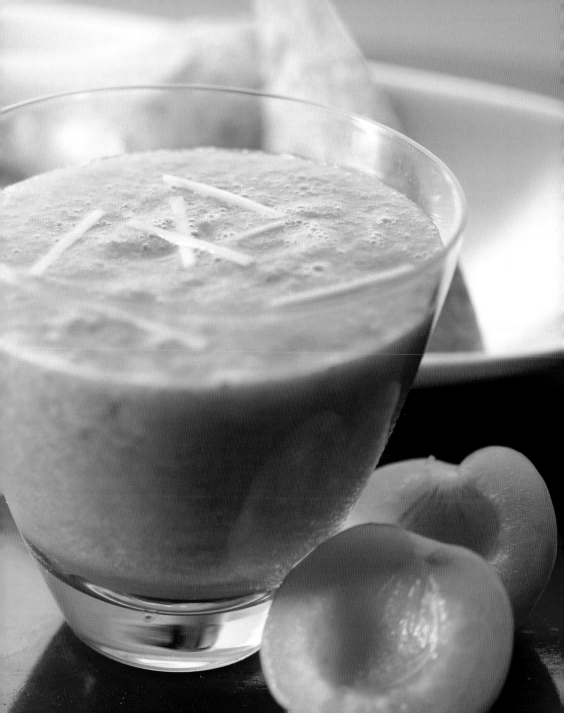

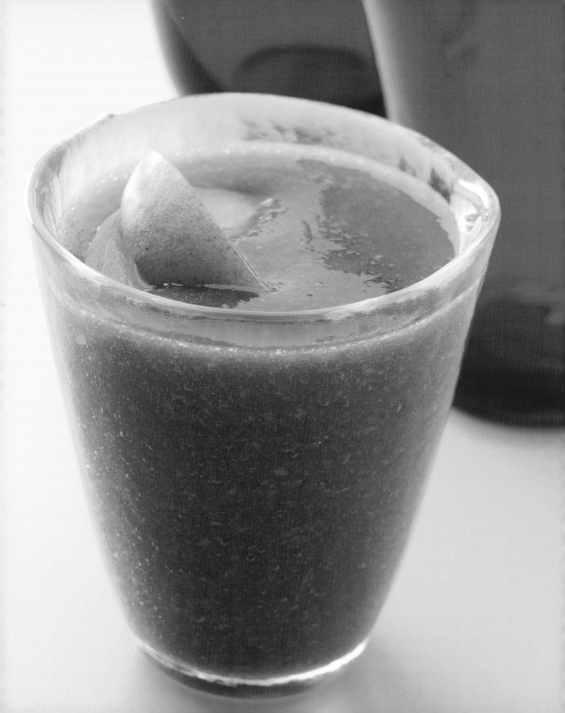

287 sweet 'n' smooth

10 apricots

juice of half a lime

10 tablespoons (150 ml) prune juice

The sweetness of these two combined is fantastic, not to mention good for keeping your guts going.

NUTRIENTS
Beta-carotene, folic acid, vitamins B3,
B5 and C; calcium, magnesium,
phosphorus, potassium, sulphur

ENERGY	★★★★★
DETOX	★☆☆☆☆
IMMUNITY	★★★★★
DIGESTION	★★★★★
SKIN	★★★★★

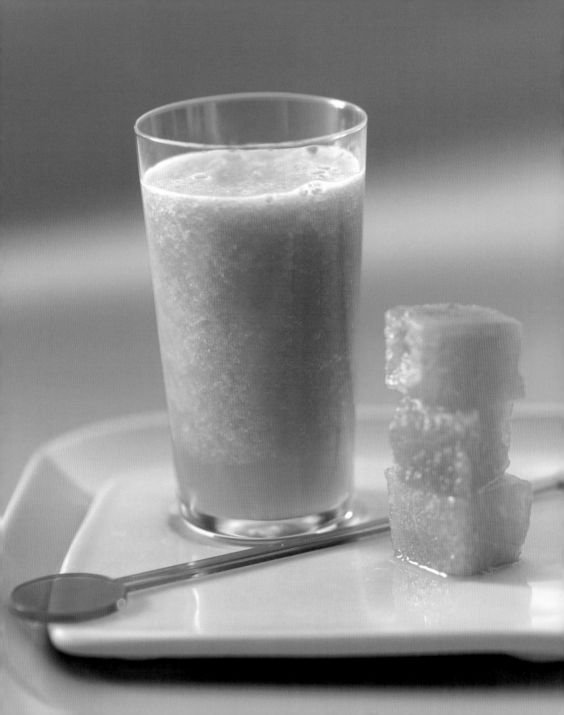

288 pure watermelon

1 small watermelon (or 4 thick slices)

The fruit, the whole fruit and nothing but the fruit. The ground-up seeds add a nutty, not to mention nutritious, touch.

NUTRIENTS
Beta-carotene, folic acid, vitamin B5, vitamin C; calcium, magnesium, phosphorus, potassium, sodium

ENERGY	★★★★★
DETOX	★★★★☆
IMMUNITY	★★★★★
DIGESTION	★★☆☆☆
SKIN	★★★★★

289   watermelon crush

½ small watermelon (or 2 thick slices)

2 handfuls raspberries

A tastebud sensation, and as for the colour…

NUTRIENTS
Beta-carotene, biotin, folic acid,
vitamin B5, vitamin C; calcium,
magnesium, manganese, phosphorus,
potassium, sodium, sulphur

ENERGY ★★★★★
DETOX ★★☆☆☆
IMMUNITY ★★★★★
DIGESTION ★☆☆☆☆
SKIN ★★★★★

290   creamy cooler

½ small watermelon (or 2 thick slices)

1 mango

Bubbling, refreshing and sweet – you can swallow this down only
in huge, noisy, full-of-goodness gulps.

NUTRIENTS
Beta-carotene, folic acid, vitamins B5,
C and E; calcium, iron, magnesium,
phosphorus, potassium, sodium,
sulphur

ENERGY	★★★★★
DETOX	★☆☆☆☆
IMMUNITY	★★★★☆
DIGESTION	★★☆☆☆
SKIN	★★★★☆

291 melon zinger

½ melon

½ pineapple

¼ inch (0.5 cm) ginger root, grated

There's something about this blend that makes the result infinitely greater than the sum of its already fantastic parts.

NUTRIENTS
Beta-carotene, folic acid, vitamin C;
calcium, magnesium, manganese,
phosphorus, potassium, sodium,
sulphur

ENERGY	★★★★★
DETOX	★★☆☆☆
IMMUNITY	★★★★☆
DIGESTION	★★★★☆
SKIN	★★★★☆

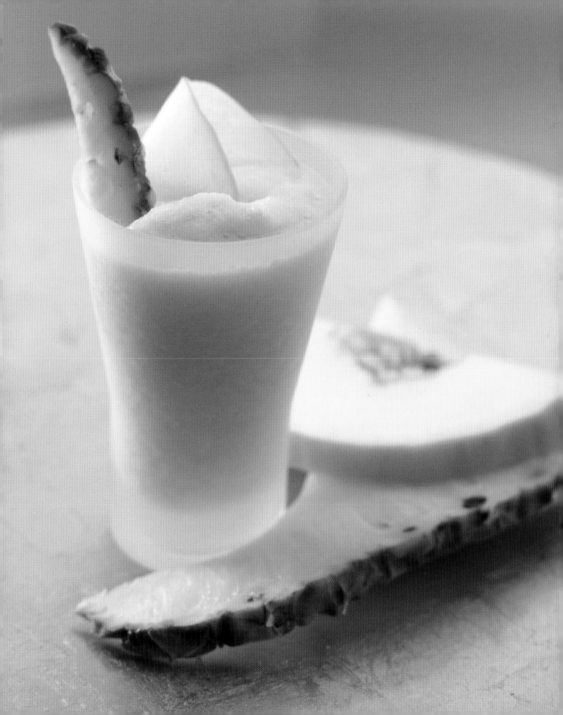

292 green sensation

½ melon

2 kiwi fruits

1 pear

juice of half a lime

4 tablespoons (60 ml) apple juice

Three refreshing fruits blended with juice to make a kicking smoothie.

NUTRIENTS
Beta-carotene, folic acid, vitamin C;
calcium, magnesium, phosphorus,
potassium, sodium, sulphur

ENERGY ★★★★★
DETOX ★★★☆☆
IMMUNITY ★★★★☆
DIGESTION ★★☆☆☆
SKIN ★★★★☆

293   melon sour

1 melon

juice of 2 limes

1 stick celery (with string well removed)

5–6 fresh mint leaves

4 tablespoons (60 ml) apple juice

A great, refreshing cocktail to awaken those sour tastebuds.

NUTRIENTS
Beta-carotene, folic acid, vitamin C;
calcium, magnesium, phosphorus,
potassium, sodium, sulphur

ENERGY	★★★★★
DETOX	★★☆☆☆
IMMUNITY	★★★★☆
DIGESTION	☆☆☆☆☆
SKIN	★★★☆☆

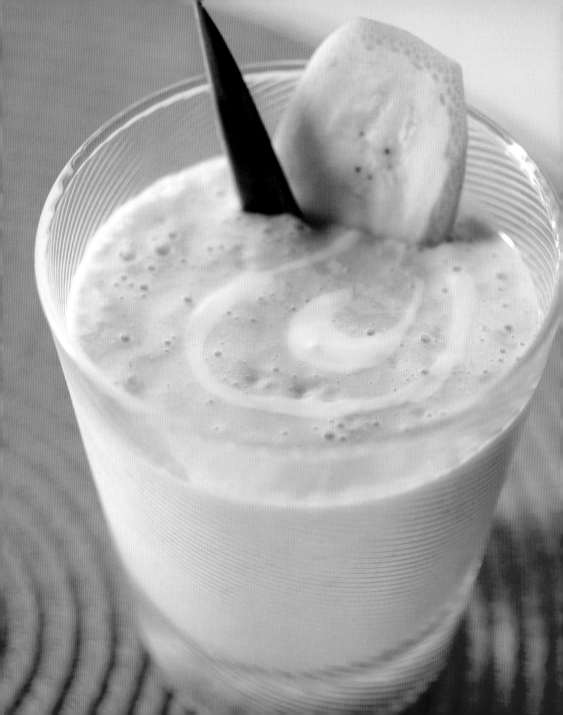

294 creamy pure banana

2 bananas

5 tablespoons (75 ml) natural yogurt

10 tablespoons (150 ml) pineapple juice

Probably the original smoothie – bananas just ask to be made up into a thick, creamy blend like this.

NUTRIENTS
Beta-carotene, folic acid, vitamins B1, B3, B6 and C; calcium, magnesium, manganese, phosphorus, potassium, sulphur, zinc; protein

ENERGY ★★★★☆
DETOX ☆☆☆☆☆
IMMUNITY ★★☆☆☆
DIGESTION ★★★★☆
SKIN ★★★☆☆

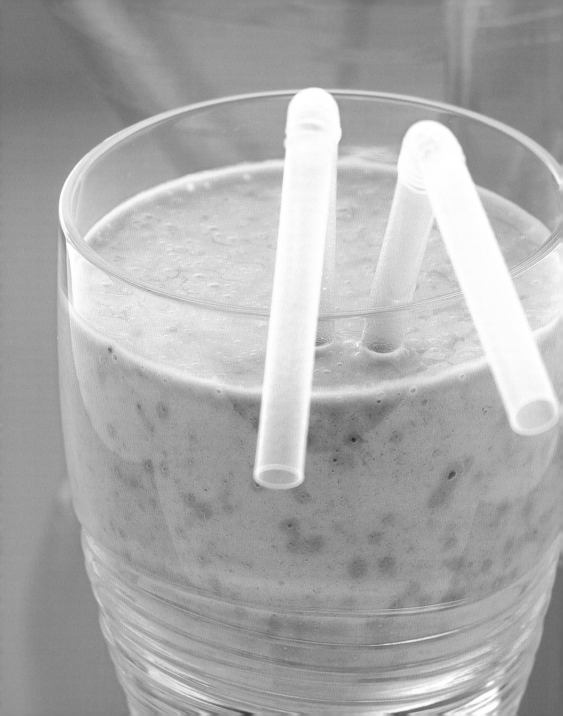

295 creamy bananacot

2 bananas

4 apricots

5 tablespoons (75 ml) natural yogurt

10 tablespoons (150 ml) apricot (or apple) juice

When a fresh apricot is ripe, it is food from the heavens. However, you can make this successfully in winter with apricots canned in juice.

NUTRIENTS
Beta-carotene, folic acid, vitamins B1, B3, B5, B6 and C; calcium, magnesium, phosphorus, potassium, sulphur, zinc; protein

ENERGY	★★★★☆
DETOX	☆☆☆☆☆
IMMUNITY	★★★☆☆
DIGESTION	★★★★☆
SKIN	★★★☆☆

296 creamy black banana

1 banana

2 heaped tablespoons blackcurrants

5 tablespoons (75 ml) natural yogurt

10 tablespoons (150 ml) apple juice (or the juice
from the blackcurrants, if they come from a can)

This is my all-time favourite combination – rich banana and
tangy blackcurrants. You can even make it throughout the winter
using blackcurrants canned in natural juice. Try crunching on the
blackcurrant seeds as they are full of healthy oils.

NUTRIENTS
Beta-carotene, biotin, vitamins B1, B3,
B5, B6, C and E; calcium, magnesium,
phosphorus, potassium, sodium,
sulphur, zinc; protein

ENERGY	★★★★☆
DETOX	☆☆☆☆☆
IMMUNITY	★★★★☆
DIGESTION	★★★☆☆
SKIN	★★★★☆

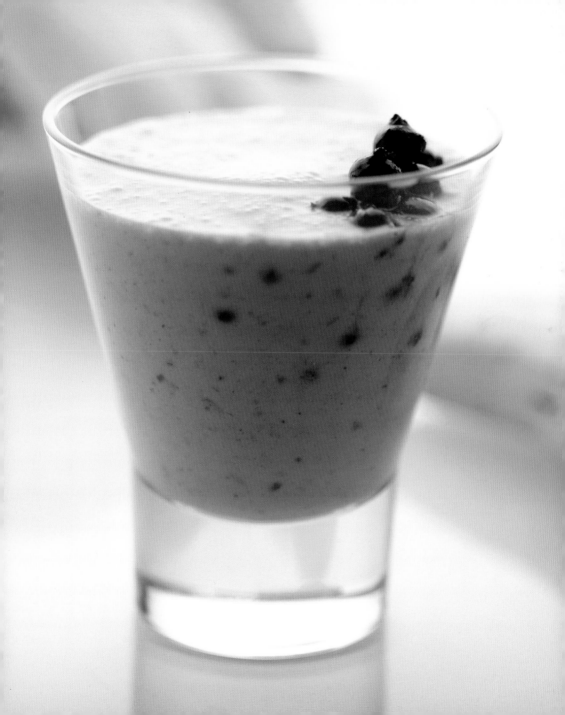

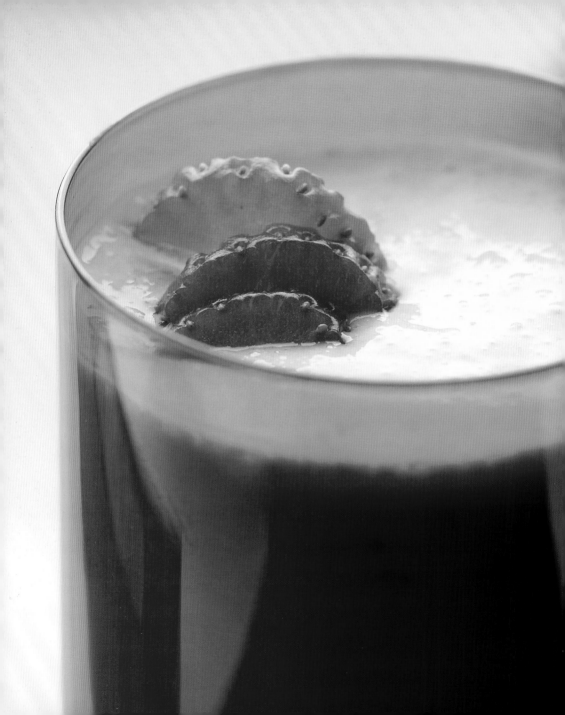

297 creamy pink banana

1 banana

2 handfuls strawberries

5 tablespoons (75 ml) natural yogurt

8 tablespoons (120 ml) apple juice

Another favourite combination of mine – best in the summer with juicy, fresh, flavoursome, organic strawberries.

NUTRIENTS
Beta-carotene, biotin, folic acid, vitamins B1, B3, B6 and C; calcium, magnesium, phosphorus, potassium, sulphur, zinc; protein

ENERGY	★★★★☆
DETOX	☆☆☆☆☆
IMMUNITY	★★★★☆
DIGESTION	★★★☆☆
SKIN	★★★★☆

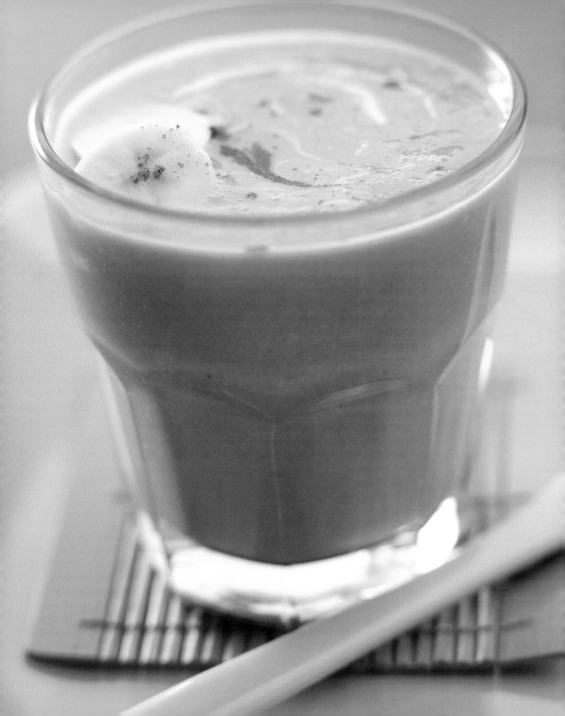

298 creamy green banana

1 banana

¼ pineapple

1 heaped teaspoon spirulina

5 tablespoons (75 ml) natural yogurt

6 tablespoons (90 ml) pineapple juice

This isn't to say you should use green bananas, but you turn a pale yellow smoothie into a pastel green by adding the spirulina.

NUTRIENTS
Beta-carotene, folic acid, vitamins B1, B3, B5, B6 and C; calcium, iron, magnesium, manganese, phosphorus, potassium, sodium, sulphur, zinc; protein; essential fatty acids

ENERGY	★★★★☆
DETOX	★★★☆☆
IMMUNITY	★★★☆☆
DIGESTION	★★★★☆
SKIN	★★☆☆☆

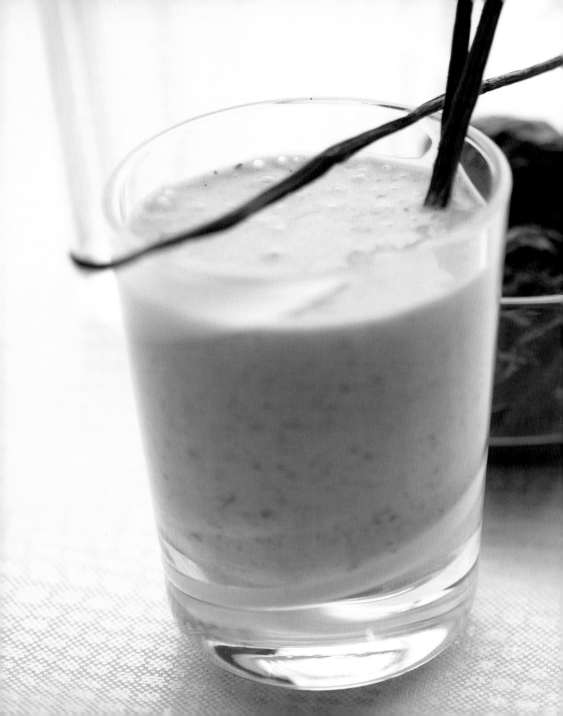

299 vanilla banana

2 bananas

8 rehydrated prunes

3 drops vanilla essence

5 tablespoons (75 ml) natural yogurt

6 tablespoons (90 ml) pineapple juice

This turns out a tasty, very sweet smoothie. If you don't have any prunes to hand or don't like them, use dried apricots instead. Both are best left to soak overnight first.

NUTRIENTS
Beta-carotene, folic acid, vitamins B1, B3, B6 and C; calcium, magnesium, manganese, phosphorus, potassium, sodium, sulphur, zinc; protein

ENERGY	★★★★★
DETOX	★☆☆☆☆
IMMUNITY	★★★★☆
DIGESTION	★★★★☆
SKIN	★★★☆☆

300 creamy passion

2 bananas

4 passion fruits

5 tablespoons (75 ml) natural yogurt

10 tablespoons (150 ml) guava juice

Surely one of the most exquisite combinations of fruit ever,
bound up with creamy yogurt to become a meal in itself.

NUTRIENTS
Beta-carotene, folic acid, vitamins B1,
B3, B6 and C; calcium, iron, magnesium,
phosphorus, potassium, sodium,
sulphur; protein

ENERGY	★★★★☆
DETOX	☆☆☆☆☆
IMMUNITY	★★★☆☆
DIGESTION	★★★☆☆
SKIN	★★☆☆☆

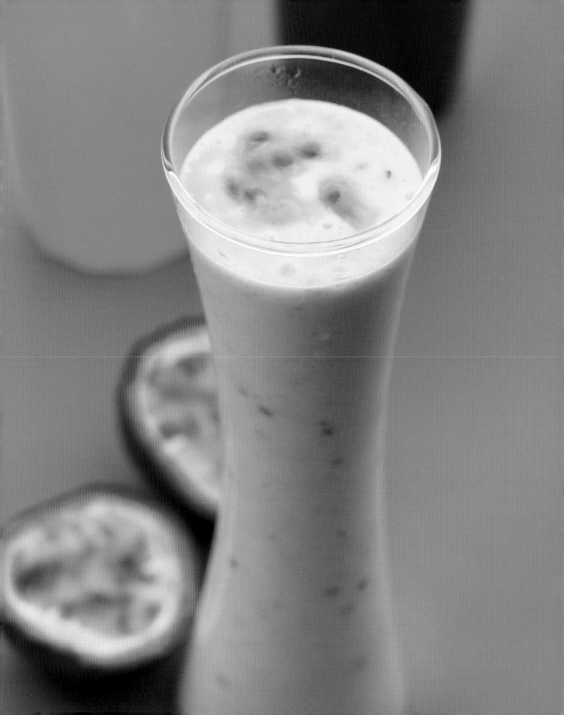

301 tropical tang

1 banana

½ mango

½ pineapple

4 tablespoons (60 ml) pineapple juice

5 tablespoons (75 ml) natural yogurt

This one reminds me of my first backpacking trip to an idyllic beach in Thailand when smoothies were on the menu for only a couple of hours a day – when the generator was turned on and the blender could be powered up.

NUTRIENTS
Beta-carotene, folic acid, vitamins B1, B3, B6, C and E; calcium, iron, magnesium, manganese, phosphorus, potassium, sodium, sulphur, zinc; protein

ENERGY	★★★★☆
DETOX	★☆☆☆☆
IMMUNITY	★★★★☆
DIGESTION	★★★★☆
SKIN	★★★☆☆

302   peachy banana dream

2 bananas

2 peaches

2 tangerines

5 tablespoons (75 ml) natural yogurt

8 tablespoons (120 ml) orange juice

Juicy, ripe peaches (or nectarines) make this one a dream combination, full of energy, with the creaminess offset by the citrus.

NUTRIENTS
Beta-carotene, folic acid, vitamins B1,
B3, B6 and C; calcium, magnesium,
phosphorus, potassium, sodium,
sulphur, zinc; protein

ENERGY	★★★★☆
DETOX	★☆☆☆☆
IMMUNITY	★★★★☆
DIGESTION	★★★☆☆
SKIN	★★★☆☆

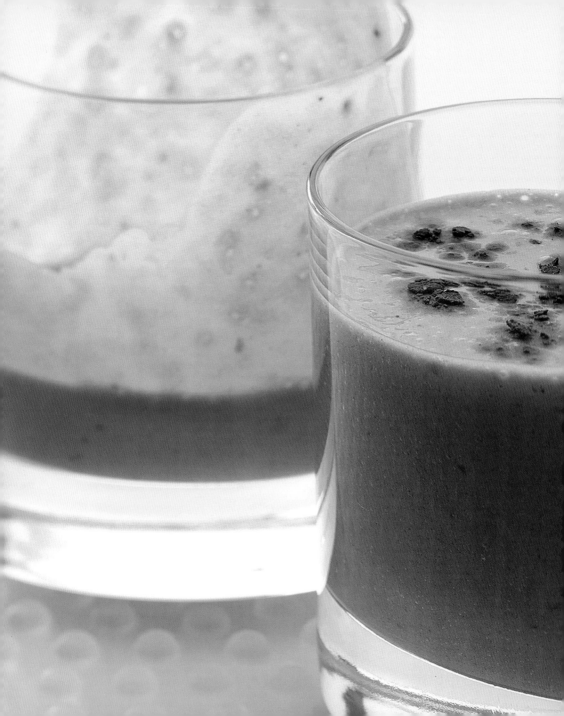

303 banana heaven

2 bananas

4 dates (pitted)

1 teaspoon cocoa powder

½ teaspoon vanilla essence

1 teaspoon honey

1 teaspoon tahini

5 tablespoons (75 ml) natural yogurt

10 tablespoons (150 ml) pineapple juice

Unbelievably good – you'll wonder whether you're actually drinking a wickedly rich ice cream.

NUTRIENTS
Beta-carotene, folic acid, vitamins B1, B3, B6 and C; calcium, magnesium, phosphorus, potassium, sulphur, zinc; protein; essential fatty acids

ENERGY	★★★★★
DETOX	☆☆☆☆☆
IMMUNITY	★★★☆☆
DIGESTION	★★★☆☆
SKIN	★★★★☆

304 creamy pure mango

2 mangoes

¼ teaspoon ground cardamom

5 tablespoons (75 ml) natural yogurt

6 tablespoons (90 ml) pineapple juice

Dense and rich, this is a high-energy blend, with a hint of my favourite spice. Just leave it out if you don't like cardamom.

NUTRIENTS
Beta-carotene, folic acid, vitamin C, vitamin E; calcium, iron, magnesium, manganese, phosphorus, potassium, sodium, sulphur, zinc; protein

ENERGY	★★★★☆
DETOX	★★☆☆☆
IMMUNITY	★★★★☆
DIGESTION	★★★☆☆
SKIN	★★★☆☆

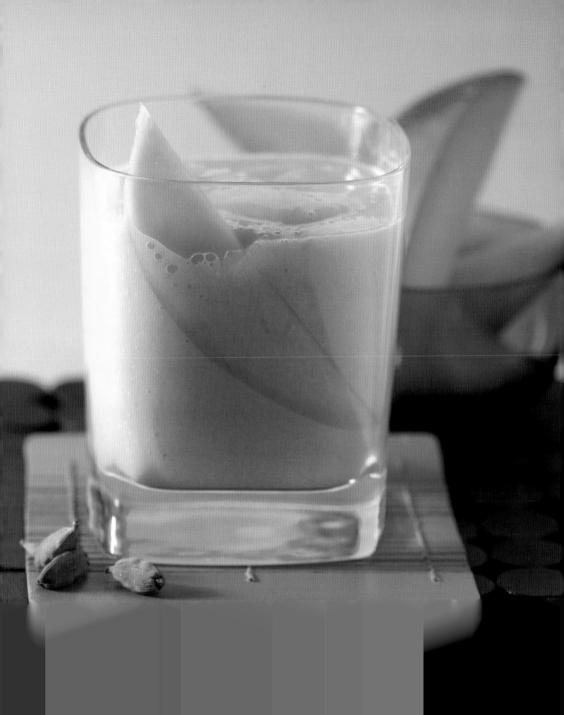

305 magical mango

1 mango

1 banana

5 tablespoons (75 ml) natural yogurt

10 tablespoons (150 ml) orange juice

Creamy and sweet – free transport to the tropics included.

NUTRIENTS
Beta-carotene, folic acid, vitamins B1,
B3, B6, C and E; calcium, iron,
magnesium, phosphorus, potassium,
sodium, sulphur, zinc; protein

ENERGY ★★★★☆
DETOX ☆☆☆☆☆
IMMUNITY ★★★☆☆
DIGESTION ★★★☆☆
SKIN ★★★☆☆

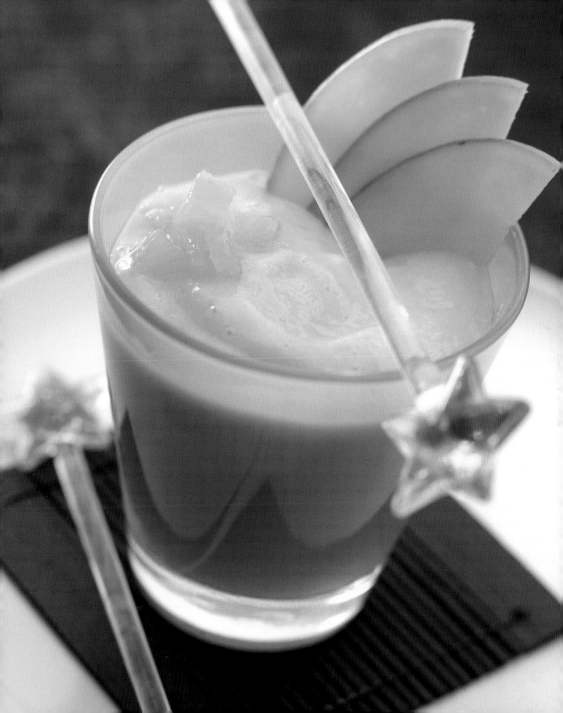

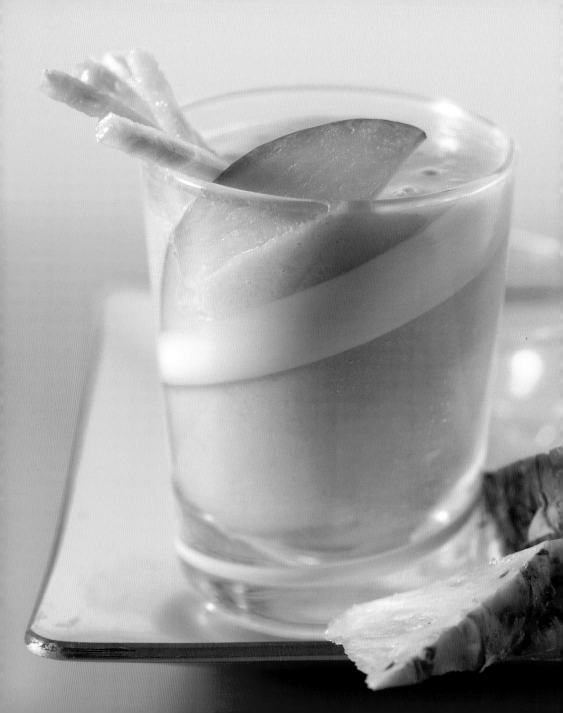

306 mango mango

2 mangoes

5 tablespoons (75 ml) natural yogurt

6 tablespoons (90 ml) pineapple juice

One of the fruits that was just made
to be blended with yogurt.

NUTRIENTS
Beta carotene, folic acid, vitamin C,
vitamin E; calcium, iron, magnesium,
manganese, phosphorus, potassium,
sodium, sulphur, zinc; protein

ENERGY	★★★★☆
DETOX	★☆☆☆☆
IMMUNITY	★★★★☆
DIGESTION	★★★★☆
SKIN	★★★☆☆

307 pango mango

2 mangoes

2 peaches

½ teaspoon vanilla essence

5 tablespoons (75 ml) natural yogurt

8 tablespoons (120 ml) orange juice

Two fantastically fruity, orange-coloured fruits taken to
another realm by the hint of vanilla, which seems to make
the smoothie even sweeter.

NUTRIENTS
Beta-carotene, folic acid, vitamins B3,
C and E; calcium, iron, magnesium,
phosphorus, potassium, sodium,
sulphur, zinc; protein

ENERGY ★★★★☆
DETOX ★☆☆☆☆
IMMUNITY ★★★★☆
DIGESTION ★★★☆☆
SKIN ★★★★☆

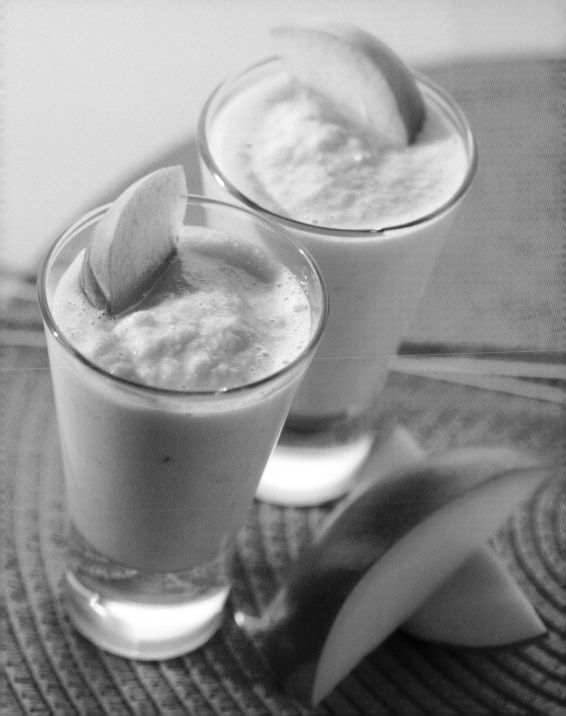

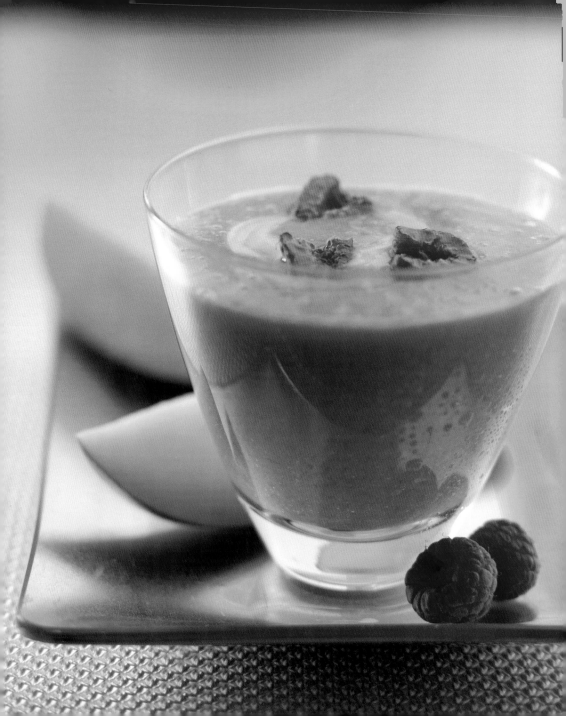

308   pinky mango

2 mangoes

2 handfuls raspberries

juice of half a lemon

5 tablespoons (75 ml) natural yogurt

8 tablespoons (120 ml) apple juice

Who said, "East is East and West is West"? The twain
meet superbly here.

NUTRIENTS
Beta-carotene, biotin, folic acid, vitamin
C, vitamin E; calcium, iron, magnesium,
manganese, phosphorus, potassium,
sodium, sulphur, zinc; protein

ENERGY	★★★★☆
DETOX	★☆☆☆☆
IMMUNITY	★★★★☆
DIGESTION	★★★☆☆
SKIN	★★★☆☆

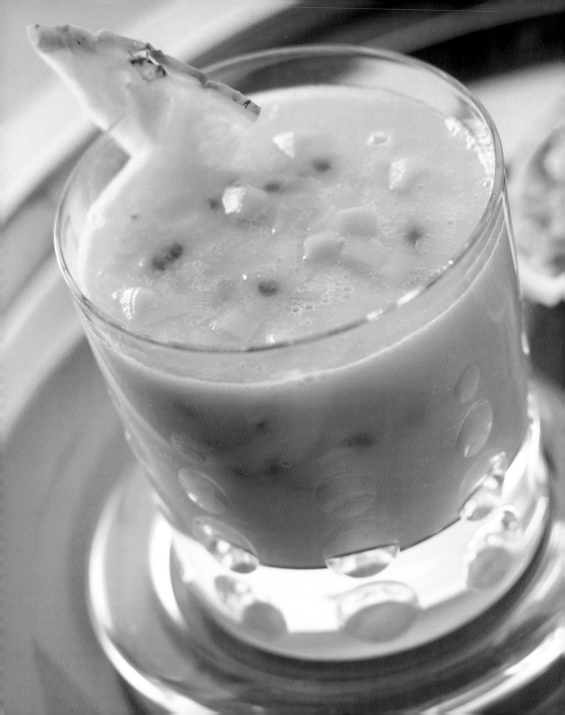

309 tropical mango medley

1 mango

½ pineapple

1 banana

1 passion fruit

5 tablespoons (75 ml) natural yogurt

6 tablespoons (90 ml) pineapple juice

A delicious, creamy drink redolent of breakfast on a palm-fringed beach.

NUTRIENTS
Beta-carotene, folic acid, vitamins B1, B3, B6, C and E; calcium, iron, magnesium, manganese, phosphorus, potassium, sodium, sulphur, zinc; protein

ENERGY	★★★★☆
DETOX	★☆☆☆☆
IMMUNITY	★★★★☆
DIGESTION	★★★★☆
SKIN	★★★☆☆

310 berry mango

1 mango

1 handful strawberries

¼ pineapple

5 tablespoons (75 ml) natural yogurt

6 tablespoons (90 ml) pineapple juice

The tangy pineapple contrasts deliciously with the creamy mango and sweet strawberries.

NUTRIENTS
Beta-carotene, folic acid, vitamin C,
vitamin E; calcium, iron, magnesium,
manganese, phosphorus, potassium,
sodium, sulphur, zinc; protein

ENERGY	★★★★☆
DETOX	★☆☆☆☆
IMMUNITY	★★★★☆
DIGESTION	★★★★☆
SKIN	★★★★☆

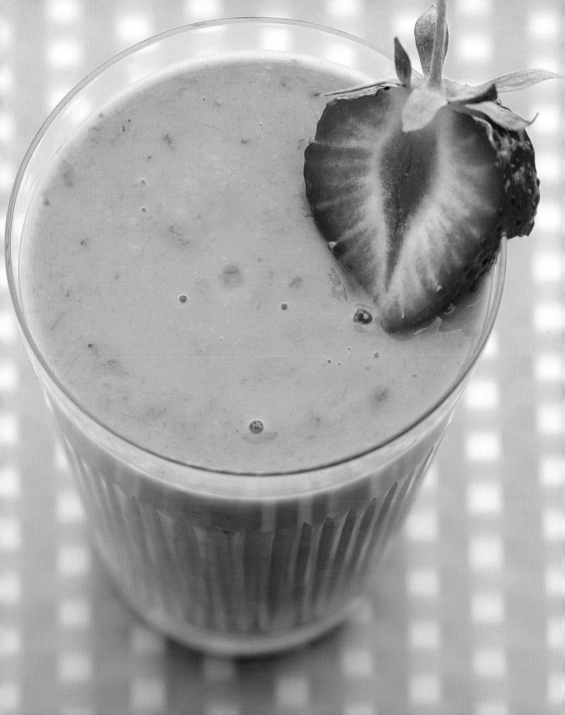

311 cocogo

2 mangoes

1 tablespoon (15 ml) coconut milk

½ teaspoon vanilla essence

5 tablespoons (75 ml) natural yogurt

6 tablespoons (90 ml) pineapple juice

A sweet, creamy drink with the tropical taste of coconut. Another one to transport you to sunny climes.

NUTRIENTS
Beta-carotene, folic acid, vitamin C, vitamin E; calcium, iron, magnesium, phosphorus, potassium, sodium, sulphur, zinc; protein

ENERGY	★★★★☆
DETOX	★☆☆☆☆
IMMUNITY	★★★★☆
DIGESTION	★★★☆☆
SKIN	★★★☆☆

312   passionate about mangoes

2 mangoes

2 tangerines

2 passion fruits

5 tablespoons (75 ml) natural yogurt

8 tablespoons (120 ml) pineapple juice

Just when you thought mangoes couldn't get any better, in jumps
passion fruit, and both are offset by the citrusy tangerines.

NUTRIENTS
Beta-carotene, folic acid, vitamins B3,
C and E; calcium, iron, magnesium,
phosphorus, potassium, sodium,
sulphur, zinc; protein

ENERGY	★★★★☆
DETOX	★☆☆☆☆
IMMUNITY	★★★★☆
DIGESTION	★★☆☆☆
SKIN	★★★☆☆

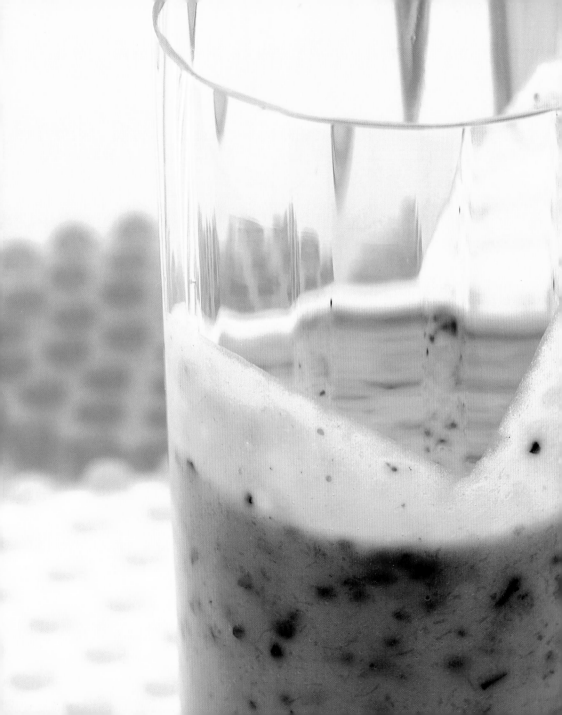

313 flecked mango

2 mangoes

2 handfuls blueberries

5 tablespoons (75 ml) natural yogurt

8 tablespoons (120 ml) apple juice

I love the flecks of blue that the skins of the berries dot throughout this drink, let alone the sublime taste they produce.

NUTRIENTS

Beta-carotene, biotin, folic acid, vitamins B1, B2, B6, C and E; calcium, chromium, iron, magnesium, phosphorus, potassium, sodium, sulphur, zinc; protein

ENERGY	★★★★☆
DETOX	★☆☆☆☆
IMMUNITY	★★★★☆
DIGESTION	★★★☆☆
SKIN	★★★☆☆

314 pink melon

2 handfuls strawberries

½ melon

5 tablespoons (75 ml) natural yogurt

6 tablespoons (90 ml) apple juice

Even though I don't normally like melon with yogurt, this blend is fantastic.

NUTRIENTS
Beta-carotene, biotin, folic acid, vitamin C; calcium, magnesium, phosphorus, potassium, sodium, sulphur; protein

ENERGY	★★★★☆
DETOX	★☆☆☆☆
IMMUNITY	★★★★☆
DIGESTION	★★★☆☆
SKIN	★★★★☆

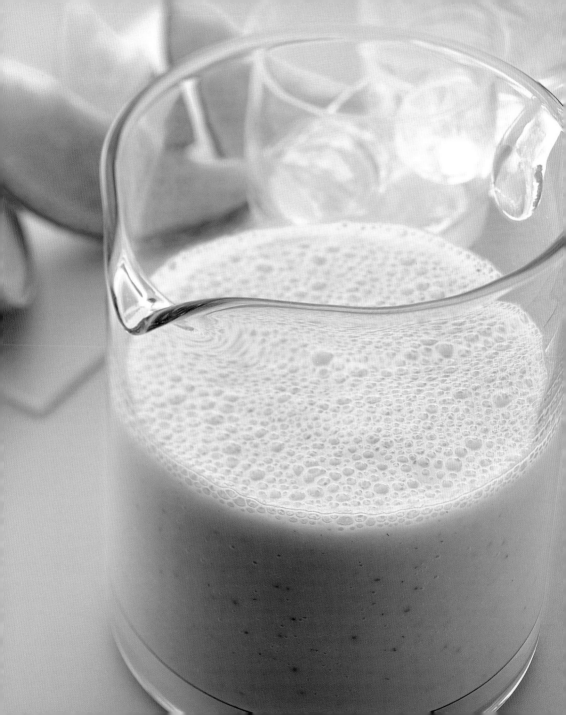

315 pure pink thickie

2 handfuls strawberries

3 handfuls raspberries

5 tablespoons (75 ml) natural yogurt

6 tablespoons (90 ml) mineral water

Everybody's summer favourites in a thick, creamy drink. Berries lend themselves perfectly to creamy smoothies.

NUTRIENTS
Beta-carotene, biotin, folic acid,
vitamin C; calcium, magnesium,
manganese, phosphorus, potassium,
sodium, sulphur; protein

ENERGY	★★★★☆
DETOX	★☆☆☆☆
IMMUNITY	★★★★☆
DIGESTION	★★☆☆☆
SKIN	★★★★☆

316   creamy pink banana II

1 handful strawberries

1 handful raspberries

1 banana

5 tablespoons (75 ml) natural yogurt

6 tablespoons (90 ml) apple juice

Pink berry treats with another firm favourite.

NUTRIENTS
Beta-carotene, biotin, folic acid,
vitamins B1, B3, B6 and C; calcium,
magnesium, manganese, phosphorus,
potassium, sodium, sulphur; protein

ENERGY ★★★★☆
DETOX ★☆☆☆☆
IMMUNITY ★★★★☆
DIGESTION ★★★☆☆
SKIN ★★★☆☆

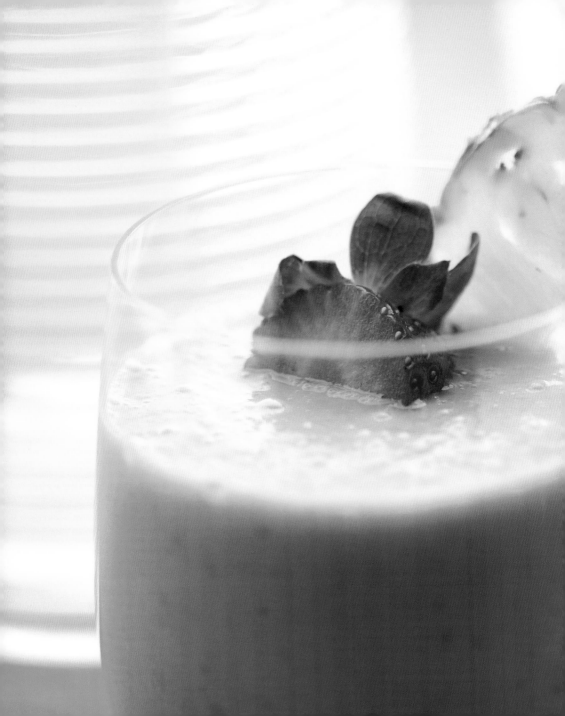

317 tropical pinkie

1 handful strawberries

1 handful raspberries

½ pineapple

5 tablespoons (75 ml) natural yogurt

6 tablespoons (90 ml) pineapple juice

Pineapple crushes up fantastically with these succulent berries.

NUTRIENTS
Beta-carotene, biotin, folic acid, vitamin C; calcium, magnesium, manganese, phosphorus, potassium, sodium, sulphur; protein

ENERGY	★★★★☆
DETOX	★☆☆☆☆
IMMUNITY	★★★★☆
DIGESTION	★★★☆☆
SKIN	★★★☆☆

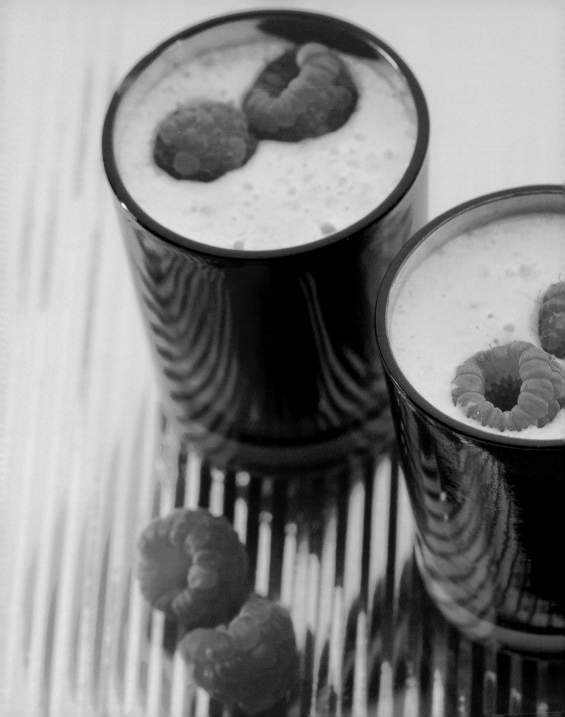

318 creamy berry tang

2 handfuls raspberries

2 oranges

5 tablespoons (75 ml) natural yogurt

6 tablespoons (90 ml) guava juice

The guava juice really brings out the flavours in this one.

NUTRIENTS
Beta-carotene, biotin, folic acid,
vitamin B3, vitamin C; calcium,
magnesium, manganese, phosphorus,
potassium, sodium, sulphur; protein

ENERGY	★★★★☆
DETOX	★☆☆☆☆
IMMUNITY	★★★★☆
DIGESTION	★★☆☆☆
SKIN	★★★★☆

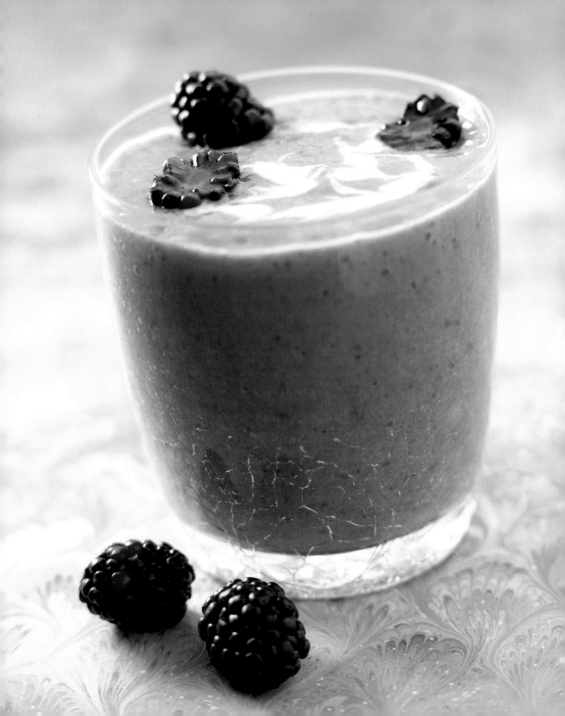

319   sweet summer brekkie

1 handful strawberries

1 handful blackberries

1 peach

1 banana

5 tablespoons (75 ml) natural yogurt

10 tablespoons (150 ml) apple juice

A great treat on a summer's morning.

NUTRIENTS
Beta-carotene, biotin, folic acid, vitamins
B3, B12, C and E; calcium, iron, magnesium,
phosphorus, potassium, sodium, sulphur,
zinc; fibre; protein

ENERGY	★★★★☆
DETOX	★★☆☆☆
IMMUNITY	★★★★☆
DIGESTION	★★☆☆☆
SKIN	★★★★☆

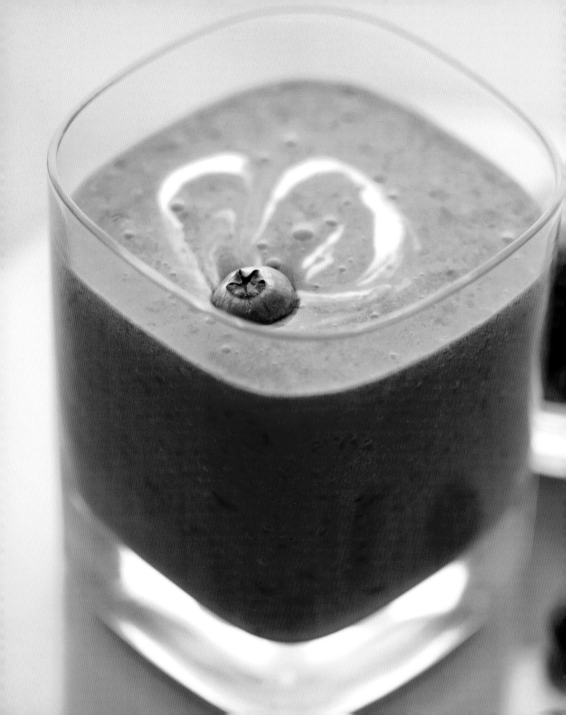

320 purple rain

1 handful blueberries

1 handful blackberries

1 handful blackcurrants

5 tablespoons (75 ml) natural yogurt

6 tablespoons (90 ml) apple juice

Pack them all in, any black or blue fruits you can get your hands on, for a powerful taste sensation, not to mention a glassful of goodness.

NUTRIENTS
Beta-carotene, biotin, folic acid, vitamins B1, B2, B5, B6, C and E; calcium, chromium, iron, magnesium, manganese, phosphorus, potassium, sodium, sulphur, zinc; protein

ENERGY	★★★★☆
DETOX	★☆☆☆☆
IMMUNITY	★★★★☆
DIGESTION	★★★☆☆
SKIN	★★★★☆

321 mighty berry

4 handfuls blueberries, blackberries, blackcurrants,
strawberries, raspberries

5 tablespoons (75 ml) natural yogurt

6 tablespoons (90 ml) cranberry juice

Purple Rain plus the red ones too – a serious berry bonanza in
a creamy base.

NUTRIENTS
Beta-carotene, biotin, folic acid, vitamins
B1, B2, B5, B6, C and E; calcium, chromium,
iron, magnesium, manganese, phosphorus,
potassium, sodium, sulphur, zinc; protein

ENERGY	★★★★☆
DETOX	★★☆☆☆
IMMUNITY	★★★★☆
DIGESTION	★★★☆☆
SKIN	★★★★☆

322 purple 'nana

3 handfuls blueberries, blackberries, blackcurrants

1 banana

5 tablespoons (75 ml) natural yogurt

6 tablespoons (90 ml) apple juice

Purple Rain with that smoothie favourite fruit – banana.

NUTRIENTS
Beta-carotene, biotin, folic acid, vitamins
B1, B2, B5, B6, C and E; calcium, chromium,
iron, magnesium, manganese, phosphorus,
potassium, sodium, sulphur, zinc; protein

ENERGY ★★★★☆
DETOX ★☆☆☆☆
IMMUNITY ★★★★☆
DIGESTION ★★★☆☆
SKIN ★★★★☆

323 mango in disguise

3 handfuls blueberries and blackberries

1 mango (or 2!)

5 tablespoons (75 ml) natural yogurt

6 tablespoons (90 ml) guava juice

You can barely discern the mango from the colour, but its taste certainly reminds you it's there, and the guava adds a different dimension altogether.

NUTRIENTS
Beta-carotene, biotin, folic acid, vitamins
B1, B2, B6, C and E; calcium, chromium,
iron, magnesium, manganese, phosphorus,
potassium, sodium, sulphur, zinc; protein

ENERGY	★★★★☆
DETOX	★☆☆☆☆
IMMUNITY	★★★★☆
DIGESTION	★★★☆☆
SKIN	★★★★☆

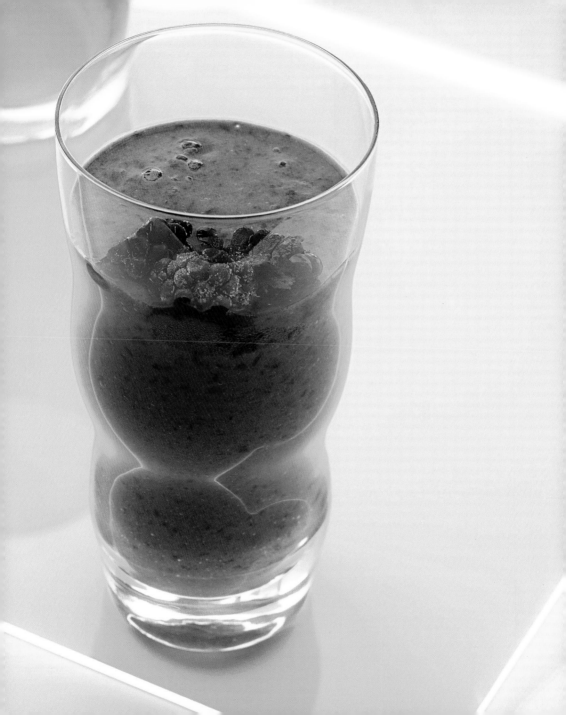

324 purple pineapple

3 handfuls blueberries, blackberries, blackcurrants

½ pineapple

5 tablespoons (75 ml) natural yogurt

6 tablespoons (90 ml) pineapple juice

The tangy, tropical taste of pineapple blends beautifully with the berries. You could even use canned fruits in the winter.

NUTRIENTS
Beta-carotene, biotin, folic acid, vitamins B1, B2, B6, C and E; calcium, chromium, iron, magnesium, manganese, phosphorus, potassium, sodium, sulphur, zinc; protein

ENERGY	★★★★☆
DETOX	★☆☆☆☆
IMMUNITY	★★★★☆
DIGESTION	★★★☆☆
SKIN	★★★★☆

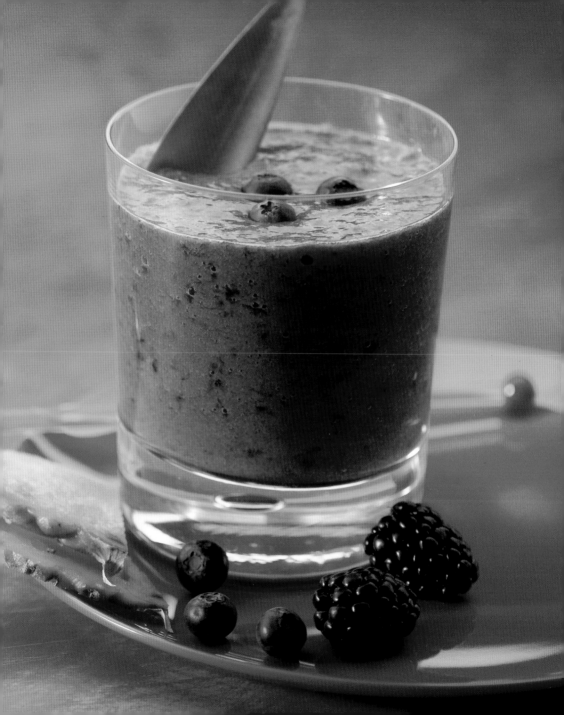

325 callie berry crush

2 handfuls blueberries

1 handful strawberries

1 banana

½ teaspoon vanilla essence

10 tablespoons (150 ml) soy (soya) milk

Of course, you can make any of the smoothie recipies vegan by replacing the yogurt with soy milk, but this particular blend is a favourite of my vegan friend Callie.

NUTRIENTS
Beta-carotene, biotin, folic acid, vitamins B1, B2, B3, B6, C and E; calcium, chromium, magnesium, phosphorus, potassium, sulphur, zinc; fibre; protein

ENERGY ★★★★★
DETOX ★☆☆☆☆
IMMUNITY ★★★☆☆
DIGESTION ★★☆☆☆
SKIN ★★★☆☆

326 dark peaches

1 handful blueberries

1 handful blackberries

2 peaches

5 tablespoons (75 ml) natural yogurt

10 tablespoons (150 ml) apple juice

This is wonderful in the autumn when you've just picked fresh blackberries in the hedgerows.

NUTRIENTS

Beta-carotene, biotin, folic acid, vitamins
B1, B2, B6, B12, C and E, calcium,
chromium, iron, magnesium, potassium,
sodium, sulphur, zinc; fibre; protein

ENERGY ★★★★☆

DETOX ☆☆☆☆☆

IMMUNITY ★★★★☆

DIGESTION ★★☆☆☆

SKIN ★★★★☆

327 passionate pine

½ pineapple

½ banana

2 passion fruits

5 tablespoons (75 ml) natural yogurt

8 tablespoons (120 ml) pineapple juice

Almost anything with passion fruit is a hit for me and this is
definitely no exception.

NUTRIENTS
Beta-carotene, folic acid, vitamins B1,
B3, B6 and C; calcium, magnesium,
manganese, phosphorus, potassium,
sodium, sulphur, zinc; protein

ENERGY ★★★★☆
DETOX ★☆☆☆☆
IMMUNITY ★★☆☆☆
DIGESTION ★★★★☆
SKIN ★☆☆☆☆

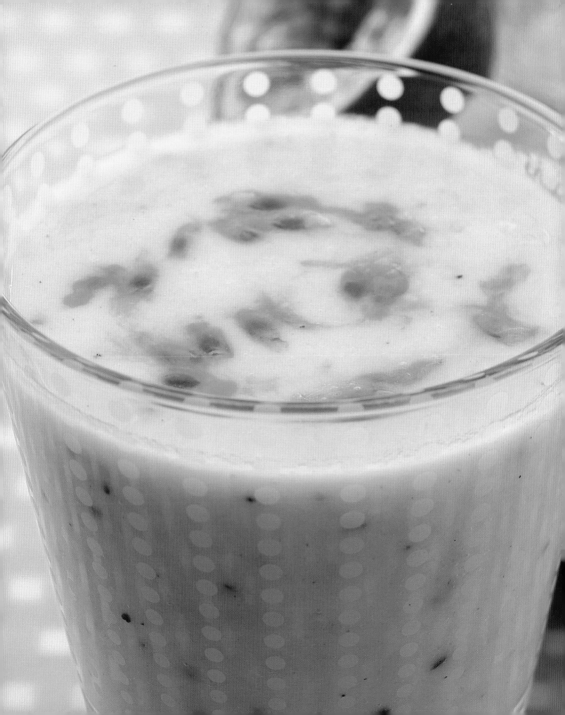

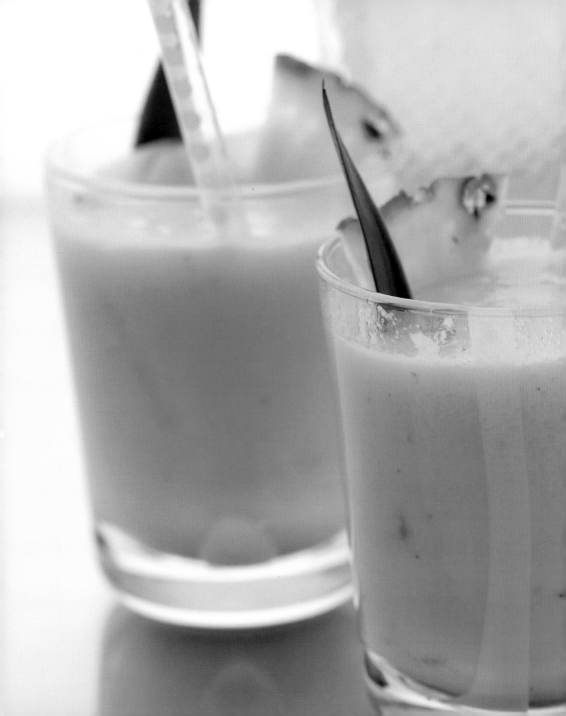

328 pure pineapple creamy

½ pineapple

5 tablespoons (75 ml) natural yogurt

8 tablespoons (120 ml) pineapple juice

Sometimes the simple ones are the best. Pick a perfectly ripe pineapple to get the optimum result.

NUTRIENTS
Beta-carotene, folic acid, vitamin C; calcium, magnesium, manganese, phosphorus, potassium, sodium, zinc; protein

ENERGY	★★★★☆
DETOX	★☆☆☆☆
IMMUNITY	★★★☆☆
DIGESTION	★★★★☆
SKIN	★★☆☆☆

329 pina banana

½ pineapple

2 bananas

2 tablespoons (30 ml) coconut milk

5 tablespoons (75 ml) natural yogurt

6 tablespoons (90 ml) pineapple juice

A truly tropical taste.

NUTRIENTS
Beta-carotene, folic acid, vitamins B1,
B3, B5, B6, C and E; calcium, magnesium,
manganese, phosphorus, potassium,
sodium, sulphur, zinc; protein

ENERGY ★★★★☆
DETOX ★☆☆☆☆
IMMUNITY ★★★☆☆
DIGESTION ★★★☆☆
SKIN ★☆☆☆☆

330   creamy blue pine

½ pineapple

2 handfuls blueberries

5 tablespoons (75 ml) natural yogurt

8 tablespoons (120 ml) pineapple juice

There's something about the delicious but gentle taste of blueberries that matches perfectly with tangy pineapple.

NUTRIENTS

Beta-carotene, biotin, folic acid, vitamins
B1, B2, B6, C and E; calcium, chromium,
magnesium, manganese, phosphorus,
potassium, sodium, zinc; protein

ENERGY	★★★★☆
DETOX	★☆☆☆☆
IMMUNITY	★★★★☆
DIGESTION	★★★★☆
SKIN	★★★★☆

331   pinkypine

½ pineapple

1 handful strawberries

5 tablespoons (75 ml) natural yogurt

8 tablespoons (120 ml) guava juice

As if the fruit combination weren't enough to make you salivate, the guava on top…

NUTRIENTS
Beta-carotene, biotin, folic acid, vitamin
B3, vitamin C; calcium, magnesium,
manganese, phosphorus, potassium,
sodium, sulphur, zinc; protein

ENERGY	★★★★☆
DETOX	★☆☆☆☆
IMMUNITY	★★★★☆
DIGESTION	★★★☆☆
SKIN	★★★★☆

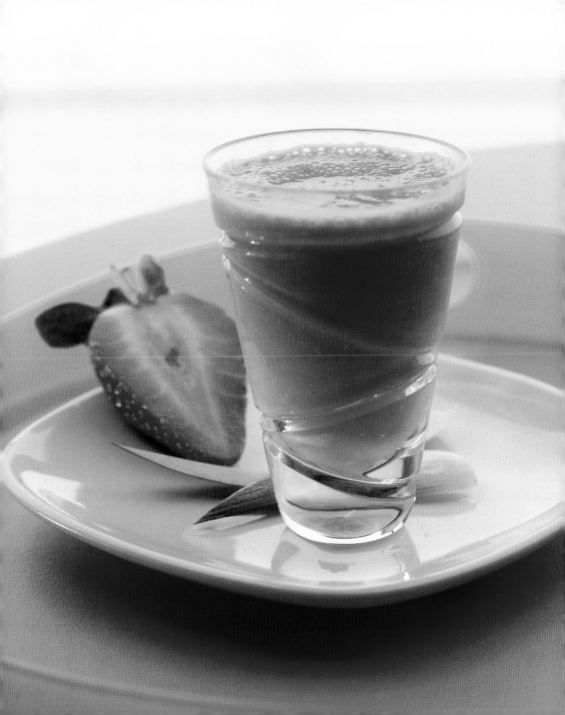

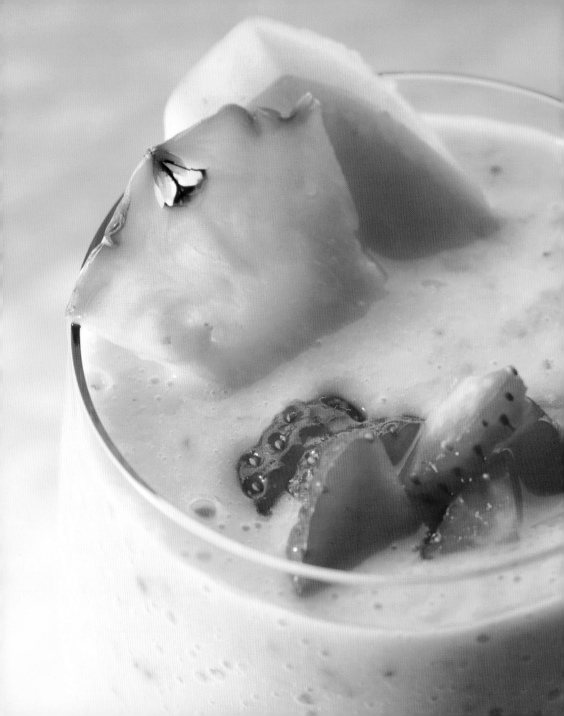

332   creamy sunset

½ pineapple

1 banana

1 handful strawberries

5 tablespoons (75 ml) natural yogurt

10 tablespoons (150 ml) pineapple (or apple) juice

This has to be one of the most simple, delicious creations.

NUTRIENTS
Beta-carotene, biotin, folic acid, vitamins B3, B12 and C; calcium, magnesium, phosphorus, potassium, sodium, sulphur, zinc; fibre; protein

ENERGY	★★★★★
DETOX	☆☆☆☆☆
IMMUNITY	★★★☆☆
DIGESTION	★★★☆☆
SKIN	★★★☆☆

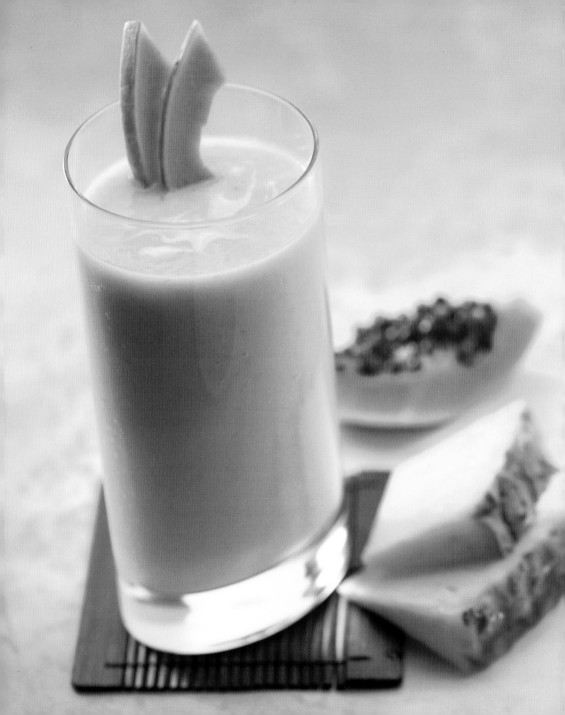

333 tropical cream

½ pineapple

½ papaya

5 tablespoons (75 ml) natural yogurt

10 tablespoons (150 ml) pineapple juice

You could be having breakfast on the beach in southern India or Thailand with this one.

NUTRIENTS
Beta-carotene, folic acid, vitamin B12, vitamin C; calcium, magnesium, phosphorus, potassium, sodium, zinc; fibre; protein

ENERGY	★★★★☆
DETOX	☆☆☆☆☆
IMMUNITY	★★★☆☆
DIGESTION	★★★★☆
SKIN	★★★★☆

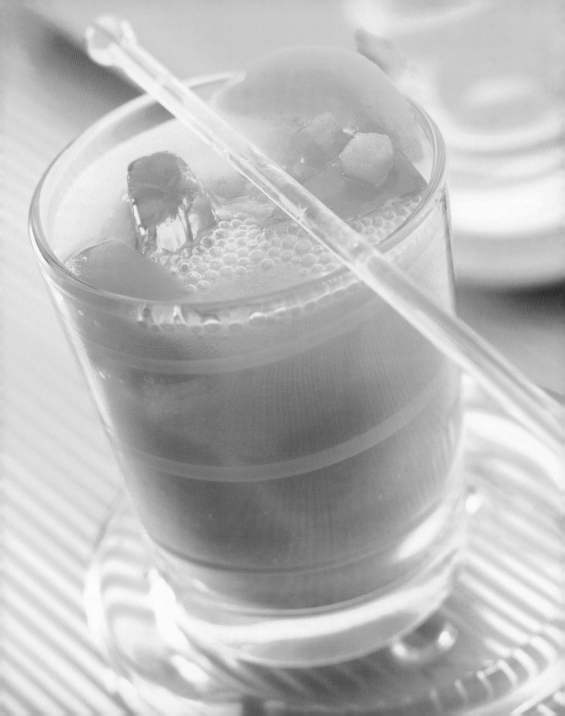

334   pure peachy cream

4 peaches

5 tablespoons (75 ml) natural yogurt

8 tablespoons (120 ml) mineral water

Some would ask, why adulterate luscious peaches with any
other fruit?

NUTRIENTS
Beta-carotene, folic acid, vitamin
B3, vitamin C; calcium, magnesium,
phosphorus, potassium, sodium,
sulphur, zinc; protein

ENERGY   ★★★★☆
DETOX   ★☆☆☆☆
IMMUNITY   ★★★★☆
DIGESTION   ★★★☆☆
SKIN   ★★★☆☆

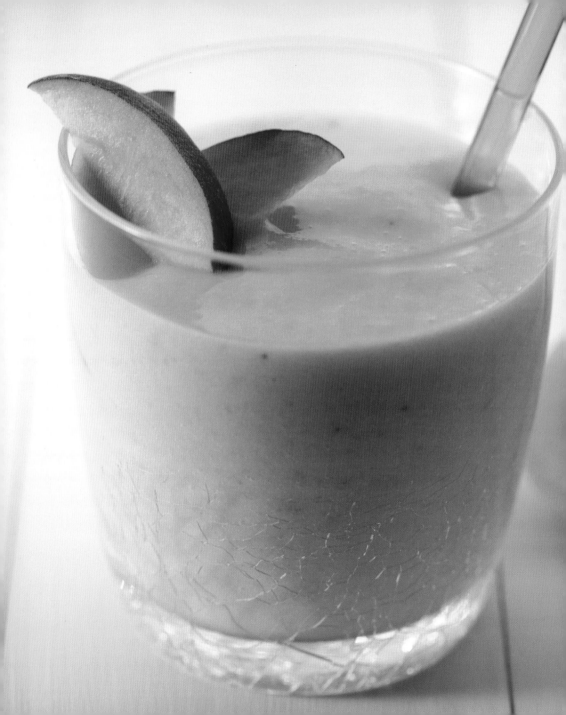

335   vanilla peach

3 peaches

1 banana

½ teaspoon vanilla essence

5 tablespoons (75 ml) natural yogurt

8 tablespoons (120 ml) pineapple juice

They're good alone, but most fruits blend well with a banana, the ultimate smoothie fruit.

NUTRIENTS

Beta-carotene, folic acid, vitamins B1, B3, B6 and C; calcium, magnesium, phosphorus, potassium, sodium, sulphur, zinc; protein

ENERGY	★★★★☆
DETOX	★☆☆☆☆
IMMUNITY	★★★☆☆
DIGESTION	★★★★☆
SKIN	★★☆☆☆

336 peachy passion

2 peaches

¼ pineapple

2 passion fruits

5 tablespoons (75 ml) natural yogurt

8 tablespoons (120 ml) pineapple juice

Another tropical and temperate blend that turns out perfectly.

NUTRIENTS
Beta-carotene, folic acid, vitamin B3,
vitamin C; calcium, iron, magnesium,
manganese, phosphorus, potassium,
sodium, sulphur, zinc; protein

ENERGY	★★★★☆
DETOX	★☆☆☆☆
IMMUNITY	★★★☆☆
DIGESTION	★★★☆☆
SKIN	★★★☆☆

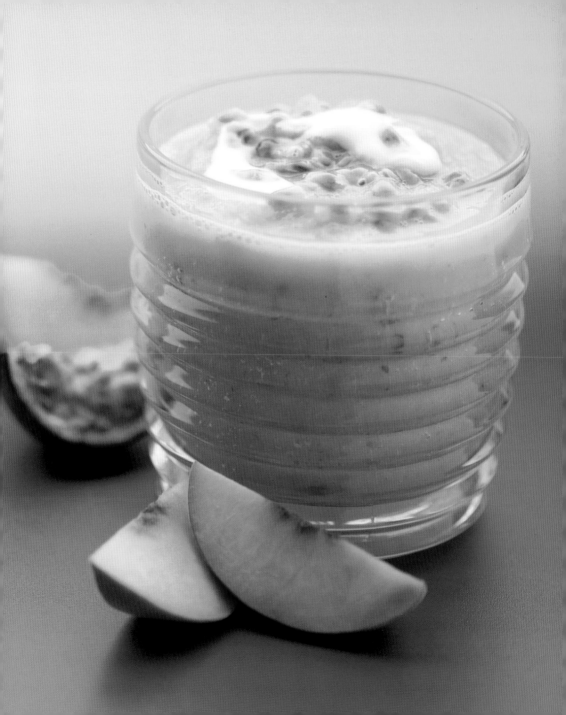

337 colour blend

2 peaches

1 banana

1 handful raspberries

5 tablespoons (75 ml) natural yogurt

8 tablespoons (120 ml) pineapple juice

Yellow and red make orange – here we have all three. Best made
in the summer with juicy, ripe peaches and raspberries.

NUTRIENTS
Beta-carotene, biotin, folic acid,
vitamins B1, B3, B6 and C; calcium,
magnesium, phosphorus, potassium,
sodium, sulphur, zinc; protein

ENERGY ★★★★☆
DETOX ★☆☆☆☆
IMMUNITY ★★★☆☆
DIGESTION ★★☆☆☆
SKIN ★★★☆☆

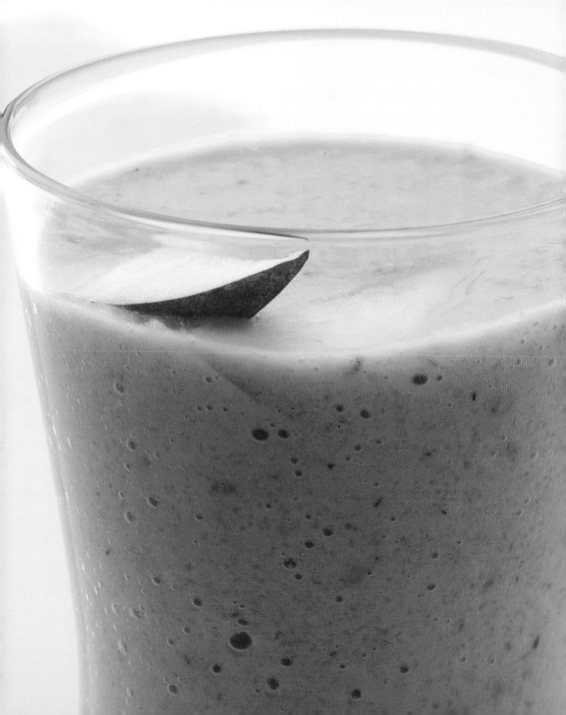

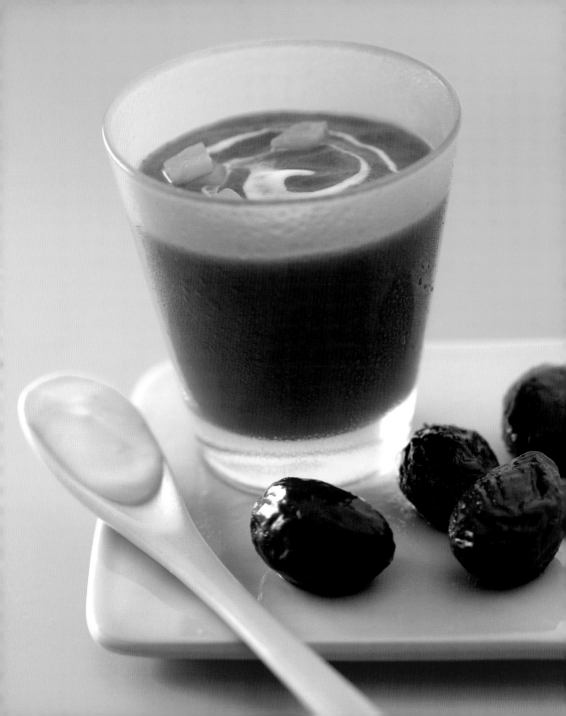

338 apricot regular

8 rehydrated dried apricots

5 rehydrated prunes

5 tablespoons (75 ml) natural yogurt

8 tablespoons (120 ml) prune juice

Of course you can use any dried fruit, but these are particularly good and extremely rich in fibre and antioxidants. It's best to soak the fruit overnight before blending it.

NUTRIENTS
Beta-carotene, folic acid, vitamins B3, B5 and C; calcium, magnesium, phosphorus, potassium, sodium, sulphur, zinc; protein

ENERGY	★★★★☆
DETOX	★☆☆☆☆
IMMUNITY	★★★★☆
DIGESTION	★★★★☆
SKIN	★★★★☆

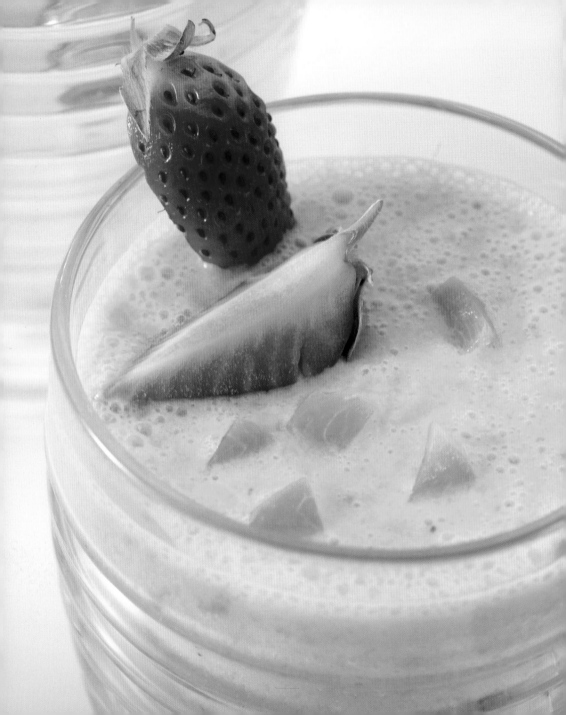

339 apricot cream

4 apricots

2 handfuls strawberries

5 tablespoons (75 ml) natural yogurt

10 tablespoons (150 ml) apple juice

Make sure the apricots are deliciously ripe
for this otherwise they won't be able to
compete with the strawberries.

NUTRIENTS
Beta-carotene, biotin, folic acid,
vitamins B3, B5, B12 and C; calcium,
magnesium, phosphorus, potassium,
sulphur, zinc; fibre; protein

ENERGY ★★★★★
DETOX ☆☆☆☆☆
IMMUNITY ★★★★☆
DIGESTION ★★☆☆☆
SKIN ★★★★★

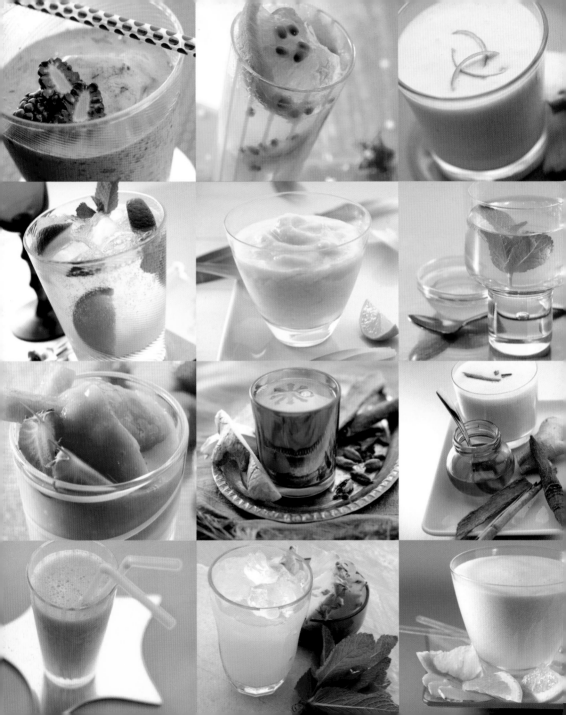

making
quenchers

4

As if all the other recipes in this book weren't refreshing enough, with quenchers we take that concept to another level. The drinks in this section are largely made with frozen fruit and ice; even the warm teas have a sensationally refreshing taste and texture.

We start with the frozen-fruit quenchers, drinks made by mixing frozen fruit pieces with juices, water, sorbets and ice in a blender to produce delicious combinations, all icy-cold on the palate. Next, the fizzy quenchers are great summer coolers, made by simply mixing all the ingredients (including sparkling mineral water) together in a jug. Finally, the tea-based recipes include home-made blends of warming spices, as well as a selection of cold teas to stimulate and revive the mind and spirit.

Guidelines for making the fizzy and tea-based quenchers are given with each recipe. All of the recipes make two generous portions.

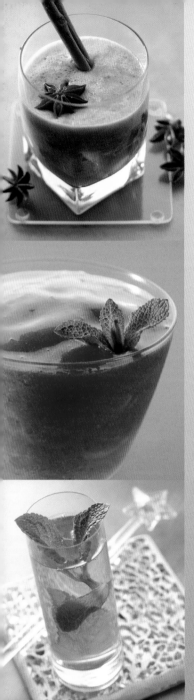

top tips

Below are a few reminders, helpful hints, tips and suggestions to enable you to get the most from making your quenchers.

1 To make frozen-fruit quenchers, drop all of the ingredients into a blender and mix them together for about a minute.

2 To make fizzy quenchers, stir all of the ingredients (including juiced or blended fruit where indicated) together in a large jug.

3 Add some pieces of chopped fruit to your fizzy quenchers to make them more like a summer cocktail.

4 If you want to make a frozen-fruit quencher but are out of frozen fruit, a time-saving alternative is to cheat by using fresh fruit blended with ice.

5 You can make bags of frozen fruit in advance – just prepare the fruit as you would for a smoothie, then chop into pieces, divide into convenient-sized portions in freezer bags and put in the freezer.

6 To freeze bananas, simply peel them and put them into a freezer bag whole – there is no need to chop them up.

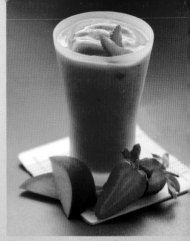

7 When a recipe lists a particular sorbet as one of the ingredients, consider this a suggestion only. Use any sorbet you may have in the freezer – the chances are it'll be delicious whatever you try.

8 Once you've made a few of the recipes, play with the different blends, changing the ingredients to suit your taste and the contents of your refrigerator, freezer or fruit bowl.

9 With the hot, brewed teas such as Ginger Brew and Full Spice, you can leave the pan on the stove and heat it up later in the day, adding a bit more water and a few more spices. This will deepen the taste and produce a lovely, rich flavour.

10 Most herbs and spices make delicious teas that are laden with health properties, so try using whatever herbs and spices you've got growing in the garden (or window box), as you're likely to be able to turn them into a refreshing, healthy tea.

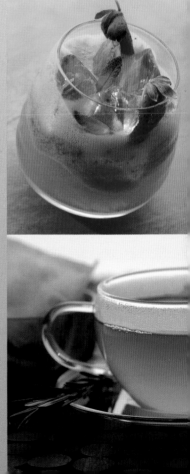

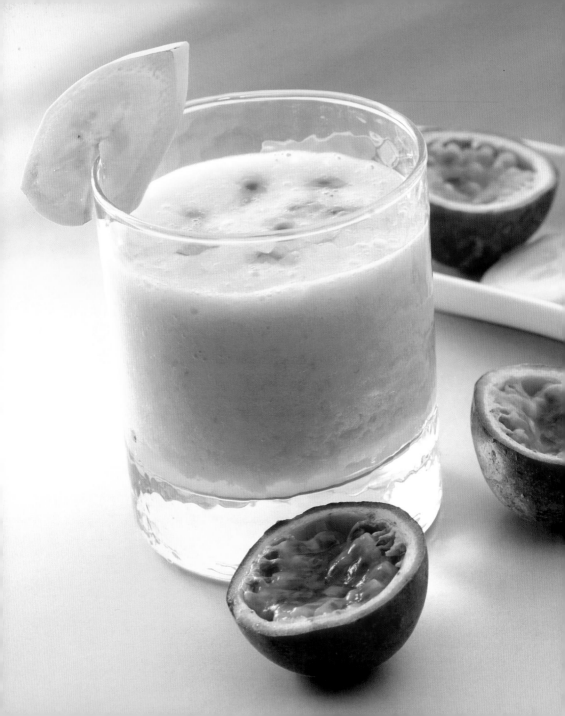

340 tangy banana freeze

2 frozen bananas

1 passion fruit

2 scoops lime sorbet

a few dashes mineral water

Just blend all of these together for a fresh taste-bomb.

NUTRIENTS
Beta-carotene, folic acid, vitamins B1, B3, B6 and C; calcium, magnesium, phosphorus, potassium, sodium, sulphur

ENERGY	★★★★★
DETOX	★☆☆☆☆
IMMUNITY	★★☆☆☆
DIGESTION	★★★☆☆
SKIN	★★★☆☆

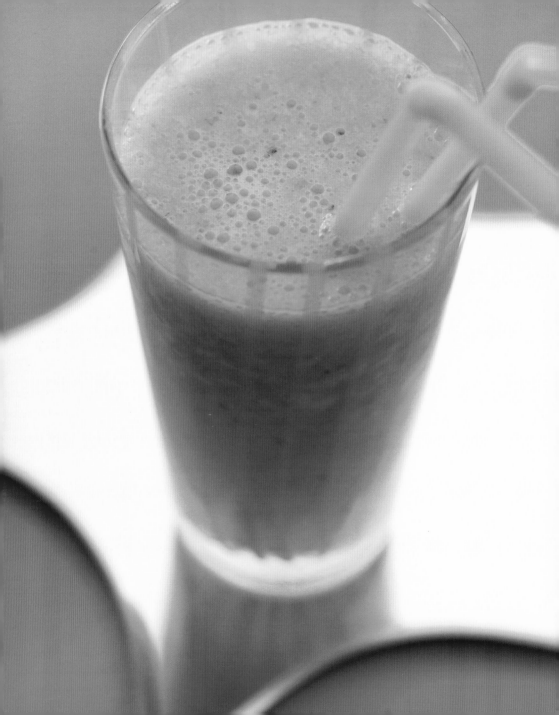

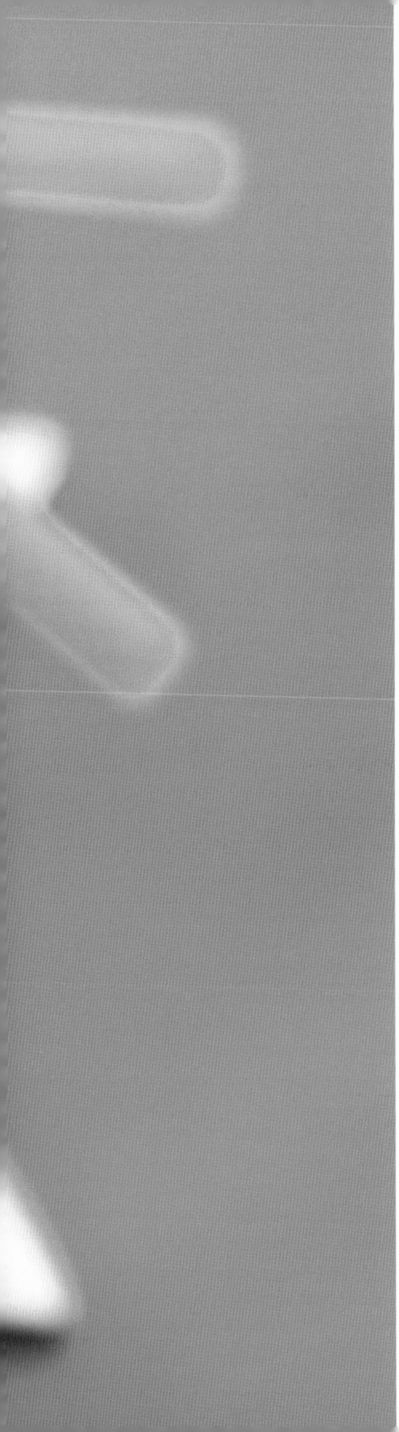

341 orange dream

2 oranges, juiced

4 nectarines

6 ice cubes

This one is like a sweet orange popsicle (ice-lolly) but even better, thanks to the nectarines.

NUTRIENTS
Beta-carotene, folic acid, vitamin C; calcium, magnesium, phosphorus, potassium

ENERGY ★★★★★
DETOX ★★☆☆☆
IMMUNITY ★★★★★
DIGESTION ★☆☆☆☆
SKIN ★★★★☆

342 lift off

2 grapefruits, juiced

½ pineapple

¼ inch (0.5 cm) ginger root, grated

6 ice cubes

This combination is a highly charged challenge to your tastebuds.

NUTRIENTS
Beta-carotene, folic acid, vitamin C;
calcium, magnesium, manganese,
phosphorus, potassium, sodium,
sulphur

ENERGY	★★★★★
DETOX	★☆☆☆☆
IMMUNITY	★★★☆☆
DIGESTION	★★★☆☆
SKIN	★★★☆☆

343 mango squeeze

2 grapefruits, juiced

2 mangoes

6 ice cubes

Mango is perfect for toning down the tanginess of the grapefruit
– all in all super-refreshing and a sweet but uplifting blend.

NUTRIENTS
Beta-carotene, folic acid, vitamin C,
vitamin E; calcium, iron, magnesium,
phosphorus, potassium, sodium,
sulphur

ENERGY	★★★★★
DETOX	★☆☆☆☆
IMMUNITY	★★★★★
DIGESTION	★★☆☆☆
SKIN	★★★★☆

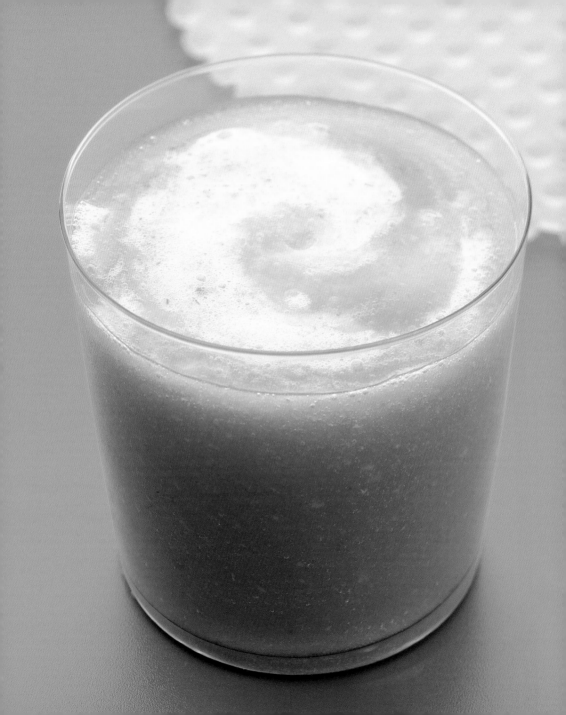

344   paw paw sharp

½ papaya

2 scoops lime sorbet

a few dashes mineral water

I just love the Australian version of papaya – paw paw – and this drink certainly does it justice.

NUTRIENTS
Beta-carotene, folic acid, vitamin C;
calcium, magnesium, phosphorus,
potassium, sodium, sulphur

ENERGY	★★★★★
DETOX	★☆☆☆☆
IMMUNITY	★★★★☆
DIGESTION	★★★★☆
SKIN	★★★☆☆

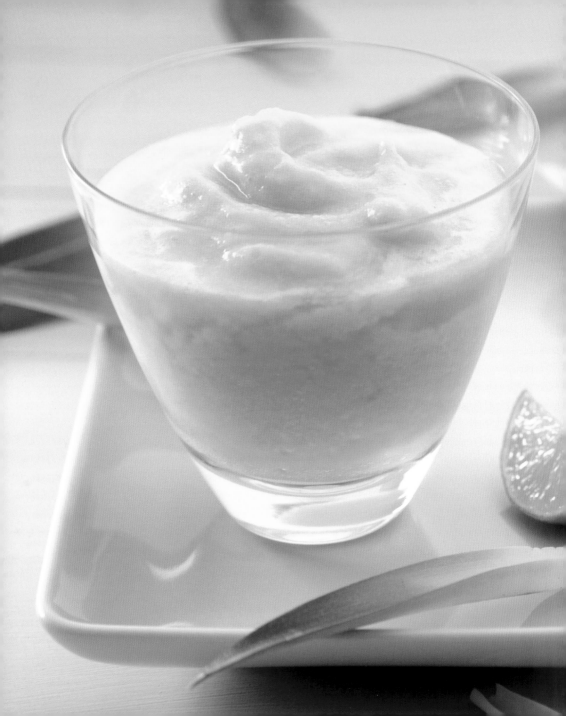

345 pure pine freeze

½ pineapple, frozen in chunks

1 scoop lime sorbet

a few dashes pineapple juice

It is hard to imagine anything more thirst-quenching than this refreshing drink.

NUTRIENTS
Beta-carotene, folic acid, vitamin C; calcium, magnesium, manganese, phosphorus, potassium, sodium, sulphur

ENERGY ★★★★★
DETOX ★☆☆☆☆
IMMUNITY ★★☆☆☆
DIGESTION ★★★★☆
SKIN ★★★☆☆

346 pine passion

½ pineapple, frozen in chunks

2 passion fruits

2 tablespoons (30 ml) natural yogurt

a few dashes pineapple juice

In my view, you can barely go wrong with passion fruit, and blended with frozen, ripe pineapple – mmm!

NUTRIENTS
Beta-carotene, folic acid, vitamins B3, B12 and C; calcium, iron, magnesium, manganese, phosphorus, potassium, sodium, sulphur, zinc; protein

ENERGY ★★★★☆
DETOX ★☆☆☆☆
IMMUNITY ★★★☆☆
DIGESTION ★★★★☆
SKIN ★★★☆☆

347 tropics at zero

½ pineapple, frozen in chunks

1 mango, frozen in chunks

1 scoop lime sorbet

a few dashes pineapple juice

You'd certainly apprecaite this one on a hot beach in the tropics.

NUTRIENTS
Beta-carotene, folic acid, vitamin C,
vitamin E; calcium, iron, magnesium,
manganese, phosphorus, potassium,
sodium, sulphur

ENERGY ★★★★★
DETOX ★☆☆☆☆
IMMUNITY ★★★★☆
DIGESTION ★★★☆☆
SKIN ★★★★☆

348 strawberries on sunbeds

½ pineapple, frozen in chunks

1 handful frozen strawberries

1 tablespoon (15 ml) coconut milk

a few dashes pineapple juice

Sit back and relax – you'd be forgiven for wondering where in the world you are with this sublime mix.

NUTRIENTS
Beta-carotene, biotin, folic acid,
vitamin C; calcium, magnesium,
manganese, phosphorus, potassium,
sodium, sulphur

ENERGY	★★★★★
DETOX	★☆☆☆☆
IMMUNITY	★★★★☆
DIGESTION	★★☆☆☆
SKIN	★★★☆☆

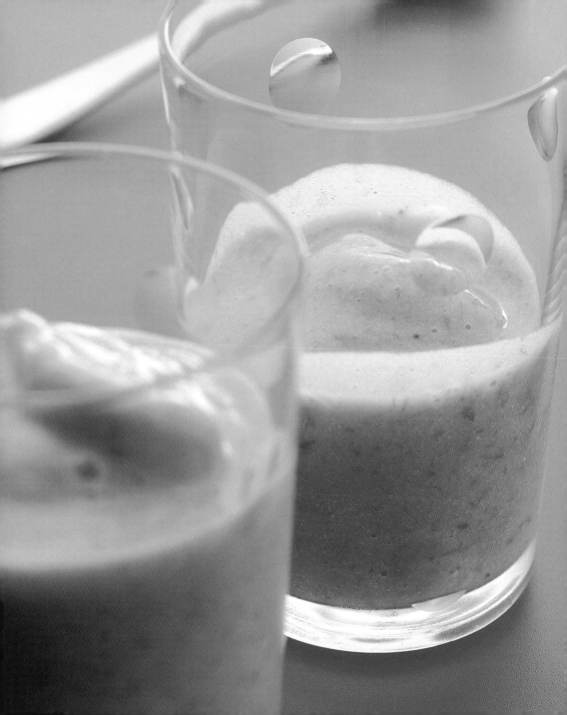

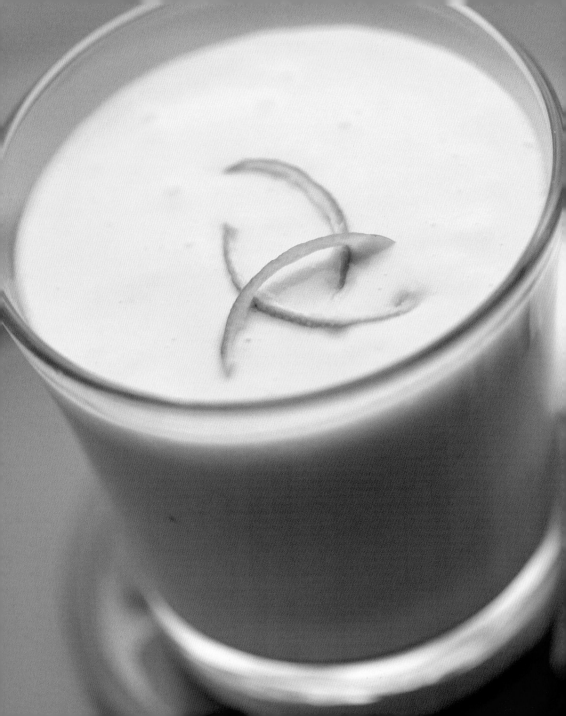

349 malibu freeze

½ pineapple, frozen in chunks

1 frozen banana

1 tablespoon (15 ml) coconut milk

juice of half a lime

a few dashes pineapple juice

Transport yourself to beneath a palm tree with this creamy cooler.

NUTRIENTS

Beta-carotene, folic acid, vitamins B1, B3, B6 and C; calcium, magnesium, manganese, phosphorus, potassium, sodium, sulphur

ENERGY ★★★★★
DETOX ★☆☆☆☆
IMMUNITY ★★☆☆☆
DIGESTION ★★★☆☆
SKIN ★★★☆☆

350 pink banana freeze

2 handfuls frozen strawberries

2 frozen bananas

a few dashes orange juice

A classic smoothie, with a frozen touch.

NUTRIENTS
Beta-carotene, biotin, folic acid,
vitamins B1, B3, B6 and C; calcium,
magnesium, phosphorus, potassium,
sulphur

ENERGY	★★★★★
DETOX	★☆☆☆☆
IMMUNITY	★★★☆☆
DIGESTION	★★☆☆☆
SKIN	★★★☆☆

351 double red

4 handfuls frozen raspberries

a few dashes cranberry juice

Tangy and sweet all at once, this bright red freezie is exquisite.

NUTRIENTS
Beta-carotene, biotin, folic acid,
vitamin C; calcium, iron, magnesium,
manganese, phosphorus, potassium,
sodium, sulphur

ENERGY	★★★★☆
DETOX	★☆☆☆☆
IMMUNITY	★★★☆☆
DIGESTION	☆☆☆☆☆
SKIN	★★★☆☆

352 double red creamy

2 handfuls frozen raspberries

2 handfuls frozen strawberries

2 tablespoons (30 ml) natural yogurt

a few dashes cranberry juice

A sweeter, creamier version of Double Red (see blend 351), made nice and thick with the addition of yogurt.

NUTRIENTS
Beta-carotene, biotin, folic acid,
vitamin B12, vitamin C; calcium, iron,
magnesium, manganese, phosphorus,
potassium, sodium, sulphur, zinc; protein

ENERGY ★★★★☆
DETOX ★☆☆☆☆
IMMUNITY ★★★☆☆
DIGESTION ★★☆☆☆
SKIN ★★★☆☆

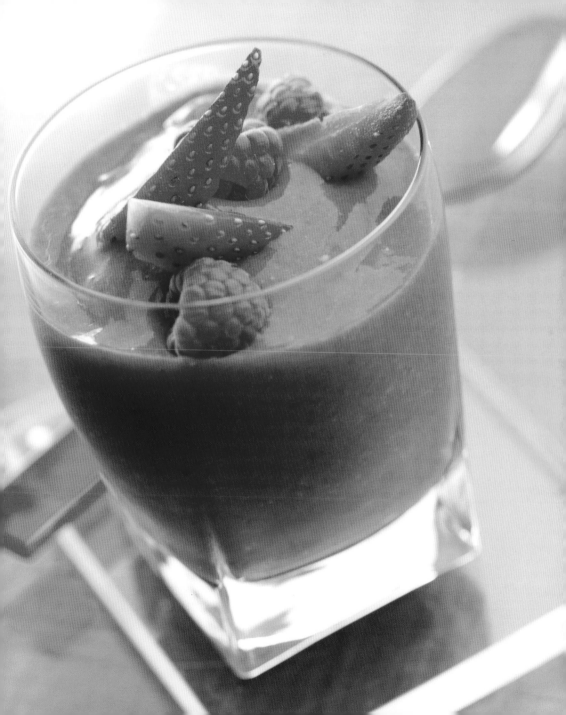

353 peachy pink cream

2 handfuls frozen strawberries

2 peaches, frozen in chunks

2 tablespoons (30 ml) natural yogurt

a few dashes orange juice

An idyllic combination with a creamy touch.

NUTRIENTS		
Beta-carotene, biotin, folic acid,	ENERGY	★★★★☆
vitamins B3, B12 and C; calcium,	DETOX	★☆☆☆☆
magnesium, phosphorus, potassium,	IMMUNITY	★★★★☆
sodium, sulphur, zinc; protein	DIGESTION	★★☆☆☆
	SKIN	★★★☆☆

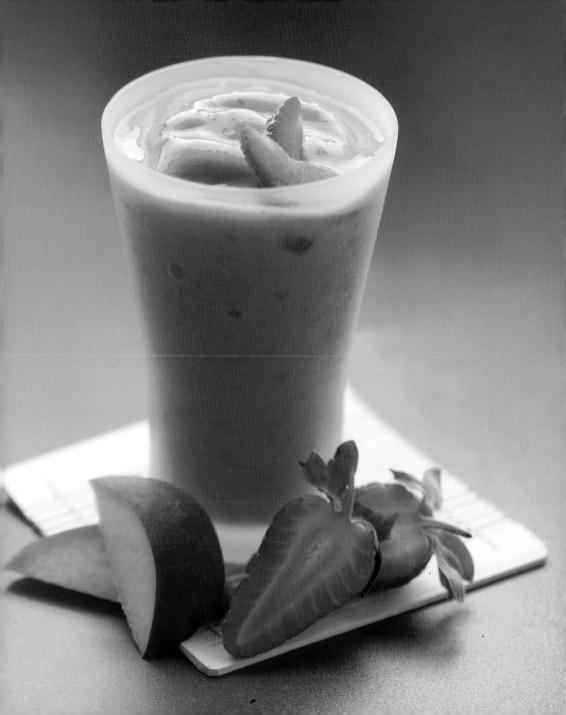

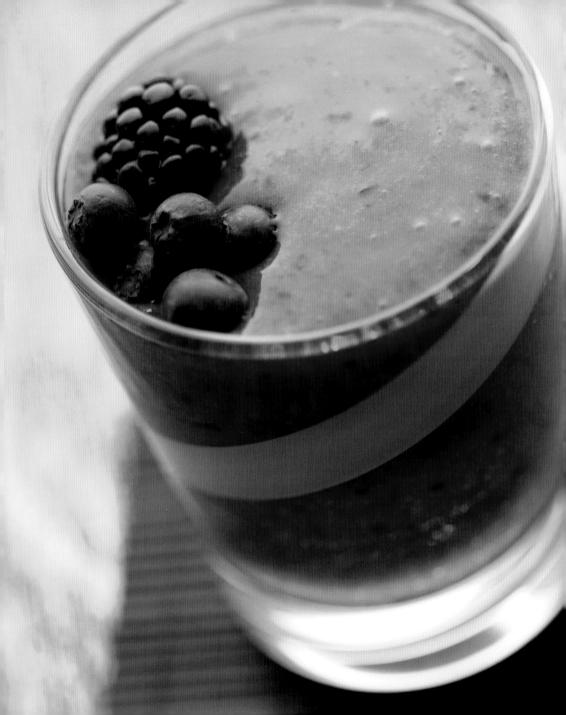

354 big black freezie

4 handfuls frozen blueberries, blackberries, blackcurrants

2 tablespoons (30 ml) natural yogurt

a few dashes apple juice

Whatever the weather, you'd almost believe it was summer when sipping this cooling refresher.

NUTRIENTS
Beta-carotene, biotin, folic acid, vitamins B1, B2, B6, B12, C and, E; calcium, chromium, magnesium, manganese, phosphorus, potassium, sodium, sulphur, zinc; protein

ENERGY	★★★★☆
DETOX	★☆☆☆☆
IMMUNITY	★★★★★
DIGESTION	★★★☆☆
SKIN	★★★★☆

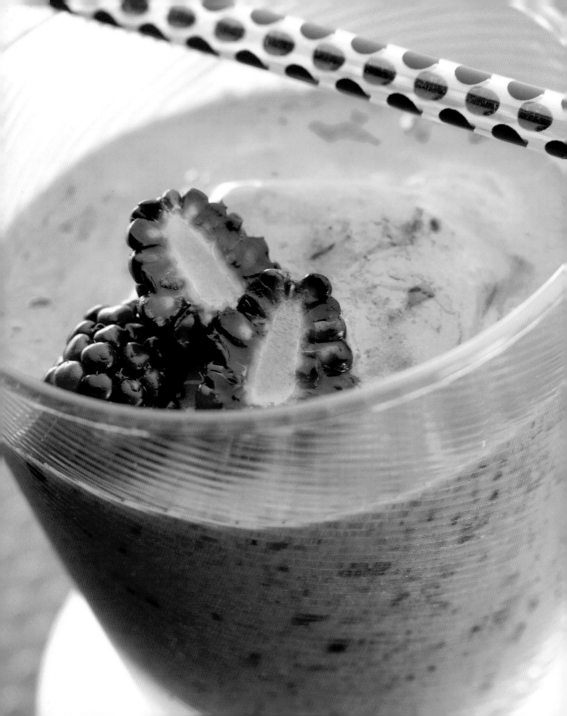

355 black & apple freezie

4 handfuls frozen blackberries

2 tablespoons (30 ml) natural yogurt

½ teaspoon vanilla essence

a few dashes apple juice

That classic English combination with a smooth vanilla undertone.

NUTRIENTS
Beta-carotene, folic acid, vitamin C,
vitamin E; calcium, iron, magnesium,
manganese, phosphorus, potassium,
sodium, sulphur; protein

ENERGY ★★★★☆
DETOX ★☆☆☆☆
IMMUNITY ★★☆☆☆
DIGESTION ☆☆☆☆☆
SKIN ★★★☆☆

356 creamy apple freezie

4 tablespoons (60 ml) frozen stewed apple

1 fresh apple, peeled, cored and chopped

4 tablespoons (60 ml) natural yogurt

¼ teaspoon ground cinnamon

½ teaspoon vanilla essence

a few dashes apple juice

This combination is especially good if you've used a sharp variety of apple such as Granny Smith.

NUTRIENTS	ENERGY	★★★★☆
Beta-carotene, folic acid, vitamin B12,	DETOX	★☆☆☆☆
vitamin C; calcium, magnesium,	IMMUNITY	★★★☆☆
phosphorus, potassium, sulphur,	DIGESTION	★★★★☆
zinc; protein	SKIN	★★☆☆☆

357 gingapple

4 tablespoons (60 ml) frozen stewed apple

2 fresh apples, peeled, cored and chopped

¼ inch (0.5 cm) ginger root, grated

2 scoops lime sorbet

a few dashes apple juice

A deliciously refreshing combination with a sharp bite from the ginger and lime.

NUTRIENTS
Beta-carotene, folic acid, vitamin C;
calcium, magnesium, phosphorus,
potassium, sodium, sulphur

ENERGY	★★★★☆
DETOX	★☆☆☆☆
IMMUNITY	★★★☆☆
DIGESTION	★★★☆☆
SKIN	★★☆☆☆

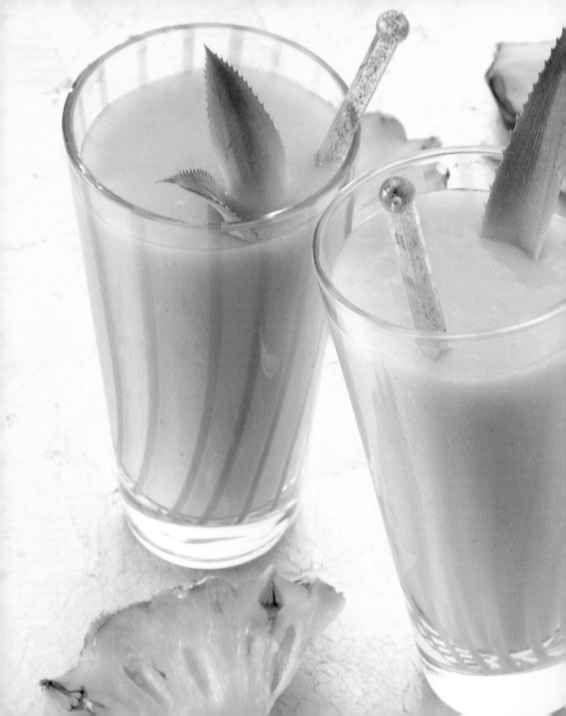

358 pine apple

4 tablespoons (60 ml) frozen stewed apple

½ pineapple, frozen in chunks

2 scoops lime sorbet

a few dashes apple juice

A wonderfully fresh blend of fruits, given
a sweet tang by the lime sorbet.

NUTRIENTS
Beta-carotene, folic acid, vitamin C;
calcium, magnesium, manganese,
phosphorus, potassium, sodium,
sulphur

ENERGY	★★★★☆
DETOX	★☆☆☆☆
IMMUNITY	★★☆☆☆
DIGESTION	★★★☆☆
SKIN	★★☆☆☆

359 apple & prune freeze

4 tablespoons (60 ml) frozen stewed apple

8 rehydrated prunes

½ teaspoon vanilla essence

4 tablespoons (60 ml) natural yogurt

a few dashes apple juice

This one is so creamy and sweet – a full meal in itself.

NUTRIENTS
Beta-carotene, folic acid, vitamin B12,
vitamin C; calcium, magnesium,
phosphorus, potassium, sulphur,
zinc; protein

ENERGY	★★★★☆
DETOX	★☆☆☆☆
IMMUNITY	★★★★☆
DIGESTION	★★★★☆
SKIN	★★☆☆☆

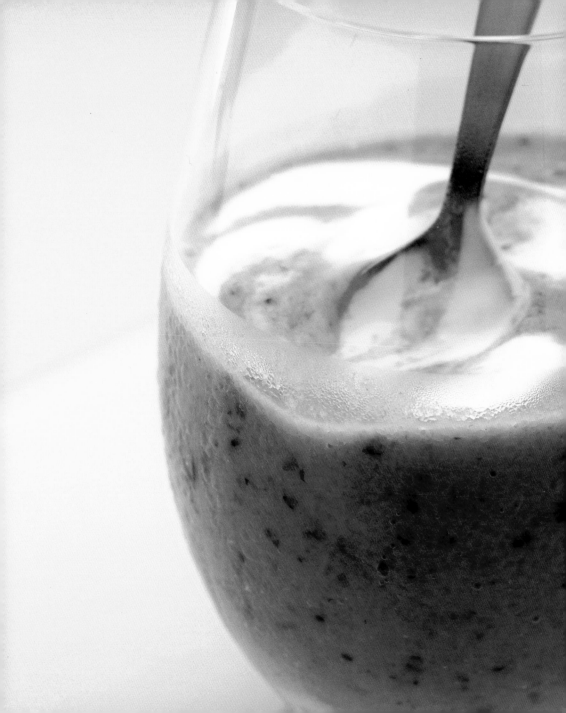

360 blue apple

4 tablespoons (60 ml) frozen stewed apple

2 handfuls frozen blueberries

2 tablespoons (30 ml) natural yogurt

a few dashes apple juice

The flecks of blue from the blueberry skins let you in on the secret of how delicious this creamy frozen-fruit quencher really is.

NUTRIENTS
Beta-carotene, folic acid, vitamin B12,
vitamin C; calcium, chromium,
magnesium, phosphorus, potassium,
sodium, sulphur, zinc; protein

ENERGY ★★★★☆
DETOX ★☆☆☆☆
IMMUNITY ★★★★☆
DIGESTION ★★★☆☆
SKIN ★★★★☆

361 watermelon tanger

½ watermelon

2 scoops lime sorbet

6 ice cubes

Watermelon is one of the most refreshing fruits, at 95 per cent water, and with the lime added it's even better. Ideal for a baking-hot day.

NUTRIENTS
Beta-carotene, folic acid, vitamin B5, vitamin C; calcium, magnesium, phosphorus, potassium, sodium, sulphur

ENERGY	★★★★★
DETOX	★☆☆☆☆
IMMUNITY	★★★★☆
DIGESTION	☆☆☆☆☆
SKIN	★★★★☆

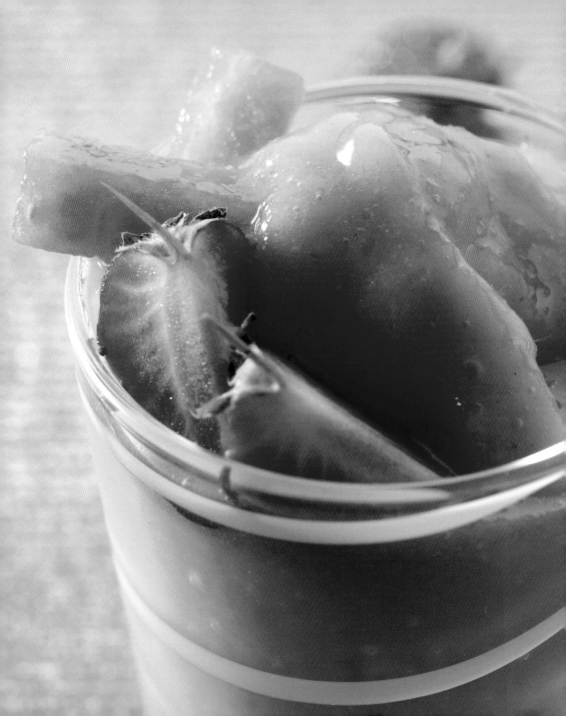

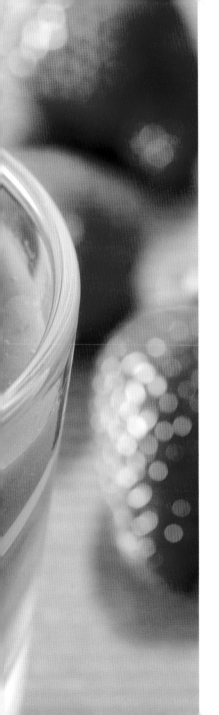

362 pink ice

½ watermelon

2 handfuls frozen strawberries

1 scoop lemon sorbet

6 ice cubes

a few dashes mineral water

Just by looking at this vision in pink, you'll know it's delicious and good for you.

NUTRIENTS
Beta-carotene, biotin, folic acid, vitamin B5, vitamin C; calcium, magnesium, phosphorus, potassium, sodium, sulphur

ENERGY	★★★★★
DETOX	★☆☆☆☆
IMMUNITY	★★★★☆
DIGESTION	★☆☆☆☆
SKIN	★★★★☆

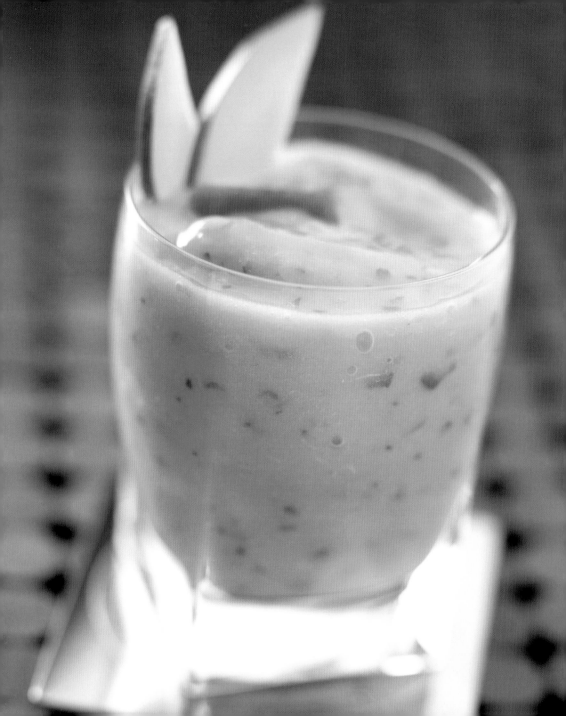

363 peachy mango ice

1 mango, frozen in chunks

3 peaches, frozen in chunks

a few dashes orange juice

Double trouble from two delicious orange fruits that blend
beautifully, especially in a frosty drink.

NUTRIENTS
Beta-carotene, folic acid, vitamins B3,
C and E; calcium, iron, magnesium,
phosphorus, potassium, sodium,
sulphur

ENERGY	★★★★★
DETOX	★★☆☆☆
IMMUNITY	★★★★★
DIGESTION	★★☆☆☆
SKIN	★★★★★

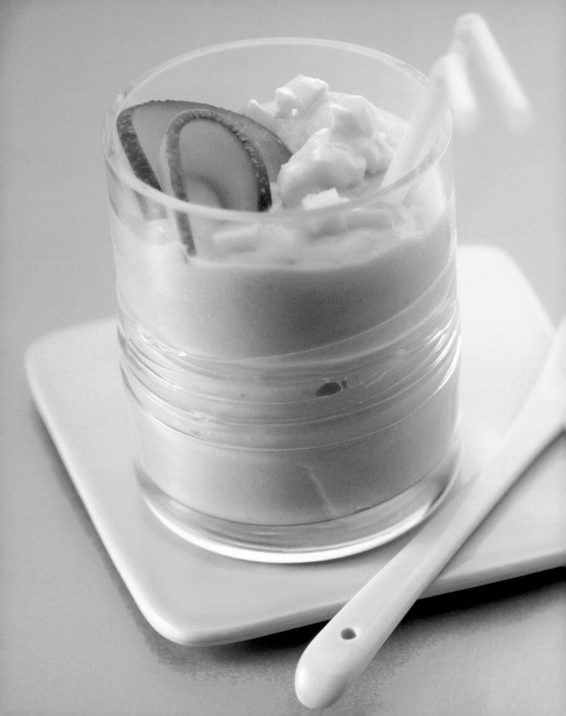

364 mango surprise

2 mangoes, frozen in chunks

juice of a lime

½ inch (1 cm) ginger root, grated

4 tablespoons (60 ml) natural yogurt

6 ice cubes

Your tastebuds won't know what hit them – smooth mango, sharp lime, zingy ginger and creamy yogurt create a winning combination.

NUTRIENTS
Beta-carotene, folic acid, vitamins B12,
C and E; calcium, iron, magnesium,
phosphorus, potassium, sodium,
sulphur, zinc; protein.

ENERGY	★★★★☆
DETOX	★☆☆☆☆
IMMUNITY	★★★☆☆
DIGESTION	★★★☆☆
SKIN	★★★☆☆

365 apricot banana ice

2 frozen bananas

6 frozen apricots

a few dashes apple juice

You have to freeze well-ripened apricots to bring out the taste in this sumptuous quencher; otherwise, freeze apricots that have been canned in juice.

NUTRIENTS
Beta-carotene, folic acid, vitamins B1, B3, B5, B6 and C; calcium, magnesium, phosphorus, potassium, sulphur

ENERGY ★★★★★
DETOX ★☆☆☆☆
IMMUNITY ★★★☆☆
DIGESTION ★★☆☆☆
SKIN ★★★☆☆

366 kiwi berry

3 kiwi fruits

2 handfuls frozen strawberries

a few dashes apple juice

4–6 ice cubes

Grab a high dose of vitamin C in this delicious combination.

NUTRIENTS
Beta-carotene, biotin, folic acid,
vitamin C; calcium, magnesium,
phosphorus, potassium, sodium,
sulphur

ENERGY	★★★★★
DETOX	★★★☆☆
IMMUNITY	★★★★★
DIGESTION	★★☆☆☆
SKIN	★★★★★

367 citrus strawberries

3 handfuls frozen strawberries

1 scoop lime sorbet

3–5 fresh mint leaves

a few dashes orange juice

This is just a splash of rum short of a daquiri!

NUTRIENTS
Beta-carotene, biotin, folic acid,
vitamin C; calcium, magnesium,
phosphorus, potassium, sulphur; fibre

ENERGY	★★★★☆
DETOX	☆☆☆☆☆
IMMUNITY	★★★☆☆
DIGESTION	★☆☆☆☆
SKIN	★★★★☆

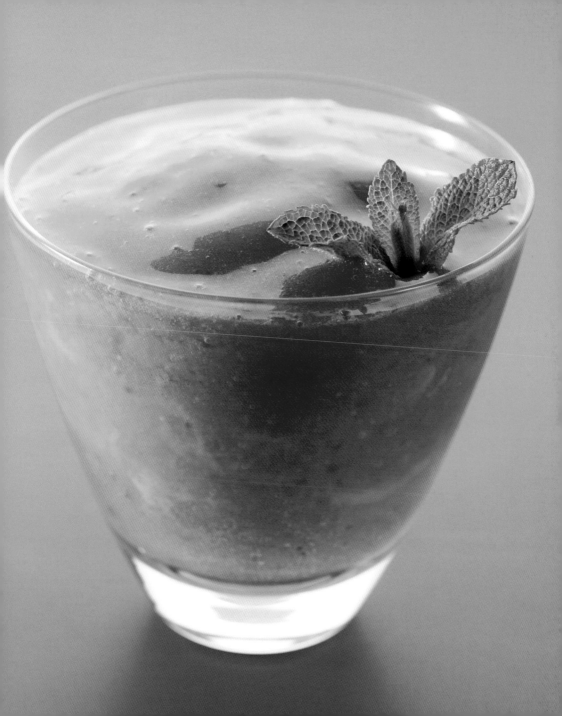

368 paw paw freezie

½ papaya

¼ pineapple, frozen in chunks

juice of a lime

¼ inch (0.5 cm) fresh ginger root, grated

a few dashes pineapple juice

6–10 ice cubes

This is a great way to enjoy perfectly ripe papaya.

NUTRIENTS
Beta-carotene, folic acid, vitamin C;
calcium, magnesium, phosphorus,
potassium, sodium, sulphur; fibre

ENERGY	★★★★☆
DETOX	★★☆☆☆
IMMUNITY	★★★★☆
DIGESTION	★★★★★
SKIN	★★★★☆

369   frozen nectar 'nana

2 nectarines, frozen in chunks

1 frozen banana

1 handful frozen strawberries

a few dashes apple juice

A wonderful trio of fruits.

NUTRIENTS
Beta-carotene, biotin, folic acid,
vitamin B3, vitamin C; calcium,
magnesium, phosphorus, potassium,
sulphur; fibre

ENERGY ★★★★★
DETOX ★☆☆☆☆
IMMUNITY ★★★☆☆
DIGESTION ★☆☆☆☆
SKIN ★★★★☆

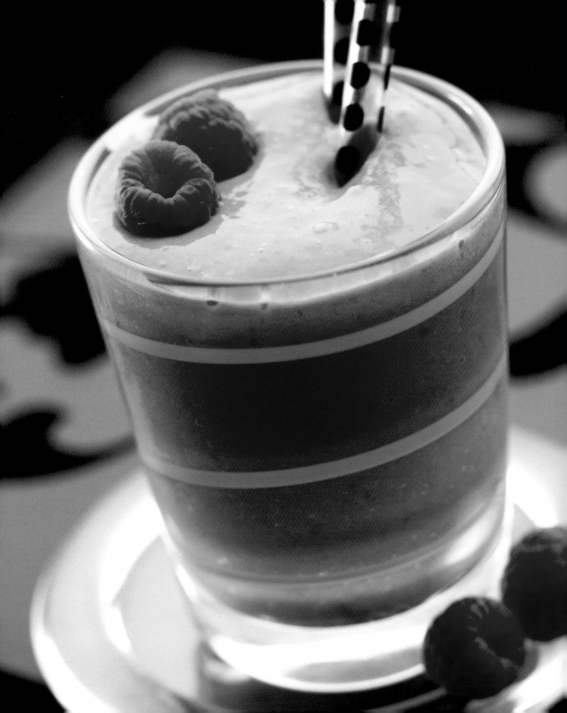

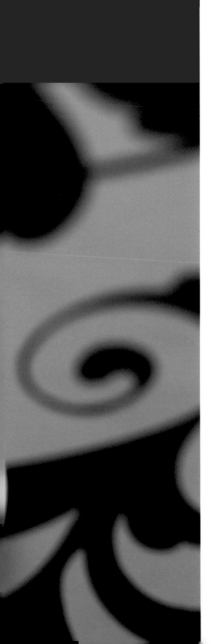

370 creamy raspanana

2 handfuls frozen raspberries

1 frozen banana

3 tablespoons (45 ml) natural yogurt

a few dashes apple juice

You can use any berries here but slightly tangy raspberries blend well with the banana.

NUTRIENTS

Beta-carotene, biotin, folic acid, vitamins B3, B12 and C; calcium, magnesium, phosphorus, potassium, sodium, sulphur, zinc; fibre; protein

ENERGY	★★★★☆
DETOX	☆☆☆☆☆
IMMUNITY	★★★☆☆
DIGESTION	★★☆☆☆
SKIN	★★★☆☆

371 lime cooler

juice of 3 limes

1 pt (500 ml) sparkling mineral water

4–6 fresh mint leaves

4–6 ice cubes

A classic, cooling summer drink, perfect in its simplicity.

NUTRIENTS
Beta-carotene, folic acid, vitamin C;
calcium, magnesium, phosphorus,
potassium, sodium, sulphur

ENERGY ★☆☆☆☆
DETOX ★★☆☆☆
IMMUNITY ★★★☆☆
DIGESTION ★☆☆☆☆
SKIN ★★☆☆☆

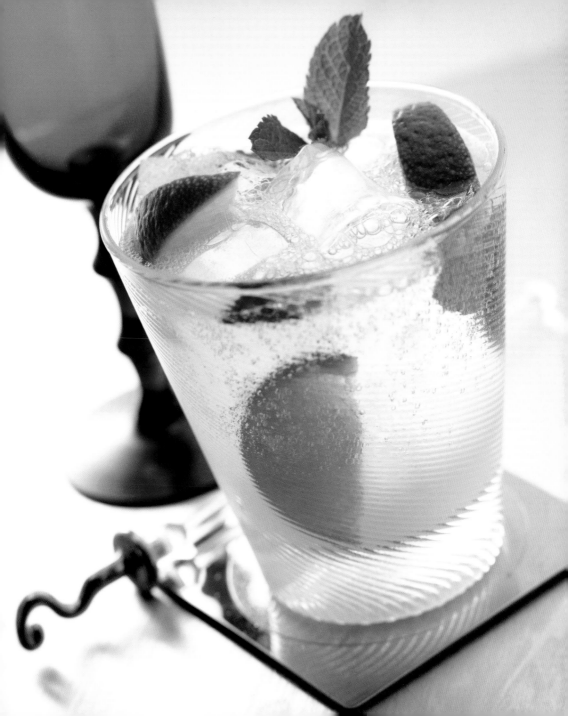

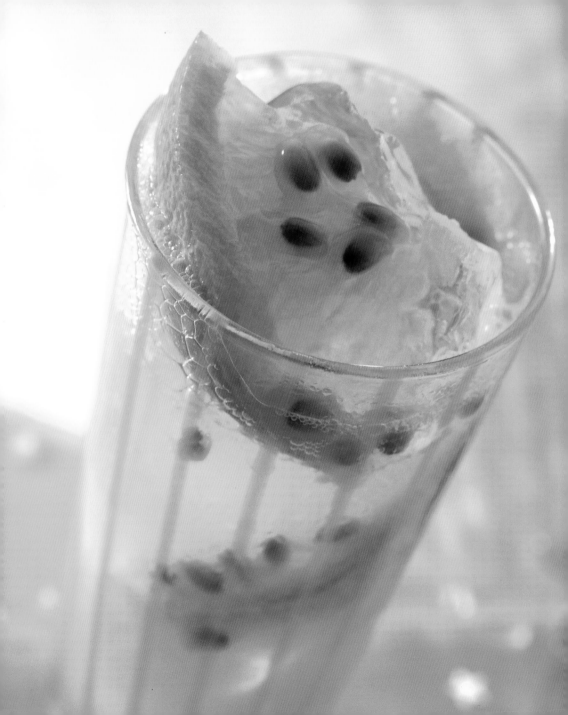

372 orange passion twinkle

juice of 4 oranges

4 passion fruits

4–6 ice cubes

sparkling mineral water to top up

Perfect on a hot summer's day. Just stir in the passion fruits or, if you don't like the seeds, pass through a strainer first.

NUTRIENTS
Beta-carotene, vitamin B3, vitamin C; calcium, magnesium, phosphorus, potassium, sodium

ENERGY	★★★★☆
DETOX	★★☆☆☆
IMMUNITY	★★★★☆
DIGESTION	☆☆☆☆☆
SKIN	★★☆☆☆

373 grape cooler

juice of 2 grapefruits

1 scoop orange sorbet

¼ inch (0.5 cm) ginger root, grated

4–6 ice cubes

sparkling mineral water to top up

Just let the sorbet melt, sweeten and froth up the freshly squeezed juice before splashing in the mineral water to give it fizz.

NUTRIENTS
Beta-carotene, folic acid, vitamin C; calcium, magnesium, phosphorus, potassium, sulphur

ENERGY ★★★★☆
DETOX ★★☆☆☆
IMMUNITY ★★★★☆
DIGESTION ★☆☆☆☆
SKIN ★★☆☆☆

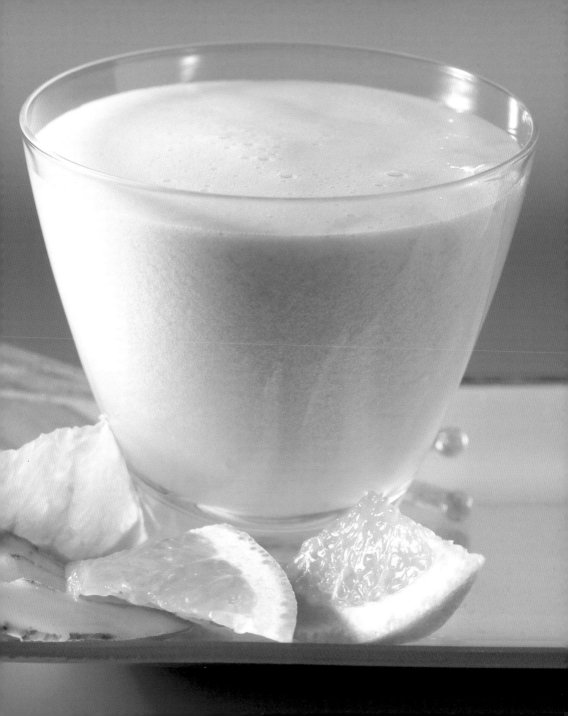

374 pine fizz

juice of half a pineapple

4–6 fresh mint leaves

4–6 ice cubes

sparkling mineral water to top up

Somehow, pineapples really suit being fizzy.

NUTRIENTS
Beta-carotene, folic acid, vitamin C;
calcium, magnesium, manganese,
phosphorus, potassium, sodium

ENERGY ★★★★☆
DETOX ★★★☆☆
IMMUNITY ★★★☆☆
DIGESTION ★★★☆☆
SKIN ★★☆☆☆

375   pick-me-up fizz

juice of half a pineapple

juice of 2 oranges

4–6 ice cubes

sparkling mineral water to top up

Fresh, tangy, sharp, juicy, fizzy – all sensations to liven you up.

NUTRIENTS
Beta-carotene, folic acid, vitamin C;
calcium, magnesium, manganese,
phosphorus, potassium, sodium

ENERGY ★★★★☆
DETOX ★★☆☆☆
IMMUNITY ★★★★☆
DIGESTION ★★☆☆☆
SKIN ★★★☆☆

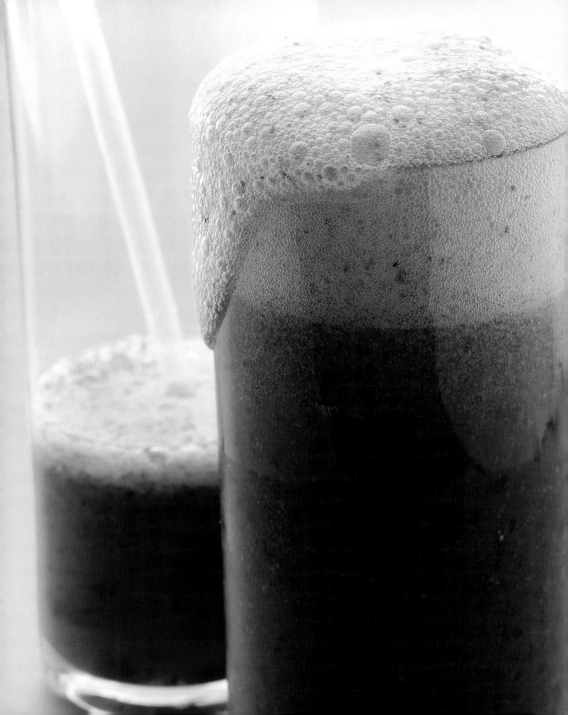

376 fizzy berry crush

2 handfuls strawberries

2 handfuls blueberries

4–6 ice cubes

sparkling mineral water to top up

Instead of fruit juice, use fruit pulp made by blending the strawberries and blueberries with the ice, so you get a fantastic texture as well as taste.

NUTRIENTS
Beta-carotene, biotin, folic acid,
vitamins B1, B2, B6, C and E; calcium,
chromium, magnesium, phosphorus,
potassium, sodium, sulphur

ENERGY	★★★★☆
DETOX	★★★☆☆
IMMUNITY	★★★★★
DIGESTION	☆☆☆☆☆
SKIN	★★★★☆

377 melon tang

1 melon

¼ inch (0.5 cm) ginger root, grated

juice of a lime

4–6 ice cubes

sparkling mineral water to top up

Blend the melon, lime juice, ginger and ice before topping up to
a fizzy cooler.

NUTRIENTS
Beta-carotene, folic acid, vitamin C;
calcium, magnesium, phosphorus,
potassium, sodium, sulphur

ENERGY	★★★★☆
DETOX	★★☆☆☆
IMMUNITY	★★★☆☆
DIGESTION	★★☆☆☆
SKIN	★★★☆☆

378 kiwi melon

½ melon

2 kiwi fruits

juice of a lime

4–6 ice cubes

sparkling mineral water to top up

Another blended fizzie – pulp the melon, kiwi, lime juice and ice before adding the mineral water for a delicious summery cocktail.

NUTRIENTS
Beta-carotene, folic acid, vitamin C;
calcium, magnesium, phosphorus,
potassium, sodium, sulphur

ENERGY	★★★★☆
DETOX	★★★☆☆
IMMUNITY	★★★★★
DIGESTION	★☆☆☆☆
SKIN	★★★★☆

379 orange strawberry fizz

4 oranges

2 handfuls strawberries

5–7 fresh mint leaves

4–6 ice cubes

sparkling mineral water to top up

Juice the oranges, then purée the strawberries in a blender with just a couple of the mint leaves and the ice. Stir the whole lot together in a big jug and garnish with the remaining mint leaves.

NUTRIENTS
Beta-carotene, biotin, folic acid,
vitamin C; calcium, magnesium,
phosphorus, potassium, sulphur; fibre

ENERGY ★★★★☆
DETOX ★★☆☆☆
IMMUNITY ★★★★☆
DIGESTION ☆☆☆☆☆
SKIN ★★★☆☆

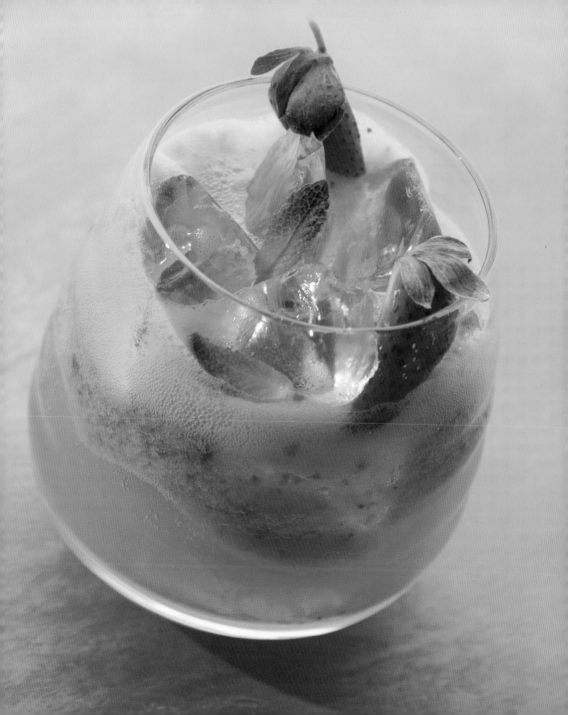

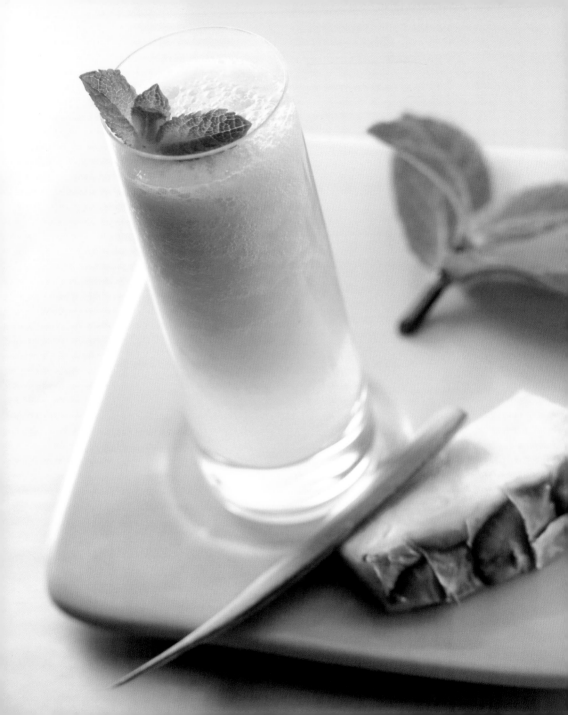

380   fiery pineapple

½ pineapple

1 inch (2.5 cm) ginger root

3–5 fresh mint leaves

4–6 ice cubes

sparkling mineral water to top up

Juice the pineapple and ginger at the same time, then stir up with the other ingredients. The hot ginger is remarkably refreshing, but use less if you prefer.

NUTRIENTS
Beta-carotene, folic acid, vitamin C;
calcium, magnesium, phosphorus,
potassium, sodium

ENERGY	★★★☆☆
DETOX	★★☆☆☆
IMMUNITY	★★★☆☆
DIGESTION	★★★★☆
SKIN	☆☆☆☆☆

381 honeyed lemonade

½ inch (1 cm) ginger root, grated

2 generous teaspoons honey

juice of 3 lemons

4–6 ice cubes

sparkling mineral water to top up

Put the ginger and honey in a mug and half fill it with boiling water, stirring to dissolve the honey. Pour the mixture in a large jug and add the other ingredients for a fabulous take on lemonade. Use more lemon juice if you want it to taste stronger.

NUTRIENTS
Vitamin C; calcium, magnesium, phosphorus, potassium, sodium, sulphur

ENERGY ★★☆☆☆
DETOX ★☆☆☆☆
IMMUNITY ★★★☆☆
DIGESTION ★★☆☆☆
SKIN ☆☆☆☆☆

382 peach cooler

4 oranges

3 peaches

4–6 ice cubes

sparkling mineral water to top up

3–5 fresh mint leaves

Juice the oranges, then mix the peaches and the ice in a blender. Stir the whole lot together in a big jug and garnish with the mint leaves.

NUTRIENTS
Beta-carotene, folic acid, vitamin
B3, vitamin C; calcium, magnesium,
phosphorus, potassium, sodium,
sulphur

ENERGY	★★★★☆
DETOX	★★☆☆☆
IMMUNITY	★★★★☆
DIGESTION	☆☆☆☆☆
SKIN	★★★★☆

383 spiky mango fizz

2 grapefruits

2 mangoes

¼ inch (0.5 cm) ginger root, grated

4–6 ice cubes

sparkling mineral water to top up

Juice the grapefruits, then mix the mangoes, ginger and ice in a blender. Stir the whole lot together in a big jug with the water.

NUTRIENTS
Beta-carotene, folic acid, vitamin C;
calcium, iron, magnesium, phosphorus,
potassium, sodium, sulphur

ENERGY	★★★★☆
DETOX	★★☆☆☆
IMMUNITY	★★★★☆
DIGESTION	★☆☆☆☆
SKIN	★★★☆☆

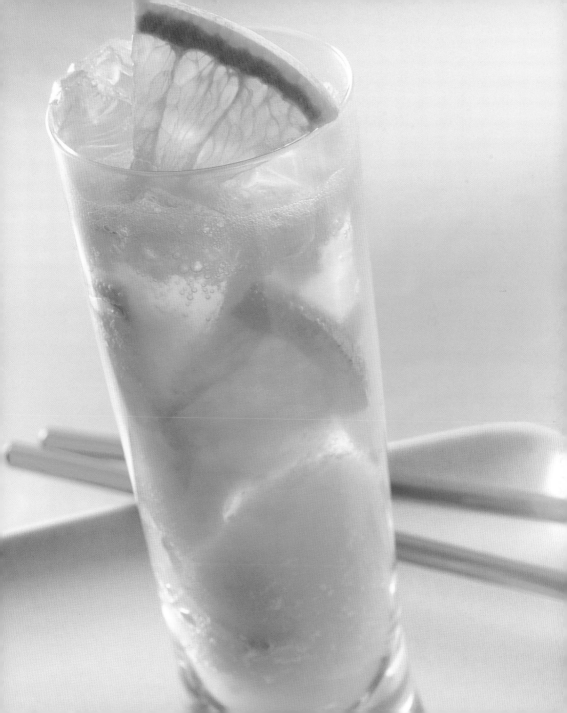

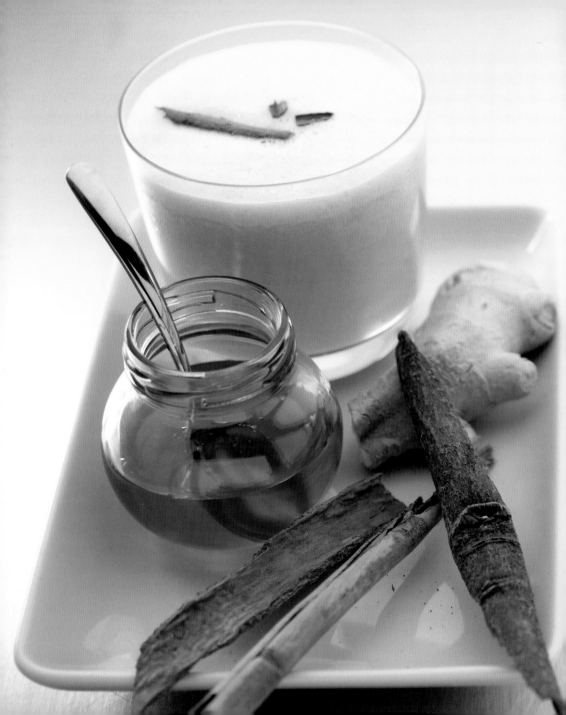

384 apple spice

7 fl oz (200 ml) water

¼ inch (0.5 cm) ginger root, grated or finely sliced

2 cinnamon sticks

1 teaspoon honey

4 tablespoons (60 ml) frozen stewed apple

7 fl oz (200 ml) apple juice

This is a delicious blend of apples and spices in a summer drink. Alternatively, you could drink it warm on a cold winter's night.

Bring the water, ginger and cinnamon to the boil and leave to simmer for at least

five minutes. Strain, add the honey and leave to cool. Meanwhile, mix the apple

and apple juice in a blender and gradually add the cooled tea.

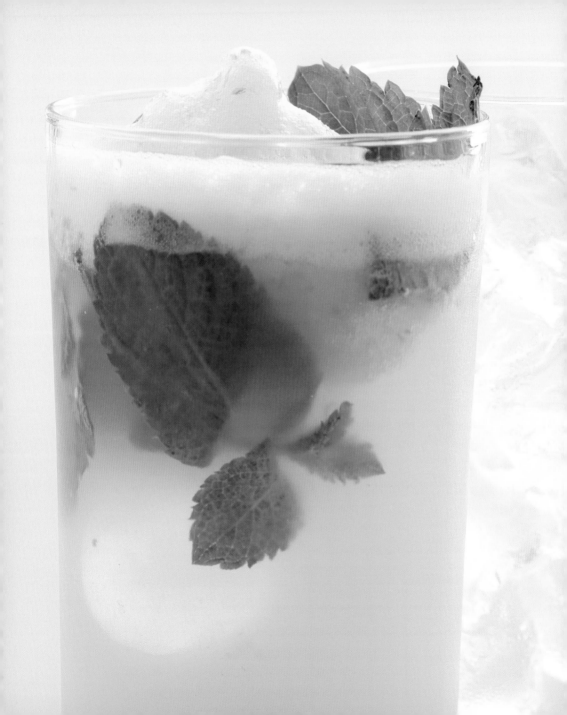

385 fresh sensation

9 fl oz (300 ml) boiling water

1 small bunch fresh mint leaves

1 inch (2.5 cm) ginger root, grated

juice of 4 oranges

1 scoop lime sorbet

4–6 ice cubes

A combination of refreshing, tangy ingredients to cool you
down on a summer's day.

Pour the boiling water over the mint leaves and grated ginger and let them steep

for five minutes. Leave to cool, then top up with freshly squeezed orange juice,

lime sorbet and ice.

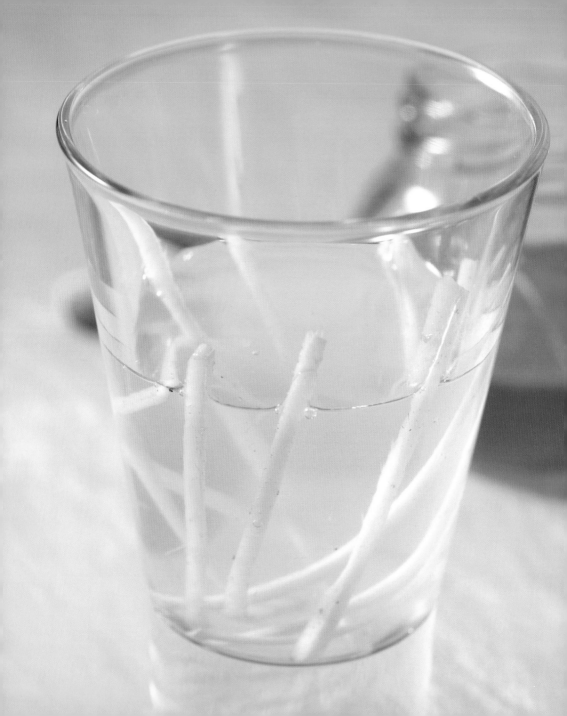

386   ginger brew

1 pt (500 ml) water

1 inch (2.5 cm) ginger root, grated

Neat ginger tea, refreshing and good
for digestion. If you find it a little
strong-tasting, add a teaspoon
of honey for a more mellow flavour.

Bring the water and ginger to the boil and then

simmer for at least five minutes. Strain and serve.

387　middle east ginger

1 pt (500 ml) water

1 inch (2.5 cm) ginger root, grated

10 cardamom pods

Ginger Brew (see blend 386) with a touch of the Middle East from the cardamom, even better for digestion.

Bring the water, ginger and cardamom to the boil and leave to simmer for at least five minutes.

Strain and serve.

388 cold soother

1 pt (500 ml) water

2 cinnamon sticks

juice of a lemon

1 teaspoon honey

A warm drink to soothe the throat on a winter's day.

Bring the water and cinnamon to the boil and leave to simmer for at least five minutes.

Strain, add the lemon juice and honey, and serve.

389 full spice

½ inch (1 cm) ginger root, grated or finely sliced

4 cardamom pods

1 cinnamon stick

5 cloves

1 pt (500 ml) water

A complete blend of delicious spices for a warming drink that's great for soothing the throat and digestion.

Bring all the ingredients to the boil and leave to simmer for at least five minutes.

Strain and serve.

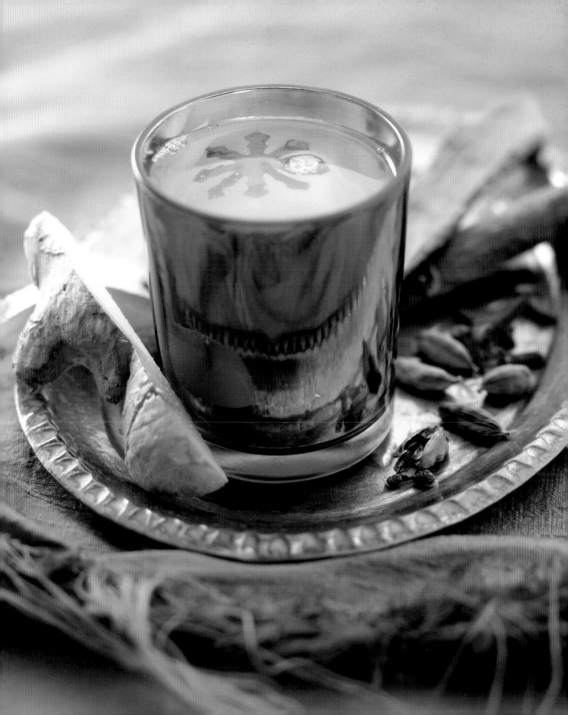

390 mint & honey

1 pt (500 ml) boiling water

1 small bunch fresh mint leaves

1 teaspoon honey

Fresh mint tea is probably the most refreshing hot drink there is, and it's good for digestion. I don't usually add honey, but to make it more like the sweet Middle Eastern version, you can stir in a spoonful.

Pour the boiling water over the mint leaves and leave to steep for five minutes.

If using honey, stir it in before serving.

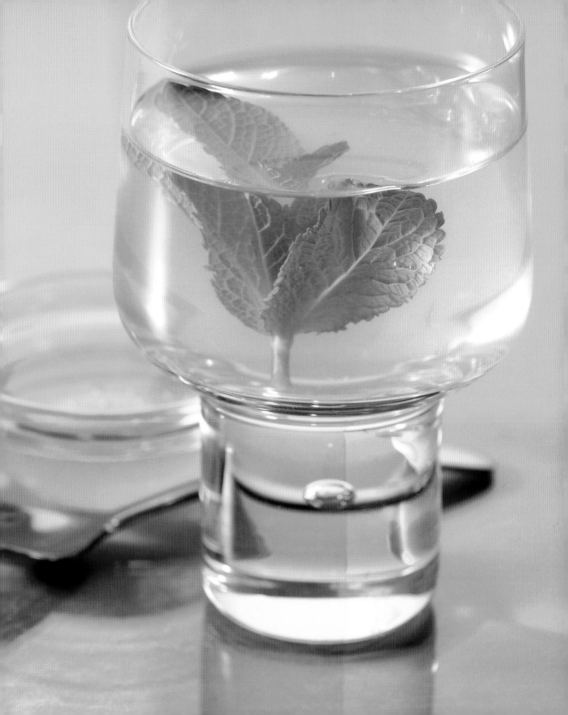

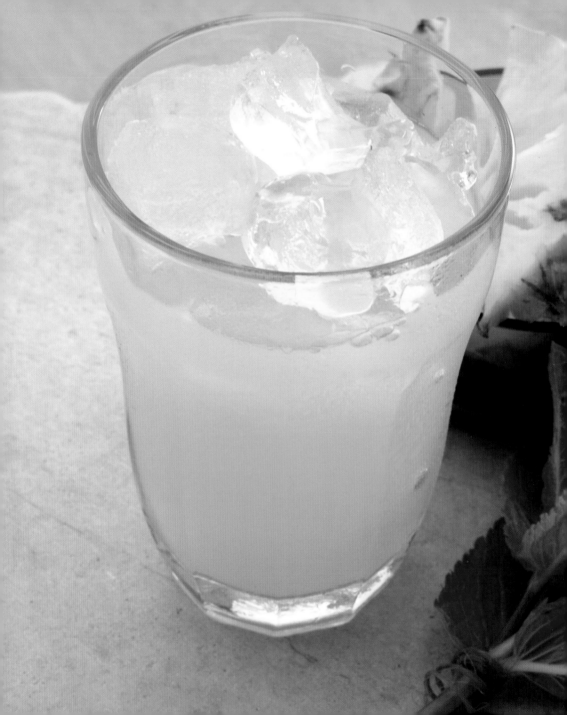

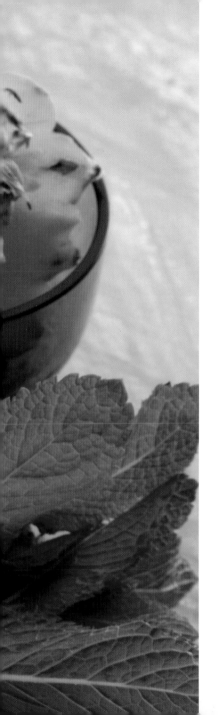

391 tangy mint cooler

1 small bunch fresh mint leaves

9 fl oz (300 ml) boiling water

7 fl oz (200 ml) pineapple juice

4–6 ice cubes

A refreshing, minty cocktail to stimulate the senses.

Make mint tea as in Mint & Honey (see blend 390),

then leave to cool. Top it up with the pineapple juice

and add ice.

392   spicy peachy cream

7 fl oz (200 ml) water

4 cardamom pods

2 cinnamon sticks

3 peaches, frozen in chunks

½ teaspoon vanilla essence

3 tablespoons (45 ml) natural yogurt

3–5 ice cubes

This one is almost a dessert in itself – a fantastic blend of eastern spices, fresh peaches and creamy yogurt.

Bring the water, cardamom and cinnamon to the boil and leave to simmer for at least five minutes.

Strain and leave to cool. Mix the peaches, vanilla and yogurt in the blender and gradually add the

cooled spice tea. Top with ice cubes and sip slowly through a straw.

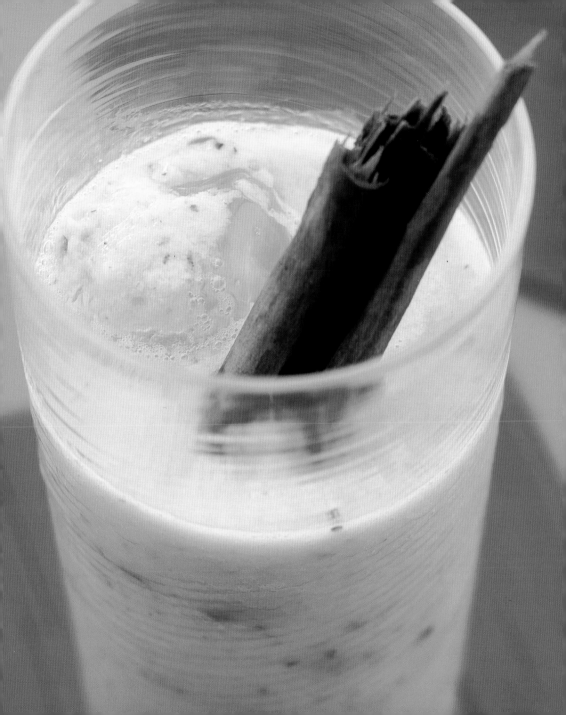

393   rosehip rasp

14 fl oz (400 ml) water

1 rosehip teabag

1 handful raspberries

2 peaches, frozen in chunks

4–6 ice cubes

Rosehip tea has a sharp, fruity, refreshing taste – the fruit contrasts with this perfectly and gives your immune system an extra boost.

Bring the water to the boil, then pour it over the teabag. Leave to steep and cool.

Meanwhile, blend the raspberries and peaches. Stir the fruit pulp into the cooled tea

and add ice cubes.

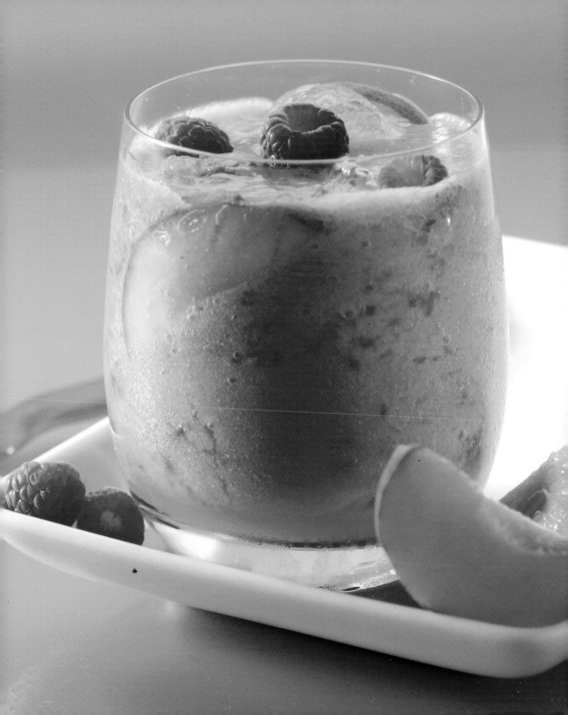

394   tummy tickler

1 pt (500 ml) water

3 star anise

1 teaspoon fennel seeds

7 cardamom pods

½ inch (1 cm) ginger root, finely sliced

1 handful fresh mint leaves

All the spices in this tea are wonderfully soothing for the digestive system – perfect after a large meal. You can make extra and leave the brew on the stove to reheat the next day.

Bring the water to the boil in a saucepan with the dried spices and ginger and leave

to simmer for at least five minutes, ideally longer. A minute or two before serving,

add the mint leaves.

395 orange spice

½ pt (250 ml) water

4–6 cinnamon sticks

8 cloves

3–4 slices orange peel

4 oranges

crushed ice (optional)

This combines the wonderful richness of the spices with the tang of the oranges.

Bring the water to the boil with the cinnamon, cloves and peel, and leave to simmer for

five minutes, ideally longer. Squeeze the oranges and add the juice just before serving.

If you prefer the tea cold, let it cool, then add the orange juice and the ice.

396 berry spice

1 pt (500 ml) water

3 star anise

5 cinnamon sticks

blackcurrant cordial to taste

crushed ice (optional)

Another refreshing combo of spices and fruit, this time with added sweetness from the cordial.

Bring the water to the boil in a saucepan with the spices and leave to simmer for at

least five minutes, ideally longer. Just before serving, add blackcurrant cordial to taste.

If you prefer the tea cold, allow it to cool, then add the cordial and ice.

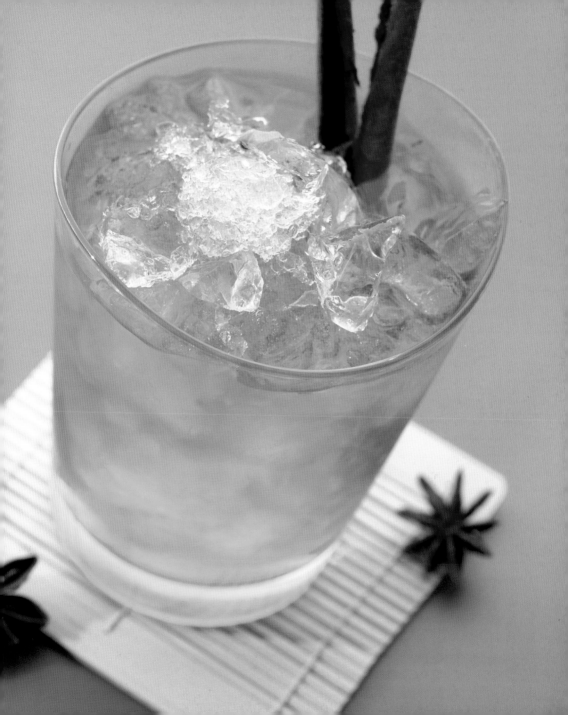

397 apple crumble

12 fl oz (350 ml) water

4–6 cinnamon sticks

8 cloves

5 fl oz (150 ml) apple juice

crushed ice (optional)

All that's missing is the topping!

Bring the water to the boil in a pan with the cinnamon and cloves. Leave to simmer for at

least five minutes. Add the apple juice a couple of minutes before serving. For a refreshing

summer drink, leave the tea to cool, then add the apple juice and lots of ice.

398 stress reliever

1 pint (500 ml) boiling water

1 teaspoon dried borage

1 teaspoon dried lemon balm

These two herbs are renowned for their calming, anti-stress properties. If you find the taste a bit too grassy, add some fresh mint and a little honey.

Put the herbs in a teapot or jug and pour the boiling water over them.

Leave to steep for 3–5 minutes and pour through a strainer before drinking.

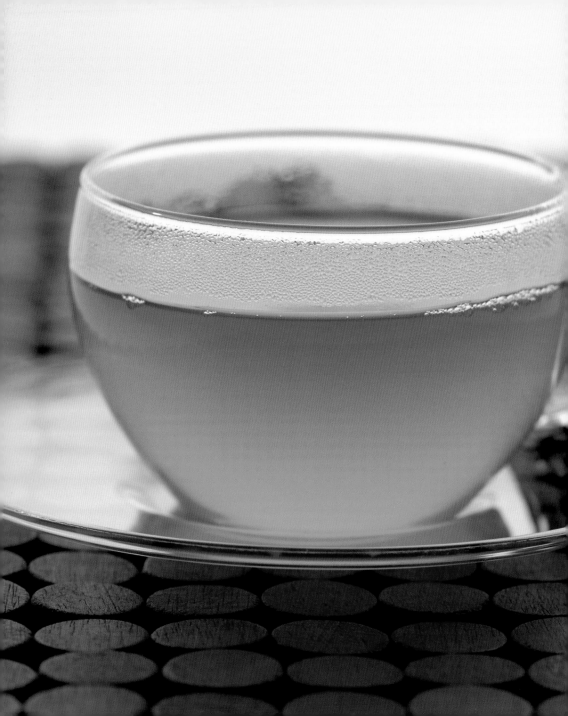

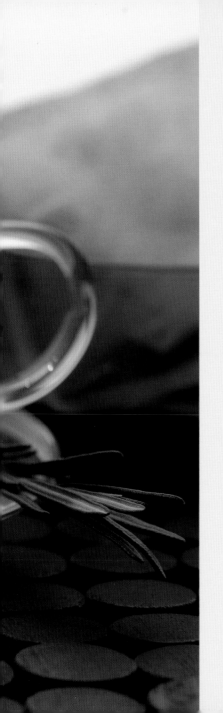

399 perky

1 level teaspoon green tea (or a teabag)

1 teaspoon dried rosemary, or 2 sprigs

1 pt (500 ml) boiling water

The gentle caffeine lift from the green tea goes well with the invigorating properties of the rosemary.

Put all the leaves in a teapot or jug and pour the boiling water over them. Leave to steep for 3–5 minutes and pour through a strainer before drinking.

400 sweet mint

1 licorice root stick

1 pt (500 ml) water

1 handful fresh mint leaves

This is a wonderfully refreshing mint tea, naturally sweetened and given a bit more depth by the licorice.

Bash the licorice root to break up the fibres a bit. Put the water and root in a saucepan,

bring to the boil and leave to simmer for about ten minutes. A minute or so before serving,

add the mint leaves.

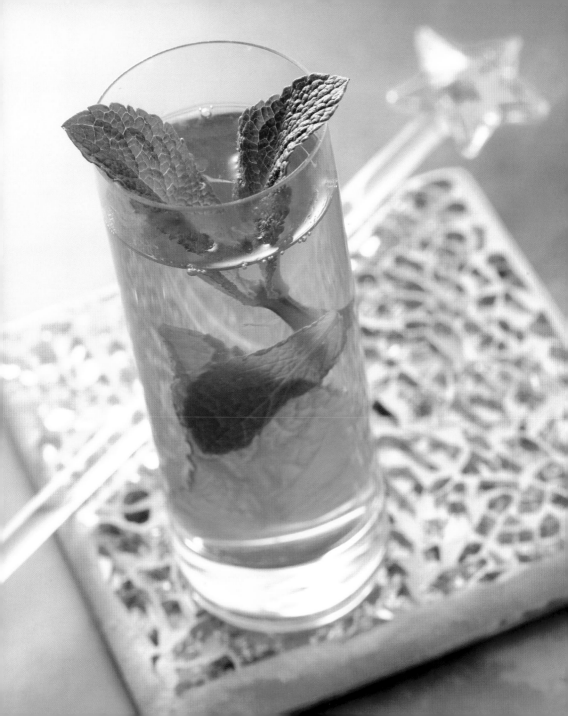

401 blackcurrant & licorice

1 licorice root stick

1 teaspoon fennel seeds

1 pt (500 ml) water

blackcurrant cordial to taste

crushed ice and fresh mint leaves (optional)

A throwback to those old-fashioned boiled sweets!

Bash the licorice root to break up the fibres. Put the root and fennel seeds in the water

and bring to the boil. Leave to simmer for ten minutes, then add the blackcurrant cordial

– or, to enjoy cold, let the tea cool and then add the cordial, ice and a few mint leaves.

402 thai tea

1 pt (500 ml) water

2 lemongrass sticks, sliced

1 inch (2.5 cm) ginger root, finely sliced

juice and sliced zest of a lime

crushed ice and fresh mint leaves (optional)

The classic combination of ginger and citrus with an Asian twist.

Bring the water to the boil with the lemongrass, ginger and lime zest. Leave to simmer for

five minutes, ideally longer. Just before serving, squeeze in the lime juice. Strain and serve.

This tea is delicious left to cool, served with ice and a few mint leaves.

403 calmer

1 pt (500 ml) water

1 lemongrass stick, sliced

8 cardamom pods

3–4 slices orange zest

1 teaspoon dried chamomile leaves (or a teabag)

1 handful fresh mint leaves

In the Far East, lemongrass has long been used to calm the nervous system; in Europe, so has chamomile.

In a saucepan, bring the water to boil with the lemongrass, cardamom pods and orange zest.

Leave to simmer for at least five minutes, ideally longer. A couple of minutes before serving,

add the chamomile and mint. Strain and serve.

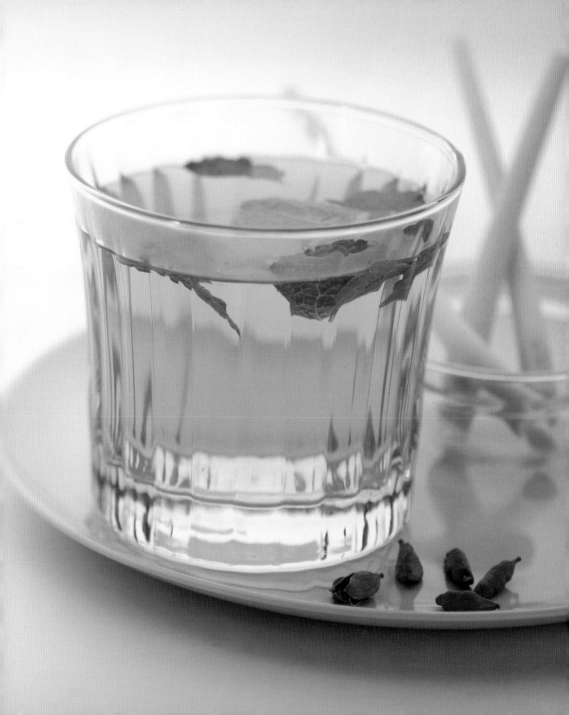

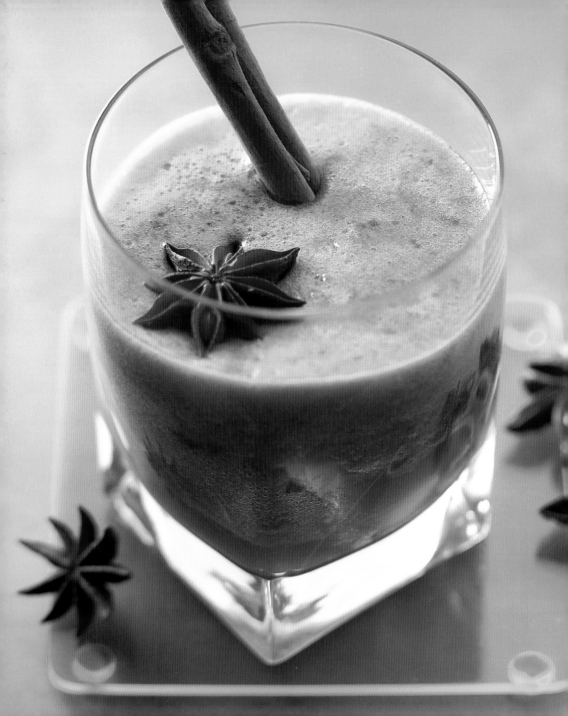

404 just peachy

14 fl oz (400 ml) water

4–6 cinnamon sticks

3 star anise

2 slices lemon zest

4 peaches

squeeze of lemon juice

4–6 ice cubes

Make sure you use really ripe peaches for this delicious, filling summer drink.

Bring the water to the boil in a saucepan with the cinnamon, anise and zest, and leave to simmer for at least five minutes, ideally longer. Allow the tea to cool before whizzing it up in a blender with the peaches (stones removed), a squeeze of lemon and the ice.

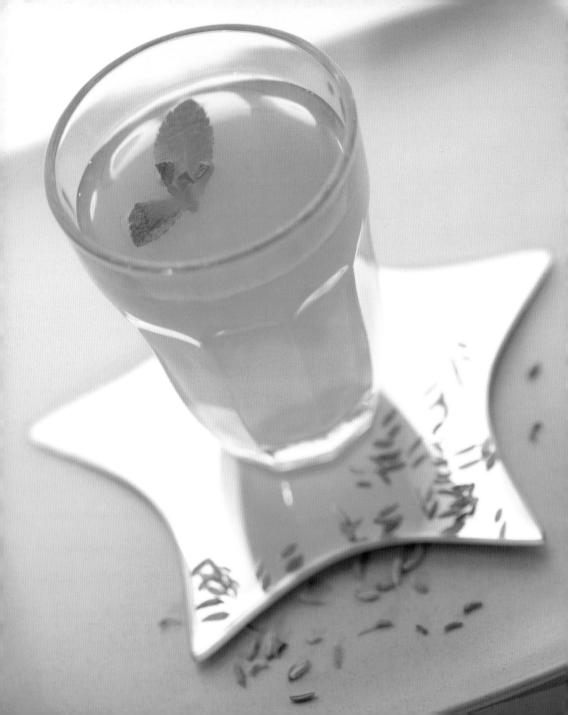

405 sweet green

1 pt (500 ml) water

1 licorice root stick

1 teaspoon fennel seeds

1 level teaspoon green tea (or a teabag)

1 handful fresh mint leaves

The slight bitterness of green tea is nicely offset by the spices
and mint.

Bash the licorice root to break up the fibres a bit. Put it in the water, in a saucepan, with the

fennel seeds. Bring to the boil and leave to simmer for about ten minutes. A couple of minutes

before serving, add the green tea and mint leaves. This tea is very refreshing cold too.

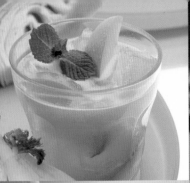
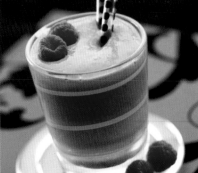
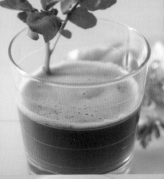
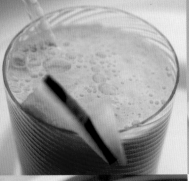
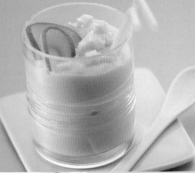
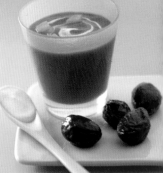
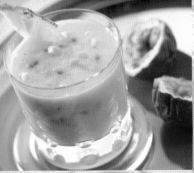
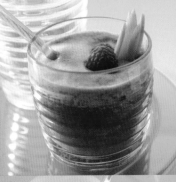
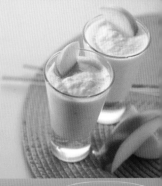
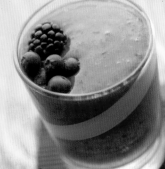
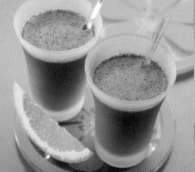
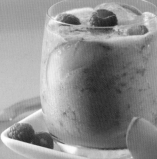

juicing
reference

This section starts with four healthful programs to make choosing your juice recipes easy. If you're just getting into the habit, begin with The Basic Intro Week to start you off gently on simple, delicious fruit and vegetable drinks. Then there's The Detox Week: juices chosen to accompany a basic detox program. If you tend to get every cough and cold going, you'd do well to give your immune system a boost by having a daily fresh juice as suggested in The Immune-Power Week. Finally, the last juice course is a wonderfully rejuvenating Juice High Weekend, where, for nearly 48 hours, you feast on nothing but juices.

Following on from the juice courses you'll find two useful charts: a list of nutrients together with their richest sources and known benefits; and an easy reference listing of common ailments with the fruit, vegetables and juice blends that can best support you in returning to perfect health.

the basic intro week

To inspire you through the maze of the countless combinations possible, this starter course introduces you to some juice recipes that are likely to become your staples. Working primarily with ingredients that you're most likely to have in your fruit bowl or refrigerator, we build up from simple fruit juices to blends you may initially have found a little challenging on the palate. Believe me, if you're not already a true juicing devotee, by the time you've got to the end of this week you will be.

Monday	Sweet C Too (blend 009)
Tuesday	Pink Pear (blend 105)
Wednesday	Gently Raspberry (blend 081)
Thursday	Pineapple Basic (blend 124)
Friday	Orange Carrot (blend 136)
Saturday	Easy Morning (blend 134)
Sunday	Apple Cleanser (blend 012)

the detox week

Many health-conscious people occasionally "go on a detox". First, it's important to remember that our bodies are constantly detoxifying, not just when we choose. Second, some of the faddy programs are, in my view, too extreme and in some cases unhealthy. However, other programs encourage us to reassess what we are consuming, and leave us feeling rejuvenated, clearer in mind and body and bursting with energy. The recipes here are particularly cleansing blends aimed at supporting you during a sensible detox program.

Monday	Apple Cleanser (blend 012)
Tuesday	Green Hit (blend 149)
Wednesday	Carrot Cleanser (blend 137)
Thursday	Beet Basic (blend 187)
Friday	Green Goddess (blend 173)
Saturday	Green 'n' Pear It (blend 175)
Sunday	Green Pines (blend 128)

the immune-power week

If you've noticed that your body's defences are not up to scratch – you pick up any passing cold and regularly suffer from throat or bladder infections – your immune system may need a hand. Even if you've always had a tendency to get ill, you should find that giving yourself a boost with fresh, raw juices and smoothies helps keep colds at bay, let alone anything more serious. These recipes are particularly powerful immunity-boosters for a concerted one-week course, but you'll feel even more benefit if you make juicing an ongoing delight.

Monday	Power-packed C (blend 059)
Tuesday	Carotene Kick (blend 193)
Wednesday	Cold War (blend 145)
Thursday	Grapefruit Blues (blend 037)
Friday	Greatfruit C (blend 039)
Saturday	Carotene Catapult (blend 141)
Sunday	Green Tomatoes (blend 202)

the juice high weekend

By consuming nothing but raw, fresh juices for a weekend, you give your body a break from the foods and drinks that normally travel through your insides. This way, the body has a chance to do a bit of its own housework and leave you rejuvenated and feeling like you're making a fresh start. It is also a good step in helping you kick a toxic habit such as smoking. This may not sound like a huge amount of fun, and it is likely to be challenging, so it's best to go on a juice fast over a weekend or two-day break, when you can relax and rest as you feel is necessary.

You'll find you get the most out of this course if you prepare yourself well beforehand by buying in all you need, and see it as treating yourself to two days of healthy calm. In addition to drinking the blends listed opposite (about 6 glasses a day in total), I suggest you incorporate the following into your weekend: plenty of spring water, several snoozes (you may feel tired, irritable or get a bit of a headache), a sauna or steam, a warm bath (sprinkle in a few drops of your favourite essential oils), a massage, gentle walks in fresh air, breathing exercises, and pastimes, such as reading, to occupy you if you are not sleeping. Avoid strenuous exercise.

Day Before	Eat light salads and fruit during the day.	
	Dinner	Green Hit (blend 149)
Day One	Breakfast	Apple Gone Loupey (blend 022)
	Late morning	Florida Blue (blend 057)
	Afternoon	Beetles (blend 188)
	Dinner	Green Goddess (blend 173)
Day Two	Breakfast	Carrot Deep Cleanser (blend 138)
	Mid-morning	Beet Basic (blend 187)
	Lunch	Large salad of fresh, raw vegetables and/or fruits.
	Dinner	Large salad of fresh, raw vegetables and/or fruits.

At the end of the program, it is crucial that you do not suddenly overload your body with large quantities of cooked or rich foods. Prepare a substantial, varied salad and dress it lightly with olive oil and lemon juice. Sit down to eat it and chew it well.

Most people are likely to feel a little tired doing the Juice High Weekend. You may also experience some bloating or flatulence, diarrhea, headaches, tiredness and sweating. These are normal; however, if they become excessive or you have other symptoms, you should visit a doctor. Do not undertake the Juice High Weekend if you are unwell, pregnant or on medication.

nutrient chart

This chart lists the main nutrients that the body needs for optimum health. The right-hand column gives all the rich food sources for each nutrient – including foods that are not used in juices or smoothies but that should nevertheless form part of your regular diet.

nutrient	benefits	rich food sources
VITAMINS		
Vitamin A	Important antioxidant, protects skin and keeps vision healthy; protects against cancer.	Butter, kidney, liver, whole milk
Beta-carotene	Important antioxidant, protects skin – including "inside skins" such as the lining of intestines, lungs, nose and throat. Beta-carotene is the plant version of vitamin A.	Apricots, asparagus, broccoli, cantaloupe melons, carrots, kale, liver, pumpkins, spinach, sweet potatoes, watermelons
Vitamin B1 (thiamine)	Needed for energy production; for the normal workings of the nervous system, muscles and heart; growth and development.	Beef kidney and liver, brewer's yeast, chickpeas, kidney beans, rice bran, salmon, soy (soya) beans, sunflower seeds, wheatgerm, wholegrain wheat and rye
Vitamin B2 (riboflavin)	Needed for the production of energy from food, and for healthy skin and mucous membranes; needed for nerves to function well and for healthy growth and development.	Almonds, brewer's yeast, cheese, chicken, eggs, fish, milk, organic meats, wheatgerm, yogurt
Vitamin B3 (niacin)	Needed for the production of energy; the health of the nervous system, digestive system and skin; and to keep cholesterol levels low.	Beef liver, brewer's yeast, chicken, fish, nuts, potatoes, pulses, sunflower seeds, turkey
Vitamin B5 (pantothenic acid)	Needed for energy production; the body's response to stress; regeneration of all cells, particularly in the nervous system; and antibodies (defenders against infections).	Blue cheese, brewer's yeast, corn, dried fruit, eggs, lentils, liver, lobster, meat, nuts, peas, soy (soya) beans, sunflower seeds, wheatgerm, wholegrain products, vegetables
Vitamin B6 (pyridoxine)	Needed for energy production; a healthy nervous system, brain and mental state; and for the body to build all types of cells, hormones and antibodies.	Avocados, bananas, bran, brewer's yeast, carrots, eggs, hazelnuts, lean meat, lentils, rice, salmon, shrimp, soy (soya) beans, sunflower seeds, tuna, wheatgerm, wholewheat flour
Vitamin B12 (cyanocobalamin)	Particularly important for the health of the brain and nervous system and the formation of red blood cells.	Cheese, clams, eggs, fish, meat, milk and milk products, poultry. NB – vitamin B12 is not found in plant foods
Folic acid	Needed for production of red blood cells, and the growth of healthy nerves, particularly in a developing fetus.	Barley, brewer's yeast, fruit, chickpeas, green leafy vegetables, lentils, liver, peas, rice, soy (soya) beans, wheatgerm
Biotin	Helps the body process sugars, carbohydrates, proteins and other vitamins; needed for healthy skin, nails and hair.	Brewer's yeast, brown rice, cashew nuts, cheese, chicken, eggs, lentils, liver, mackerel, meat, milk, oats, peanuts, peas, soy (soya) beans, sunflower seeds, tuna, walnuts

nutrient	benefits	rich food sources
Vitamin C (ascorbic acid)	Countless uses: promotes healthy blood capillaries and gums, and healthy skin and healing; aids absorption of iron and production of hemoglobin; boosts the body's defences against illnesses, helps protect against cancer, heart disease, allergies, infections, colds, stress and even aging.	Blackcurrants, broccoli, Brussels sprouts, grapefruits, green bell peppers, guavas, kale, kiwi fruits, lemons, oranges, papayas, potatoes, spinach, strawberries, tomatoes, watercress
Vitamin D	Helps control use of calcium, needed for strong bones and teeth.	Cod liver oil, eggs, herrings, mackerel, salmon, sardines
Vitamin E	Antioxidant; helps protect skin, circulation, brain, hormones and much more against effects of pollution; anti-clotting properties protect against heart disease.	Almonds, corn oil, hazelnuts, sunflower seeds and oil, walnuts, wheatgerm, wholewheat flour
Vitamin K	Needed to ensure the blood can clot normally.	Broccoli, Brussels sprouts, green cabbage, spinach, Camembert cheese, cauliflower, Cheddar cheese, green tea, oats, soy (soya) beans

MINERALS

Calcium	Best-known for building healthy bones, so particularly important for growing children and women reaching menopause at risk of osteoporosis. Also needed for muscles to contract and relax properly (including the heart muscle) and for healthy nerve function.	Almonds, Brazil nuts, cheese, green leafy vegetables, kelp, milk, molasses, salmon (canned), sardines (canned), sesame seeds, shrimp, soy (soya) beans, yogurt
Chromium	Helps processing of sugars and carbohydrates; works with the hormone insulin to balance blood sugar levels and hence energy, concentration and appetite.	Beef, brewer's yeast, cheese, chicken, eggs, fish, fruit, liver, molasses, potatoes, seafood, whole grains
Copper	Needed in tiny amounts in the body for proper transport and production of red blood cells, and for triggering the release of iron to form hemoglobin.	Barley, cocoa, honey, lentils, molasses, mushrooms, mussels, nuts, oats, oysters, salmon, seeds, wheatgerm
Iodine	Forms part of the thyroid hormone that controls metabolism.	Cod liver oil, fish, oysters, table salt (iodized), seaweed, sunflower seeds
Iron	Part of hemoglobin – the red blood cell substance which carries oxygen from the lungs around the body to all the cells. Also needed as a catalyst for other processes in the body including cell reproduction.	Cashew nuts, cheese, egg yolks, chickpeas, green leafy vegetables, lean meat, lentils, molasses, mussels, offal, pumpkin seeds, sardines, seaweed, walnuts, wheatgerm
Magnesium	Works with calcium in many body functions, such as the transmission of messages down nerve cells; contraction and relaxation of muscles; growth and development of bones; also for the production of energy.	Almonds, fish, green leafy vegetables, molasses, nuts, soy (soya) beans, sesame and sunflower seeds, wheatgerm

nutrient	benefits	rich food sources
Manganese	An antioxidant, needed for healthy nerves and brain; sex hormone production.	Avocados, barley, blackberries, brown rice, buckwheat, chestnuts, ginger, hazelnuts, oats, peas, pecans, seaweed, spinach
Potassium	Works with sodium to control normal nerve function and muscle contraction, including a regular heartbeat. The two also help balance the flow of water and nutrients in and out of cells, preventing water retention.	Avocados, bananas, citrus fruits, lentils, milk, molasses, nuts, parsnips, potatoes, raisins, sardines (canned), spinach, whole grains
Selenium	Works with vitamin E as a powerful antioxidant to protect against aging and degenerative diseases including certain cancers and heart disease.	Avocados, broccoli, cabbage, celery, chicken, egg yolks, garlic, lentils, liver, milk, mushrooms, onions, seafood, wheatgerm, whole grains
Sodium	Alongside potassium, helps control the water balance in the body. Important for regulating blood pressure, healthy nervous function and normal muscle contraction and relaxation.	Table salt and most commercially processed and packaged foods, as well as bacon, bread, butter, ham, milk, canned vegetables
Sulphur	Antioxidant; also helps the liver release bile and detoxify various substances; needed for the production of collagen, our cellular "glue", so it is important for skin health and the repair of injured skin.	Cabbage, clams, eggs, fish, garlic, milk, onions, wheatgerm
Zinc	Acts as an antioxidant; is needed for normal taste; also needed for the growth and regeneration of new cells (particularly important in fetal development and teenagers); helps skin heal; needed for healthy reproductive organs, especially in men.	Egg yolks, fish, milk, molasses, oysters, peanuts, red meat, sesame seeds, soy (soya) beans, sunflower seeds, turkey, wheatgerm, whole grains
OTHER IMPORTANT NUTRIENTS		
Essential fatty acids	Needed for brain power, healthy nerves, smooth skin, hormone balance and more, these fats are incorporated into the membrane or skin of every cell in the body to keep each one working optimally.	Fish such as herrings, mackerel, salmon and sardines; nuts; seeds such as hemp, flaxseeds (linseed), pumpkin, sesame and sunflower
Protein	The basic material of all living cells – not just those that form the structure of our bodies but also blood cells, hormones and much more. Dietary sources are essential for rebuilding and regeneration, and for all body systems to function.	Eggs, fish, meat, milk, poultry, soy (soya)

juices for ailments

This chart lists the best foods to eat to help your body fight a range of common ailments, and offers a selection of the juice recipes that are rich in such foods. However, drinking the juices suggested is intended as a supplement to, and not a replacement for, professional medical advice.

ailment	foods to eat	blend no.	title
Acne	All greens (such as broccoli, kale, parsley, spinach, watercress), fruit and vegetable fibre, garlic, seeds and their oils, yogurt	178 181 267 324	Green Waldorf Super Defender Heaven Scent Purple Pineapple
Anemia	All greens (such as broccoli, kale, parsley, spinach, watercress), beets (beetroot), berries, kiwi fruits, citrus fruits, molasses	182 197 188 067	Grape & Green Tabouleh Beetles Blackcurrant Twist
Angina	Broccoli, citrus fruits, fruit and vegetable fibre, kale, kiwi fruits, seeds and their oils, strawberries, watercress, wheatgerm	175 178 253 268	Green 'n' Pear It Green Waldorf Mango Blues Globe Trotter
Arthritis	Apricots, berries, broccoli, carrots, garlic, ginger, kiwi fruits, mangoes, pineapples, red bell peppers, seeds and their oils, watercress, wheatgerm	113 130 160 083 380	Breakfast Pear Joint Aid Carrot Jointaid Berry Bonanza Fiery Pineapple
Asthma	Apricots, berries, broccoli, carrots, ginger, kale, mangoes, melons, red bell peppers, seeds and their oils, sweet potatoes, watercress, watermelons	122 183 139 271	Ginger Zinger Creamy Green Carrot Crunch Peachy Strawbs
Bladder problems	Blueberries, broccoli, citrus fruits, cranberries, garlic, kiwi fruits, strawberries, watermelons, yogurt	028 141 277 289	Cranapple Carotene Catapult Cranapple Crush Watermelon Crush
Boils	All greens (such as broccoli, kale, parsley, spinach, watercress), berries, citrus fruits, fruit and vegetable fibre, garlic, kiwi fruits	073 174 138 250	Orange Pepper Green Apple Carrot Deep Cleanser Summer Mango Special
Bronchitis	Apricots, broccoli, carrots, citrus fruits, garlic, kale, kiwi fruits, mangoes, melons, red bell peppers, seeds and their oils, strawberries, sweet potatoes, watercress, watermelons	039 119 145 141	Greatfruit C Black Pineapple Cold War Carotene Catapult
Burns, cuts & bruises	Apricots, broccoli, cabbages, carrots, citrus fruits, garlic, kale, kiwi fruits, mangoes, milk, red bell peppers, seeds and their oils, strawberries, watercress, yogurt	056 066 269 308	Bright Orange Muddy Puddle Supreme Strawberry Pinky Mango

ailment	foods to eat	blend no.	title
Bursitis	Apricots, broccoli, cabbages, carrots, citrus fruits, garlic, ginger, kale, kiwi fruits, mangoes, pineapples, red bell peppers, seeds and their oils, strawberries, watercress	122 130 084 272	Ginger Zinger Joint Aid Sharp Citrusberry Pink Berry Crush
Candidiasis	All greens (such as broccoli, kale, parsley, spinach, watercress), yogurt	175 138 144 328	Green 'n' Pear It Carrot Deep Cleanser Veggie Carotene Catapult Pure Pineapple Creamy
Cardiovascular disease	Broccoli, citrus fruits, fruit and vegetable fibre, kale, kiwi fruits, seeds and their oils, strawberries, watercress, wheatgerm	059 130 227 269	Power-packed C Joint Aid Take Heart Supreme Strawberry
Chronic catarrh	Apricots, berries, carrots, citrus fruits, mangoes, melons, papayas, pineapples, watermelons	140 155 119 267	Carrot Digestif Florida Carrot Black Pineapple Heaven Scent
Chronic fatigue	All greens (such as broccoli, kale, parsley, spinach, watercress), bananas, berries, citrus fruits, kale, kiwi fruits, seeds and their oils, watercress, wheatgerm, yogurt	168 173 298 320	Salad Cooler Green Goddess Green Banana Creamy Purple Rain
Cold sores	Apricots, berries, broccoli, carrots, citrus fruits, garlic, kale, kiwi fruits, mangoes, red bell peppers, strawberries, tomatoes, watercress	059 145 144 202	Power-packed C Cold War Veggie Carotene Catapult Green Tomatoes
Colitis	Apples, apricots, broccoli, cabbages, carrots, citrus fruits, fruit and vegetable fibre, kale, kiwi fruits, mangoes, melons, papayas, pineapples, seeds and their oils, strawberries, watercress, wheatgerm	012 144 179 264	Apple Cleanser Veggie Carotene Catapult Sweet Green Melon Papaya Pure
Common cold & 'flu	Apricots, broccoli, carrots, citrus fruits, garlic, ginger, kale, kiwi fruits, mangoes, melons, nectarines, red bell peppers, strawberries, watercress, watermelons	059 145 252 273	Power-packed C Cold War Nectargo Citrus Strawbs
Constipation	Fruit and vegetable fibre, plenty of water and juices, seeds and their oils	002 188 242 338	Apple Basic Beetles Regular Banana Apricot Regular
Cough	Apricots, berries, broccoli, carrots, citrus fruits, garlic, ginger, kale, kiwi fruits, mangoes, melons, papayas, pineapples, red bell peppers, sweet potatoes, watercress, watermelons	040 119 141 265	Surprising Sweetie Black Pineapple Carotene Catapult Papaya Salad

ailment	foods to eat	blend no.	title
Cystitis	Broccoli, citrus fruits, cranberries, garlic, kiwi fruits, strawberries, pineapples, watermelons, yogurt	028 277 289 331	Cranapple Cranapple Crush Watermelon Crush Pinkypine
Dermatitis	Apples, apricots, berries, broccoli, carrots, celery, citrus fruits, garlic, kale, kiwi fruits, mangoes, melons, red bell peppers, seeds and their oils, watercress, watermelons	022 137 213	Apple Gone Loupey Carrot Cleanser Creamy Crunch Any juice/smoothie with seeds/seed oil
Diabetes	All greens (such as broccoli, kale, parsley, spinach, watercress), fruit and vegetable fibre, seeds and their oils	140 182 181 261	Carrot Digestif Grape & Green Super Defender Pineberry
Diarrhea	Apples, carrots, celery, pears	001 027 112 213	Eve's Downfall Apple Zing Pear Basic Creamy Crunch
Diverticulitis	Fruit and vegetable fibre, garlic, ginger, yogurt	004 126 268 328	Basic with a Boost Digestaid Globe Trotter Pure Pineapple Creamy
Dry skin	Apricots, berries, broccoli, carrots, citrus fruits, garlic, kale, kiwi fruits, mangoes, melons, red bell peppers, seeds and their oils, watercress, watermelons	155 083	Florida Carrot Berry Bonanza Any juice/smoothie with seeds/seed oil
Ear infection	Apricots, berries, broccoli, carrots, citrus fruits, garlic, kale, kiwi fruits, mangoes, melons, red bell peppers, seeds and their oils, watercress, watermelons	072 145 144 083	Water Cooler II Cold War Veggie Carotene Catapult Berry Bonanza
Eczema	Berries, broccoli, carrots, garlic, kale, kiwi fruits, mangoes, melons, red bell peppers, seeds and their oils, watercress, watermelons	130 141 183 275	Joint Aid Carotene Catapult Creamy Green Blue Healer
Endometriosis	All fruit and vegetable juices and fibre, seeds and their oils, soy (soya) milk, yogurt	071 137 260	Orange Aniseed Twist Carrot Cleanser Apple Squared Any smoothie with soy (soya) milk
Eyesight problems	Apricots, berries, carrots, kale, mangoes, melons, pineapples, red bell peppers, watercress, watermelons	133 159 275 330 186	What's Up, Doc? Capple and Black Blue Healer Blue Pine Creamy Eye Opener

ailment	foods to eat	blend no.	title
Fatigue	All fruit and vegetable juice and fibre, bananas, berries, carrots, pears, molasses, yogurt	113	Breakfast Pear
		137	Carrot Cleanser
		298	Green Banana Creamy
		321	Mighty Berry
		399	Perky
		405	Sweet Green
Fever	All fresh fruit and vegetable juices (especially apricots, berries, broccoli, carrots, citrus fruits, kale, kiwi fruits, mangoes, melons, red bell peppers, sweet potatoes, watercress and watermelons), garlic, seeds and their oils	061	Orange Medley
		145	Cold War
		193	Carotene Kick
		288	Pure Watermelon
Fibroids	All greens (such as broccoli, kale, parsley, spinach, watercress), celery, citrus fruits, fennel, fruit and vegetable fibre, pears, soy (soya) milk, seeds and their oils	071	Orange Aniseed Twist
		175	Green 'n' Pear It
			Any smoothie with soy milk and seeds/seed oil
Food poisoning	Apples, carrots, celery, ginger, pears	002	Eve's Downfall
		027	Apple Zing
		103	Pear Basic
		213	Creamy Crunch
Fractures	All greens (such as broccoli, kale, parsley, spinach, watercress), milk, molasses, peaches, pineapples, seeds and their oils, soy (soya) milk, yogurt	066	Muddy Puddle
		173	Green Goddess
		302	Peachy Banana Dream
		330	Creamy Blue Pine
Gallbladder disorders	Apples, beet (beetroot), grapefruits, yogurt	137	Carrot Cleanser
		188	Beetles
		189	Blood 'n' Grape
		170	Bloody Cuke
Gout	Cabbages, carrots, celery, cherries, kale, strawberries	096	Cherry Pie
		100	Cherry Cooler
		151	Carrot Lift
		222	Soft and Sharp
Hemorrhoids	Apricots, berries, broccoli, carrots, citrus fruits, fruit and vegetable fibre, kale, kiwi fruits, mangoes, melons, red bell peppers, watercress, watermelons, wheatgerm	016	Black Orchard Berry Buster
		057	Florida Blue
		159	Capple and Black
		258	Pastel Perfect
Hangover	All greens (such as broccoli, kale, parsley, spinach, watercress), apples, bananas, carrots, celery, ginger, yogurt	027	Apple Zing
		137	Carrot Cleanser
		290	Creamy Cooler
		298	Green Banana Creamy
Hay fever	Apricots, berries, broccoli, carrots, citrus fruits, kale, kiwi fruits, mangoes, melons, seeds and their oils, strawberries, sweet potatoes, watercress, watermelons	059	Power-packed C
		177	Green Grapefruit
		141	Carotene Catapult
		269	Supreme Strawberry

ailment	foods to eat	blend no.	title
Heartburn	Cabbages, papayas, pineapples	030	Bellyful
		115	Gut Soother
		126	Digestaid
		264	Papaya Pure
Herpes	Berries, broccoli, carrots, citrus fruits, garlic, kale, kiwi fruits, seeds and their oils, tomatoes, watercress	059	Power-packed C
		145	Cold War
		144	Veggie Carotene Catapult
		202	Green Tomatoes
High blood pressure	All fresh fruit and vegetables, especially greens (such as broccoli, kale, parsley, spinach, watercress), apples, garlic, seeds and their oils, wheatgerm	022	Apple Gone Loupey
		149	Green Hit
		222	Soft and Sharp
		227	Take Heart
Hives (urticaria)	Apricots, berries, broccoli, carrots, citrus fruits, garlic, kale, kiwi fruits, mangoes, melons, red bell peppers, sweet potatoes, watercress, watermelons	059	Power-packed C
		079	Citrusberry
		193	Carotene Kick
		307	Pango Mango
Hypoglycemia	All fresh fruit and vegetable juices and fibre, cucumbers, mangoes, seeds and their oils, yogurt	182	Grape & Green
		163	Cucumber Refresher
		310	Berry Mango
		320	Purple Rain
Indigestion	Cabbages, papayas, pineapples	030	Bellyful
		115	Gut Soother
		126	Digestaid
		387	Middle East Ginger
		394	Tummy Tickler
Irritable bowel syndrome	All fruit and vegetable juices and fibre, all greens (such as broccoli, kale, parsley, spinach, watercress), bananas, cabbages, papayas, pineapples	178	Green Waldorf
		115	Gut Soother
		264	Papaya Pure
		298	Green Banana Creamy
Kidney problems	All greens (such as broccoli, kale, parsley, spinach, watercress), apricots, carrots, celery, cranberries, cucumbers, melons, molasses, pears, pumpkins, red bell peppers, sweet potatoes, watermelons	106	Pink Pear II
		219	Pink Punch
		166	Water, Water Everywhere
		173	Green Goddess
Memory problems	All fresh fruit and vegetable juices, especially berries, broccoli, citrus fruits, kale, kiwi fruits, watercress, seeds and their oils, wheatgerm	065	Orange Winter Crumble
		178	Green Waldorf
		253	Mango Blues
			Any smoothie with seeds/ seed oil
Menopause-related problems	All fruit and vegetable juices and fibre, apples, celery, fennel, garlic, soy (soya), seeds and their oils, wheatgerm	012	Apple Cleanser
		071	Orange Aniseed Twist
		217	Crunch Morning Favourite
			Any smoothie with soy (soya) milk

ailment	foods to eat	blend no.	title
Menstrual problems	All fruit and vegetable juices and fibre, beets (beetroot), celery, fennel, garlic, seeds and their oils, soy (soya)	071 181 187	Orange Aniseed Twist Super Defender Beet Basic Any smoothie with soy (soya) milk
Motion sickness	Cabbages, carrots, ginger, peppermint	139 140 390 386	Carrot Crunch Carrot Digestif Mint & Honey Ginger Brew
Muscle cramps	All greens (such as broccoli, kale, parsley, spinach, watercress), molasses, seeds and their oils, wheatgerm	012 156 215 173	Apple Cleanser Chlorophyll Carrot Savoury Fruit Green Goddess
Obesity	All fruit and vegetable juices and fibre	019 137 217 256	Waldorf Salad Carrot Cleanser Crunch Morning Favourite Pineapple Zing
Osteoporosis prevention	All greens (such as broccoli, kale, parsley, spinach, watercress), garlic, milk, molasses, peaches, seeds and their oils, soy (soya), yogurt	128 175 178 336	Green Pines Green 'n' Pear It Green Waldorf Peachy Passion
Premenstrual syndrome	All greens (such as broccoli, kale, parsley, spinach, watercress), celery, fennel, garlic, seeds and their oils, soy (soya)	069 175 178	Muddy Tonic Green 'n' Pear It Green Waldorf Any smoothie with soy (soya) milk
Prostate problems	Celery, fennel, fruit and vegetable fibre, garlic, molasses, soy (soya), seeds and their oils, tomatoes	196 211 178 296	Ginger Tom Tomorange Green Waldorf Creamy Black Banana
Psoriasis	Apricots, broccoli, carrots, fruit and vegetable fibre, mangoes, pumpkins, red bell peppers, seeds and their oils, sweet potatoes, watercress	122 141 183 252	Ginger Zinger Carotene Catapult Creamy Green Nectargo
Shingles	Apricots, berries, broccoli, carrots, citrus fruits, garlic, kale, kiwi fruits, mangoes, melons, red bell peppers, sweet potatoes, seeds and their oils, watercress, watermelons	059 145 141 181	Power-packed C Cold War Carotene Catapult Super Defender

ailment	foods to eat	blend no.	title
Sinusitis	Apricots, berries, broccoli, carrots, citrus fruits, kale, kiwi fruits, mangoes, melons, red bell peppers, sweet potatoes, seeds and their oils, watercress, watermelons	119 145 183 275	Black Pineapple Cold War Creamy Green Blue Healer
Sleeping problems	All greens (such as broccoli, kale, parsley, spinach, watercress), apples, bananas, milk, molasses, seeds, soy (soya) milk, yogurt	024 180 295 303	Apple Lullaby Green Lullaby Creamy Bananacot Banana Heaven
Sprains, strains & other injuries	All greens (such as broccoli, kale, parsley, spinach, watercress), garlic, milk, molasses, seeds and their oils, soy (soya), yogurt	030 066 173 298	Bellyful Muddy Puddle Green Goddess Creamy Green Banana
Stomach ulcers	Cabbages, carrots, melons, papaya	030 140 179 264	Bellyful Carrot Digestif Sweet Green Melon Papaya Pure
Stress	All fruit and vegetable juices and fibre, all greens (such as broccoli, kale, parsley, spinach, watercress), berries, carrots, citrus fruits, milk, molasses, pineapples, red bell peppers, seeds and their oils, soy (soya) milk, wheatgerm, yogurt	137 178 298 331 398	Carrot Cleanser Green Waldorf Creamy Green Banana Pinkypine Stress Reliever
Sunburn	Apricots, berries (especially blackcurrants), broccoli, carrots, citrus fruits, garlic, kiwi fruits, mangoes, pumpkins, red bell peppers, strawberries, sweet potatoes, watercress	064 002 290 292	Bitter Melon Apple Basic Creamy Cooler Green Sensation
Tonsillitis	Apricots, berries, broccoli, carrots, citrus fruits, garlic, kale, kiwi fruits, mangoes, melons, pineapples, red bell peppers, seeds and their oils, sweet potatoes, watercress, watermelons	119 116 145 275	Black Pineapple Pink Pineapple Cold War Blue Healer
Varicose veins	All fruit and vegetable juices and fibre, berries, broccoli, citrus fruits, kale, kiwi fruits, seeds and their oils, watercress, wheatgerm	002 057 083 338	Apple Basic Florida Blue Berry Bonanza Apricot Regular
Water retention	Celery, cucumbers, melons, watermelons	214 165 221 166	Cool 'n' Pale II Mellow Melon Salty Sharp Melon Water, Water Everywhere

Index

References are to page numbers, not recipes. This index should be used in conjunction with the index of ailments on pages 713–19 and the suggested juice courses on pages 706–709.